Getting to Know Semaglutide and Other GLP-1–Based Medications

Richard Skiba

AFTER MIDNIGHT
PUBLISHING

Skiba, Richard (Author)

Getting to Know Semaglutide and Other GLP-1–Based Medications

ISBN 978-1-7643896-6-2 (Paperback) 978-1-7643896-7-9 (eBook) 978-1-7643896-8-6 (Hardcover)

Non-fiction

Contents

Introduction

Over the past decade, few medical therapies have reshaped public health, clinical practice, and global conversation as profoundly as semaglutide. What began as a targeted treatment for type 2 diabetes has rapidly evolved into a transformative therapy for obesity, metabolic disease, cardiovascular risk reduction, and potentially much more. As scientific understanding grows and real-world experience expands, semaglutide now stands at the forefront of a revolution in how we treat chronic metabolic conditions—moving beyond the outdated notion of willpower and toward a modern, biological understanding of appetite, energy regulation, and long-term health.

This book was written to provide a clear, comprehensive, and evidence-based guide to semaglutide: what it is, how it works, who it helps, and what patients and clinicians can realistically expect throughout treatment. Across the chapters that follow, we explore not only the pharmacology and clinical data behind semaglutide but also its broader impact on healthcare systems, ethics, public attitudes, and the lived experiences of those using the medication. We examine the landmark STEP, SUSTAIN, PIONEER, and SELECT trials; emerging next-generation incretin therapies; long-term treatment considerations; and the rapidly changing global landscape of access, affordability, and regulation.

Semaglutide's rise has brought unprecedented benefits—significant weight loss, improved metabolic health, reduced cardiovascular events—but also complex challenges. Supply shortages, misinformation, inappropriate prescribing, and the growth of unsafe compounded products have created new risks. At the same time, shifting social narratives about obesity, body image, and medication use have generated both hope and stigma. Understanding these dynamics is essential for ensuring that semaglutide is used safely, ethically, and effectively.

Whether you are a healthcare professional seeking clarity, a patient beginning your treatment journey, or a policymaker navigating the broader implications of these therapies, this book aims to provide practical guidance grounded in science—not hype. Semaglutide is not a miracle drug, nor a cosmetic shortcut; it is a powerful medical tool for a chronic medical condition, and its success relies on thoughtful prescribing, realistic expectations, and supportive lifestyle change.

As we look ahead, the future of incretin-based therapies is expanding rapidly. New agents—dual and triple agonists, oral multi-incretins, and amylin combination therapies—promise even greater impact. Understanding semaglutide today prepares us for the therapies of tomorrow.

Chapter 1

What Is Semaglutide?

Semaglutide has rapidly emerged as one of the most influential medications in modern metabolic medicine, reshaping long-standing approaches to treating type 2 diabetes, obesity, and cardiometabolic disease. Its development marks a major advancement in our understanding of the incretin system and the therapeutic potential of GLP-1 receptor agonists. What began as a targeted effort to improve glycaemic control has expanded into a broad clinical tool capable of producing meaningful, sustained weight loss and reducing the risk of serious cardiovascular events. As global demand and scientific interest continue to rise, semaglutide now represents a cornerstone therapy across multiple areas of chronic disease management.

This chapter introduces semaglutide within its broader clinical and scientific context, outlining what the medication is, how it works, and why it has become so widely used. It provides an overview of its mechanisms of action, its effects on glucose regulation and appetite, and its therapeutic roles in diabetes, obesity, and cardiovascular risk reduction. In doing so, the chapter sets the foundation for deeper exploration in the sections that follow, including dosing strategies, clinical outcomes, safety considerations, and real-world patient experiences. Whether readers are new to GLP-1–based therapies or seeking a comprehensive reference, this chapter serves as the essential starting point for understanding semaglutide's place in contemporary healthcare.

Overview of Semaglutide as A GLP-1 Receptor Agonist

Semaglutide Overview

Semaglutide is a novel medication classified as a glucagon-like peptide-1 (GLP-1) receptor agonist, primarily utilized in managing two significant chronic conditions—type 2 diabetes and obesity. For individuals with type 2 diabetes, semaglutide enhances glycaemic control by supporting the body's natural insulin response while concurrently reducing glucagon levels and delaying gastric emptying, leading to increased satiety [1, 2]. In studies, semaglutide demonstrated significant reductions in glycated haemoglobin levels, indicating its effectiveness in managing blood sugar [3]. This action is critical, as sustained glycaemic control lowers the risk of diabetes-related complications, thus repositioning diabetes medications from merely glucose-intensive treatments to agents that may modify the disease [4].

In the context of obesity, semaglutide serves as a long-term weight management therapy by suppressing appetite and adjusting energy intake. Clinical trials reveal that individuals using semaglutide can achieve substantial weight loss, thus reducing obesity-related health risks [5, 6]. Notably, the SELECT trial underscored semaglutide's efficacy in reducing severe adverse cardiovascular events (MACE) in overweight or obese patients with pre-existing cardiovascular conditions and highlighted its potential role beyond diabetes management [7]. This broadened therapeutic significance emphasizes semaglutide's status as a landmark advancement in metabolic medicine.

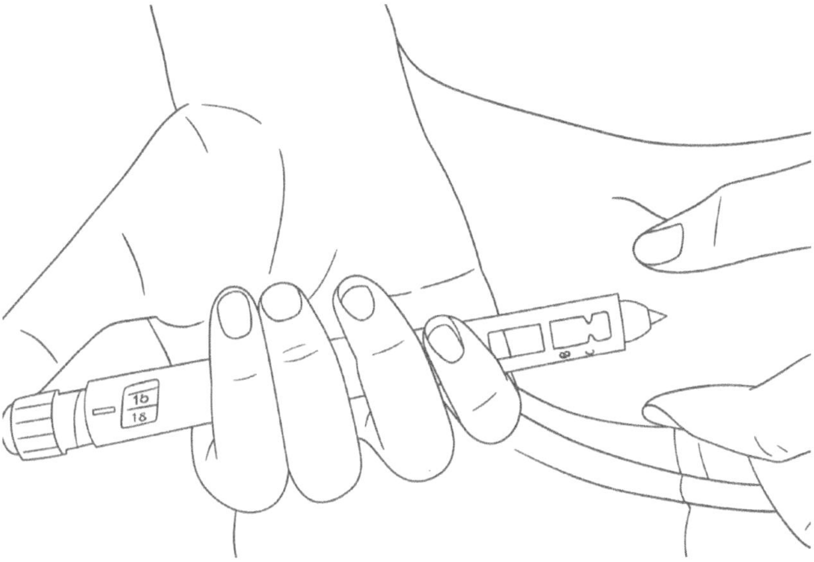

Figure 1: Using a Semaglutide Injector Pen.

Mechanistically, semaglutide mimics the effects of GLP-1 by enhancing insulin secretion in response to meals, decreasing gastric mucosal function, and bolstering signals of fullness conveyed to the brain [8]. Its unique modification allows for prolonged action in the body, facilitating less frequent dosing schedules—available as a weekly injection or a daily oral tablet [9]. Notably, differences in delivery mechanisms have broadened the accessibility of semaglutide among patients, allowing for more personalized treatment preferences [10].

Beyond its applications for diabetes and obesity, semaglutide also presents cardiovascular protective benefits. Evidence from clinical trials indicates that patients treated with semaglutide experience a significant decrease in risk for cardiovascular-related events, including heart attacks and strokes, particularly in those with heightened cardiovascular risk profiles [6, 7]. The observed benefits are attributed to improvements in cardiovascular and renal health parameters, including better lipid profiles and reduced oxidative stress [11]. This comprehensive effect on patient health has led to its inclusion in essential medicine lists, signifying its critical role in contemporary health care systems [12].

Side effects of semaglutide are predominantly gastrointestinal, reflecting the drug's natural mechanism of action by slowing digestion and affecting appetite [13]. These effects typically manifest during the initiation or dose escalation of the medication, though they tend to diminish as patients titrate to their maintenance doses [11].

Semaglutide has become an essential therapeutic agent in managing type 2 diabetes, aiding in weight reduction, and offering significant cardiovascular protection. The multifaceted benefits of semaglutide underscore its pivotal role in modern metabolic therapy, marking a transformative step in the treatment paradigms for chronic diseases.

Semaglutide as A GLP-1 Receptor Agonist

Semaglutide is a synthetic analogue of glucagon-like peptide-1 (GLP-1), a naturally occurring incretin hormone produced in the gut. It plays a crucial role in regulating glucose metabolism, appetite, and gastrointestinal function following food intake. The incretin effect is characterized by increased insulin secretion, decreased glucagon release, and slowed gastric emptying, all of which contribute to glucose homeostasis [14-16]. By mimicking GLP-1, semaglutide enhances these physiological pathways, providing a significant therapeutic approach in managing conditions like type 2 diabetes and obesity.

Glucagon-Like Peptide-1 (GLP-1)
GLP-1 is a natural hormone made in the gut after eating.
It helps the body by:

- increasing insulin (to lower blood sugar)
- reducing glucagon (which raises blood sugar)
- slowing digestion
- sending signals to the brain that you are full

Medications like semaglutide copy the action of GLP-1.

Incretin
Incretins are a group of hormones released from the gut when you eat. Their job is to help manage blood sugar by telling the pancreas to release insulin.
GLP-1 is one of the main incretin hormones.

Type 2 Diabetes
Type 2 diabetes is a long-term condition where the body:

- doesn't use insulin properly (insulin resistance), and
- may not make enough insulin
  This causes high blood sugar over time, which can lead to health problems such as heart disease, eye disease, kidney issues, and nerve damage.

Obesity
Obesity is a medical condition where a person has too much body fat that can harm their health.

It is influenced by many factors, such as genetics, hormones, environment, stress, and metabolism—not just diet and exercise. Obesity increases the risk of diabetes, heart disease, some cancers, and other health issues.

The physiological action of GLP-1 involves three main mechanisms: it stimulates insulin secretion from the pancreas in a glucose-dependent manner, reduces appetite by acting on central nervous system pathways to signal satiety, and slows gastric emptying to prolong the digestive process [14, 15]. These actions are vital because they help maintain blood glucose levels within a normal range while reducing the likelihood of postprandial hyperglycaemia, a common challenge in diabetes management. Semaglutide, with its prolonged half-life compared to native GLP-1, allows for less frequent administration without compromising efficacy [17, 18]. This long-acting property is particularly beneficial as it enhances treatment adherence and clinical outcomes [16, 19].

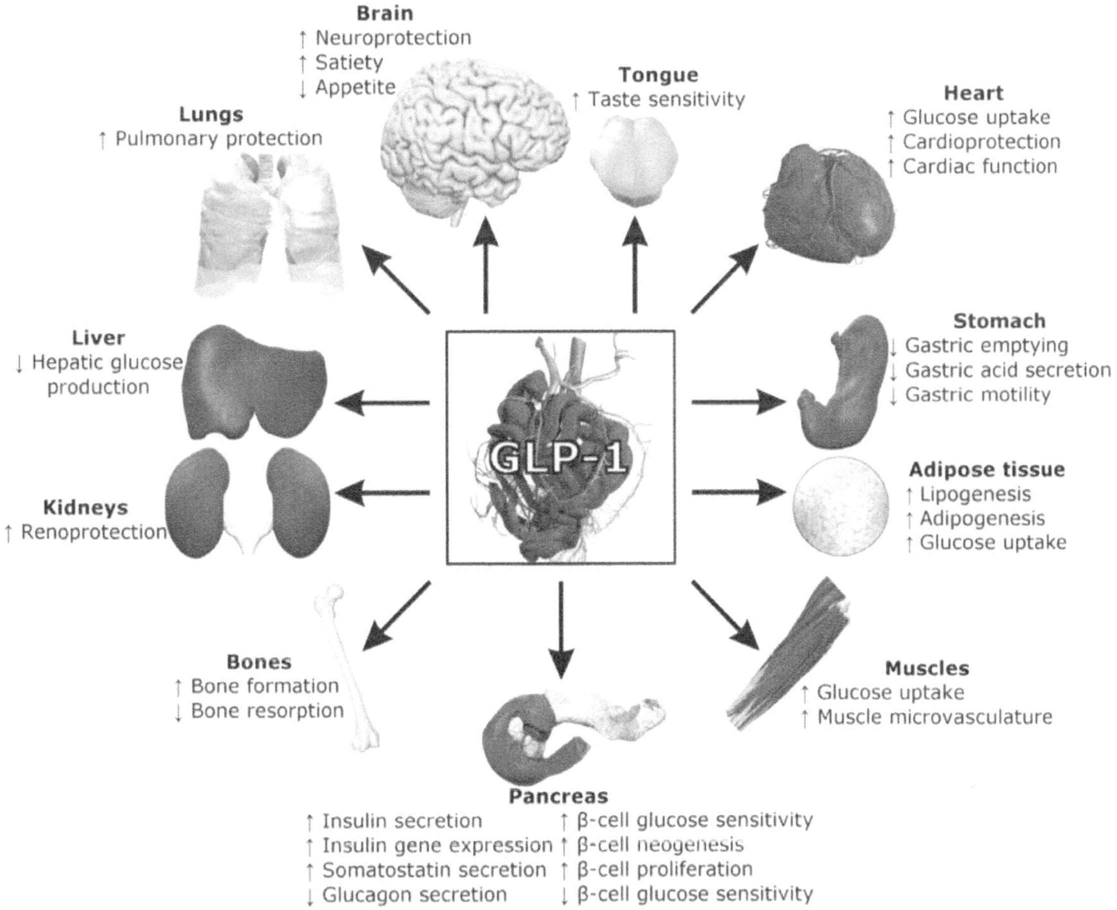

Figure 2: The physiological actions of glucagon-like peptide-1 (GLP-1). Lthoms11, CC BY 4.0, via Wikimedia Commons.

Numerous studies have established the efficacy of semaglutide. For instance, the SUSTAIN trials demonstrated significant reductions in HbA1c and body weight among participants with type 2 diabetes using semaglutide [18, 20]. This has positioned semaglutide as one of the leading treatments for type 2 diabetes and obesity, highlighting its beneficial effects not only on blood sugar control but also on weight management [18, 19]. Through its mechanisms, semaglutide acts on the same physiological pathways utilized naturally by the body, amplifying the effects of natural GLP-1 and contributing to improved overall metabolic health.

Semaglutide helps your body keep your blood sugar steady and your appetite lower, using the same pathways your body already uses after eating. This is why it has become such an important treatment for people with type 2 diabetes and for those trying to lose weight.

As a GLP-1 receptor agonist, semaglutide plays a crucial role in glucose regulation by binding to and activating GLP-1 receptors located in several key tissues throughout the body, including the pancreas, brain, and gastrointestinal (GI) tract. Upon activation, these receptors stimulate insulin secretion from pancreatic beta cells in a glucose-dependent manner, thus mitigating hyperglycaemia during elevated blood glucose levels while concurrently suppressing glucagon, a hormone that typically raises blood glucose levels. Research indicates that this glucose-dependent mechanism significantly reduces the risk of hypoglycaemia associated with semaglutide use when it is administered in isolation [21, 22].

The insulinotropic effect of GLP-1 receptor activation can be attributed to its ability to enhance the sensitivity of beta cells to glucose, resulting in a moderated insulin release only when blood sugar levels are high. Concurrently, semaglutide's inhibition of glucagon secretion from alpha cells plays a vital role in its glucose-lowering effect, with studies suggesting that the suppression of glucagon contributes substantially to the overall efficacy of GLP-1 receptor agonists in managing type 2 diabetes [23-25]. Furthermore, the medication's impact on gastric emptying slows the rate at which food leaves the stomach, contributing to a more gradual increase in postprandial blood glucose levels and prolonging feelings of satiety [22, 26].

GLP-1 Receptor Agonist

A GLP-1 receptor agonist is a type of medicine that works by copying the actions of the natural hormone GLP-1 in the body.

It "activates" GLP-1 receptors—special switches found in the pancreas, brain, and digestive system.

When these switches are turned on, the body:

- releases insulin when blood sugar is high
- reduces hunger
- slows digestion

Semaglutide is an example of a GLP-1 receptor agonist.

Insulinotropic Effect
The insulinotropic effect means "the ability to increase insulin release."
A medicine (or hormone) with an insulinotropic effect helps the pancreas release more insulin only when blood sugar rises.
GLP-1 and semaglutide have this effect, making them helpful for controlling blood sugar without causing low blood sugar when used alone.

The actions of semaglutide reflect those of the natural hormone GLP-1. This hormone is secreted by the intestines in response to food intake, subsequently activating GLP-1 receptors that facilitate glucose homeostasis. By modulating both insulin and glucagon levels, semaglutide provides a dual approach to managing diabetes symptoms: it directly lowers blood sugar levels while addressing hunger and cravings, thereby assisting patients in managing their weight [27-29]. Evidence suggests that the multifaceted mechanisms of GLP-1 agonists like semaglutide render them advantageous over other diabetes medications, particularly regarding their lower risk of causing hypoglycaemia and their ability to improve appetite regulation—features that are particularly beneficial for individuals with obesity and type 2 diabetes [22, 30].

Semaglutide operates through an intricate network of physiological pathways, promoting insulin secretion while suppressing glucagon, and slowing gastric emptying. This complex interplay ultimately leads to enhanced glycaemic control, reduced hunger, and prevention of significant blood sugar spikes after meals, thereby providing a sophisticated method of diabetes management grounded in existing hormonal systems [21, 22].

Semaglutide helps your body control blood sugar more smoothly, reduces hunger, and prevents big sugar spikes after eating—using the same pathways your body already has.

Semaglutide, a glucagon-like peptide-1 (GLP-1) receptor agonist, exerts a significant impact on central appetite regulation, particularly within the hypothalamus, a crucial region for integrating hunger and satiety signals. Evidence suggests that semaglutide enhances satiety by acting directly on GLP-1 receptors in the hypothalamus, modulating key pathways involved in appetite control [31-33]. This central action results in notable reductions in reported hunger and food intake, supported by clinical trials where participants showed decreased energy consumption and diminished food cravings following semaglutide treatment [31, 32].

Hypothalamus
The hypothalamus is a small but very important part of the brain that controls many basic body functions.
It acts like the body's "control centre," helping regulate:

- hunger and fullness
- body temperature

- thirst
- sleep
- hormones
- stress responses

When it comes to appetite, the hypothalamus receives signals from the gut and hormones like GLP-1.
This helps the brain decide when you feel hungry and when you feel full.

Clinically, increased satiety signals allow individuals to feel satisfied more quickly during meals and maintain a sense of fullness longer, thereby aiding in the natural reduction of caloric intake [31, 32]. In controlled studies, participants receiving semaglutide displayed significant weight loss, emphasizing the drug's efficacy in managing both obesity and diabetes [34, 35]. These findings highlight how semaglutide not only modulates appetite but also improves glycaemic control, distinguishing it from previous incretin therapies that lacked this dual effectiveness [34, 36].

Research indicates that semaglutide's appetite-suppressive effects are complemented by its ability to enhance insulin secretion and decrease glucagon levels, leading to improved metabolic outcomes [37]. Specifically, participants often experience significant reductions in blood glucose levels alongside the weight loss achievements attributed to semaglutide use [34, 35]. This dual mechanism of improving glycaemic control while significantly reducing appetite and caloric intake enables semaglutide to stand out as a pivotal treatment option for individuals with type 2 diabetes and obesity [38].

Semaglutide operates through a multifaceted mechanism that targets appetite regulation in the hypothalamus, enhancing satiety while concurrently improving glycaemic control. This effective combination promotes significant, sustainable weight loss, thereby supporting its increased application in clinical practice for managing obesity and type 2 diabetes [31, 32, 34, 35].

Semaglutide helps your brain feel full and your body control blood sugar at the same time. This is why it has become so widely used for treating both diabetes and obesity.

Semaglutide, a modified glucagon-like peptide-1 (GLP-1) analogue, has been engineered to achieve an extended half-life, facilitating once-weekly injections and a unique oral formulation that allows for once-daily dosing. The structural modifications to the native GLP-1 molecule include key alterations designed to enhance its stability against enzymatic degradation and improve its pharmacokinetics. Specifically, semaglutide exhibits high lipophilicity and a substantial binding affinity to serum albumin, functioning as a carrier that prolongs its systemic circulation and ensures a consistent therapeutic effect over time [39-41].

The necessity for infrequent dosing of semaglutide arises from these structural adaptations. The incorporation of an acylated fatty acid chain, which enhances albumin binding, results in a significantly extended half-life of approximately one week in humans, as well as a smooth pharmacokinetic profile that supports therapeutic dosing schedules without the burden of daily injections [39, 41, 42]. These modifications allow semaglutide to maintain effective plasma levels with a reduced risk of fluctuations that often accompany more frequently dosed medications [40, 41, 43].

Orally, semaglutide is co-formulated with sodium N-(8-2-hydroxybenzoyl amino) caprylate (SNAC), an absorption enhancer that promotes transcellular delivery of the peptide across the gastric epithelium. This formulation helps to circumvent the inherent challenges of peptide bioavailability, such as enzymatic degradation and limited absorption, which are typical for orally administered peptide-based drugs. Consequently, the oral form of semaglutide can be taken once daily, complementing its injectable form [44-46].

These advancements significantly lower the treatment burden for patients, allowing for a stable administration rhythm that promotes adherence. Semaglutide's capability of providing consistent therapeutic levels while being easy to administer further affirms its role in improving treatment outcomes in conditions such as type 2 diabetes [46-48]. In summary, semaglutide's design enhances patient convenience and treatment efficacy by ensuring sustained plasma concentrations with minimal dosing frequency, thus simplifying management protocols in diabetes care [42, 46, 49].

Semaglutide is built to last longer in the body, so it works steadily and doesn't need frequent dosing—making treatment much easier for patients.

Semaglutide has rapidly established itself as a fundamental therapy for managing several significant health conditions, including Type 2 Diabetes (T2D), obesity, and cardiovascular risk reduction. The efficacy and safety of semaglutide are well-supported by robust clinical evidence derived from large-scale trials such as SUSTAIN, PIONEER, STEP, and SELECT. These trials have shown consistent benefits across a range of outcomes, demonstrating significant improvements in glycaemic control and broader metabolic health advantages. For example, semaglutide has been associated with reductions in body mass index (BMI), waist circumference, and systolic blood pressure, with positive impacts on lipid profiles noted as well [50-52].

SUSTAIN Trials

The SUSTAIN trials were a series of large clinical studies that tested injectable semaglutide in people with Type 2 Diabetes.

These studies looked at how well semaglutide:

- lowers blood sugar
- helps with weight loss
- reduces the risk of heart problems

The results showed strong improvements in glucose control and metabolic health.

PIONEER Trials
The PIONEER trials were clinical studies that tested oral semaglutide tablets (Rybelsus) for Type 2 Diabetes.
These trials examined:

- effectiveness of the pill version
- safety
- how it compares to other diabetes medications

They proved that oral semaglutide can work as well as many injectable treatments.

STEP Trials
The STEP trials focused on semaglutide for weight management in people with obesity or overweight.
These studies showed that high-dose semaglutide can lead to significant and sustained weight loss, far greater than most previous medications.
STEP trials are the main evidence behind Wegovy (the weight-loss version of semaglutide).

SELECT Trial
The SELECT trial tested whether semaglutide could reduce major heart problems—such as heart attack, stroke, or death—in people who were overweight or obese *but did NOT have diabetes*.
The study found that semaglutide significantly reduced cardiovascular risk, making it one of the first weight-loss medications to show this benefit.

In particular, the SUSTAIN trials, especially SUSTAIN 6, provided compelling evidence of semaglutide's ability to improve glycaemic control while significantly reducing cardiovascular events. In SUSTAIN 6, semaglutide was associated with a 26% reduction in major adverse cardiovascular events compared to placebo, showcasing its dual utility in managing diabetes and reducing cardiovascular risk [40, 53]. The PIONEER studies indicated that oral semaglutide is effective, demonstrating similar results to subcutaneous formulations, which enhances its therapeutic appeal [52].

Moreover, semaglutide's role extends beyond diabetes management; it has emerged as a promising treatment for obesity, where it has demonstrated sustained weight loss results due to its appetite-suppressing effects [54]. This property is critical for patients with T2D who often struggle with weight management. The STEP trials specifically underscored semaglutide's efficacy in obesity management, reinforcing its utility as an anti-obesity agent [55].

Beyond its central role in glucose regulation and weight management, semaglutide has demonstrated improvements in blood pressure regulation and cholesterol levels, which are essential for comprehensive metabolic health [56]. The broader implications of these findings suggest that semaglutide's therapeutic benefits are multifaceted, impacting various aspects of health typically compromised in patients with T2D and obesity.

Semaglutide has evolved into a cornerstone therapy for managing Type 2 Diabetes, obesity, and related cardiovascular risks, supported by substantial clinical evidence indicating its safety and effectiveness across a range of health outcomes. The significant findings from major clinical trials solidify its role not only as a glucose-lowering agent but also as an integral component of a comprehensive strategy aimed at improving overall metabolic health.

Semaglutide has become a major treatment because strong scientific studies show it helps people manage diabetes, lose weight, and lower their risk of heart problems—all at the same time.

Identification and Characteristics

Semaglutide can be pronounced in two widely accepted ways: *sem-AG-luu-tyde* or *SEM-ə-GLOO-tyde*. Both versions are commonly used by healthcare professionals, reflecting slight differences in regional speech patterns rather than medical correctness.

Semaglutide is marketed under several trade names, each associated with specific therapeutic uses. Ozempic is the injectable form approved for the treatment of type 2 diabetes, while Rybelsus is the oral tablet version used for the same condition. Wegovy, also an injectable formulation, is approved for weight management and obesity treatment. Although the formulations may differ, all contain the same active ingredient—semaglutide—delivered at doses appropriate to the approved indication.

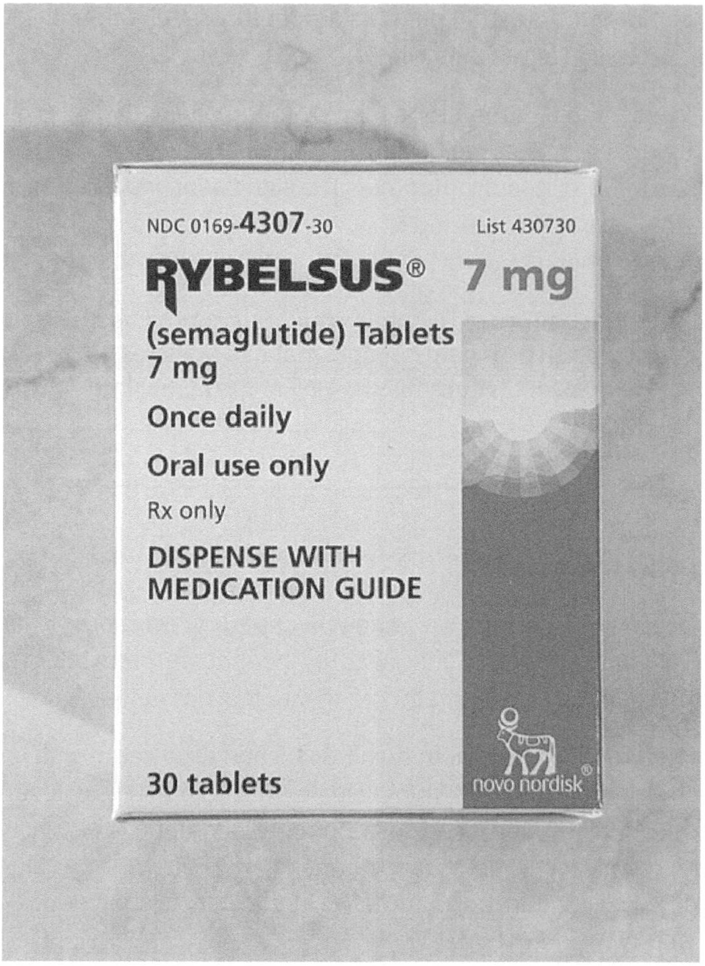

Figure 3: A box of Rybelsus (semaglutide) 7mg, seen from the front. Grendelkhan, CC BY-SA 4.0, via Wikimedia Commons.

A range of trusted medical information platforms provide authoritative details about semaglutide. Resources such as the AHFS Drug Information database, Drugs.com, and MedlinePlus offer clinician- and patient-friendly overviews. In addition, DailyMed, the official U.S. repository for FDA-approved drug labels, contains the full prescribing information for all semaglutide-containing products.

In Australia, semaglutide is classified under Pregnancy Category D, meaning there is evidence of human foetal risk. For this reason, it is not recommended for use during pregnancy, and women planning to conceive are advised to discontinue semaglutide well in advance because of its long half-life.

Semaglutide can be administered in two different routes: subcutaneous injection and oral tablet. The injectable form is used for both Ozempic and Wegovy, while Rybelsus offers a rare peptide medication that can be taken orally. This dual-route availability makes semaglutide unique among similar therapeutic agents.

In the World Health Organization's ATC (Anatomical Therapeutic Chemical) classification system, semaglutide is coded as A10BJ06. This classification identifies it as a medication for diabetes (A10) and specifically as a GLP-1 receptor agonist (BJ).

Across major global jurisdictions, semaglutide is strictly prescription-only. In Australia it is categorized as an S4 prescription medicine, in Canada as Schedule D, in the UK as POM (Prescription Only Medicine), and in both the United States and the European Union as prescription-only (℞). This consistent regulatory stance underscores the need for medical supervision due to its potency and clinical significance.

From a pharmacokinetic perspective, semaglutide, a glucagon-like peptide-1 (GLP-1) receptor agonist, exhibits significant variations in bioavailability when administered through different routes. Specifically, subcutaneously administered semaglutide achieves a bioavailability of approximately 89%, indicating that most of the administered dose enters systemic circulation effectively [57]. In contrast, the bioavailability of oral semaglutide is markedly lower, estimated to be between 1% to 2% [42, 58]. This low absorption rate necessitates specific dosing instructions whereby the oral formulation must be taken on an empty stomach to maximize absorption and avoid interference from food [42, 58].

The metabolism of semaglutide is primarily facilitated through proteolytic processes rather than conventional liver pathways, which distinguishes it from many other pharmacological agents [59]. The drug's prolonged elimination half-life, approximately 7 days, allows for its convenient once-weekly subcutaneous administration [57, 59]. Following administration, semaglutide continues to exert effects lasting around 63.6 hours, demonstrating its extended action profile that is well-suited for the chronic treatment of conditions such as type 2 diabetes [46, 60]. Moreover, semaglutide is gradually excreted via both urine and faeces, underscoring its stable pharmacokinetic profile, which is crucial for maintaining steady therapeutic levels during weekly dosing regimens [42, 60].

In consideration of the pharmacokinetic profiles of both oral and injectable forms of semaglutide, it is apparent that the choice of administration route significantly influences bioavailability and overall efficacy. Key studies highlight the critical role of dosing strategies in optimizing the therapeutic outcomes of semaglutide, particularly in managing type 2 diabetes [42, 46, 57]. As dosing regimens are refined, the implications of pharmacokinetics on patient adherence to medication and overall treatment success remain an important area of research [46, 57, 60].

Semaglutide's chemical and identification data help researchers and regulators ensure accuracy in scientific communication. Its CAS Number (910463-68-2), PubChem CID (56843331), DrugBank ID (DB13928), ChemSpider ID (34981134), UNII (53AXN4NNHX), KEGG designation (D10025), and ChEBI entry (CHEBI:167574) allow for precise referencing across chemical, pharmacological, and regulatory databases. The molecule has a very large and complex structure, reflected in its chemical formula $C_{187}H_{291}N_{45}O_{59}$ and an unusually high molar mass of 4113.641 g/mol. Such size and complexity explain why peptide-based medications like semaglutide typically cannot be taken orally unless specially formulated and protected against digestive breakdown. Structural codes such as SMILES and InChI are used by scientists and software systems to model and analyse the molecule in three dimensions.

Overall, semaglutide is a prescription-only medication used worldwide for type 2 diabetes, long-term weight management, and the reduction of cardiovascular risk. It is available as a weekly injection or a daily pill, has a long duration of action, and has been rigorously studied and approved globally. While highly effective, its use requires professional oversight—particularly due to pregnancy risks and the need for careful dose management—making it a powerful but carefully regulated tool in modern metabolic medicine.

Table 1: Summary of Semaglutide Properties.

Category	Information
Pronunciation	*sem-AG-luu-tyde* (/sɛmˈæglʊtaɪd/); *SEM-ə-GLOO-tyde* (/ˌsɛməˈgluːtaɪd/)
Trade Names	Ozempic (injectable, type 2 diabetes); Rybelsus (oral, type 2 diabetes); Wegovy (injectable, weight management/obesity; MASLD/NASH treatments emerging)
Drug Class	GLP-1 receptor agonist
Therapeutic Uses	Type 2 diabetes treatment; long-term weight management; obesity treatment; reduction of major cardiovascular risk; investigational uses in liver disease (MASH)
Pregnancy Category (AU)	Category D – evidence of foetal risk; avoid in pregnancy
Routes of Administration	Subcutaneous injection (weekly); Oral tablet (daily)
ATC Code (WHO)	A10BJ06
Global Legal Status	Prescription only (AU: S4; CA: Schedule D; UK: POM; US: Rx-only; EU: Rx-only)
Bioavailability	89% (subcutaneous) ; 1–2% (oral)
Metabolism	Proteolysis (enzyme-based breakdown of peptides)
Elimination Half-Life	~7 days
Duration of Action	~63.6 hours

Category	Information
Excretion	Urine and faeces
IUPAC Name	Long systematic peptide name (abbreviated in most clinical references)
CAS Number	910463-68-2
PubChem CID	56843331
DrugBank ID	DB13928
ChemSpider ID	34981134
UNII	53AXN4NNHX
KEGG	D10025
ChEBI	CHEBI:167574
Molecular Formula	$C_{187}H_{291}N_{45}O_{59}$
Molar Mass	4113.641 g/mol
Structural Codes	SMILES, InChI (used for computational modelling)

The History Of GLP-1 Discovery and Diabetes/Obesity Treatments

Early Research and Discovery of GLP-1 (1970s–1980s)

The scientific foundations for semaglutide began in the 1970s, when researchers Jens Juul Holst and Joel Habener were investigating hormones involved in digestion, initially focusing on duodenal ulcer disease. Their work explored the substances released by the gut during eating and how these hormones influenced the pancreas. In animal studies using pig pancreases, they discovered that one of these hormones—glucagon-like peptide-1 (GLP-1)—had a potent effect on stimulating insulin [61]. This critical discovery, made in 1988, provided the biochemical basis for what would eventually become an entirely new class of medications for diabetes and obesity. Decades later, the contributions of Holst and Habener, along with Daniel J. Drucker, were recognized with the 2021 Warren Alpert Foundation Prize, highlighting the profound impact their early research had on metabolic medicine [62].

From Hormone to Therapeutic Candidate (1990s)

In 1993, researcher Michael Nauck conducted studies demonstrating that the infusion of glucagon-like peptide-1 (GLP-1) into individuals with type 2 diabetes could effectively normalize blood glucose levels by enhancing insulin secretion and suppressing glucagon release. Specifically, his research indicated that administration of GLP-1 (7-36 amide) resulted in a significant reduction in fasting hyperglycaemia, primarily due to increased insulin levels triggered by enhanced glucose sensitivity in patients with type 2 diabetes [63]. However, despite these encouraging results, GLP-1's therapeutic potential was hampered by its rapid degradation in the bloodstream, limiting its utility as a long-term treatment option [63, 64] . This instability necessitated alternative strategies to harness GLP-1's benefits for clinical application without the unwanted gastrointestinal side effects that direct administration of natural GLP-1 often caused [64, 65].

Hyperglycaemia
Hyperglycaemia means high blood sugar.
It occurs when the body does not have enough insulin or cannot use insulin properly, causing glucose to build up in the bloodstream. Symptoms can include increased thirst, frequent urination, tiredness, and blurry vision. Long-term hyperglycaemia can damage organs such as the heart, kidneys, nerves, and eyes.

Insulin
Insulin is a hormone made by the pancreas that allows glucose (sugar) in the blood to enter cells, where it is used for energy. Without enough insulin—or if the body becomes resistant to it—blood sugar levels rise. Insulin is essential for maintaining healthy metabolism and preventing hyperglycaemia.

Glycaemic Control
Glycaemic control refers to how well a person manages their blood-sugar levels over time. Good glycaemic control means keeping blood glucose within a healthy range through a combination of medication, diet, physical activity, and monitoring. HbA1c blood tests are commonly used to measure long-term glycaemic control.

Liraglutide
Liraglutide is a GLP-1 receptor agonist, similar to semaglutide.
It mimics the natural hormone GLP-1 to increase insulin, reduce glucagon, slow digestion, and promote feelings of fullness. Liraglutide is used to treat type 2 diabetes (brand name Victoza) and obesity/weight management (brand name Saxenda). It is an older, once-daily medication compared to semaglutide's once-weekly dosing.

The research challenges regarding GLP-1 led to innovations, particularly with the support of Novo Nordisk, aiming to create a modified version of the peptide that retained its efficacy while being more stable and manageable for patients. Significant progress was made by a team led by Lotte Bjerre Knudsen at Novo Nordisk, culminating in the development of liraglutide in 1998. This analogue proved to be a breakthrough in diabetes management, as it not only enhanced glycaemic control through increased insulin secretion and decreased glucagon but also necessitated less frequent dosing compared to previous GLP-1 formulations [62, 64]. Liraglutide eventually emerged as one of the most widely prescribed treatments for type 2 diabetes and was later used in obesity management [62, 64, 66].

Following liraglutide, further refinements in GLP-1 analogue development led to semaglutide, engineered for extended half-life and more convenient administration with just a once-weekly dosage [62, 64]. The innovative contributions by researchers like Jesper Lau, Thomas Kruse, and Paw Bloch facilitated this advance, establishing semaglutide's role as not only a key treatment for diabetes but also an effective agent for long-term weight control [62, 66]. Clinical trials have demonstrated semaglutide's efficacy in managing blood glucose and providing weight reduction, thereby expanding the therapeutic options available for patients [40, 66].

Clinical Trials and Early Regulatory Approvals for Diabetes

The development of semaglutide as a long-acting therapy for type 2 diabetes has marked a significant advancement in diabetes management. Originally entering phase II clinical trials in June 2008, semaglutide was evaluated for its efficacy as a once-weekly therapy, establishing itself as a preferable alternative to liraglutide, which required daily administration [66] . Eventually branded as Ozempic, semaglutide progressed to phase III clinical trials starting in January 2016, concluding in May 2017, and these trials provided robust data supporting its safety and effectiveness [40].

The FDA's approval of semaglutide was based on results from the SUSTAIN clinical trial program, which consisted of several pivotal trials involving thousands of participants across multiple countries, comparing its performance against standard anti-diabetic medications and placebo. The trials consistently demonstrated significant improvements in key outcomes such as HbA1c reduction, enhanced blood glucose control, and considerable weight loss compared to the control groups [50, 67]. Notably, the SUSTAIN trials (1 to 6) assessed the comparative efficacy of semaglutide against other treatment options and confirmed its superior glycaemic efficacy and safety profile [66, 68].

Two key trials, identified by clinical trial registration numbers NCT02054897 and NCT02305381, were designed as randomized, double-blind, placebo-controlled studies. Each trial enrolled participants who received semaglutide treatment for 30 weeks, ensuring reliable outcomes regarding its safety and efficacy [66]. Additionally, the SUSTAIN 6 trial notably included 3,297 individuals at high cardiovascular risk and found that semaglutide not only effectively managed glycaemic levels but also significantly reduced the incidence of cardiovascular events, aligning with current treatment goals of improving both diabetes control and reducing cardiovascular risk [69, 70].

Moreover, outside of its glycaemic control capabilities, the cardiovascular outcome trials (CVOTs) have shed light on the broader implications of semaglutide's benefits. For instance, semaglutide demonstrated a substantial reduction in rates of major cardiovascular events within the SUSTAIN 6 trial, further validating its comprehensive therapeutic role in managing diabetes [69]. The extensive evidence from these trials underscores semaglutide's standing as an effective long-acting therapy for type 2 diabetes, combining both efficacy in glucose management and cardiovascular protection, thereby enhancing overall patient outcomes [68, 71].

Development as a Long-Acting Therapy

In June 2008, a significant milestone was achieved in diabetes research when semaglutide entered phase II clinical trials aimed at evaluating its potential as a once-weekly therapeutic option for type 2 diabetes. This new drug was designed to offer a prolonged effect compared to liraglutide, which was already established in the market. Semaglutide later became known by its brand name, Ozempic. Following the successful completion of phase II studies, phase III clinical trials commenced in January 2016 and concluded in May 2017, producing robust evidence supporting the drug's safety and efficacy in managing type 2 diabetes [20, 72, 73]. The trials encompassed a comprehensive cohort of over 4,000 participants across 33 countries, highlighting the global interest and engagement in semaglutide research [73, 74].

The FDA's evaluation of semaglutide for type 2 diabetes treatment was largely founded on the outcomes from major clinical trials. Specifically, semaglutide's efficacy was compared against placebo and other standard anti-diabetic medications, demonstrating superior results in reducing HbA1c levels and improving blood glucose control across various demographics [20, 73]. Notably, pivotal randomized, double-blind, placebo-controlled trials (NCT02054897 and NCT02305381) provided solid foundations for the FDA's approval, as they kept participants and healthcare providers unaware of treatment allocations, thus minimizing bias in the results. These trials involved administering semaglutide for 30 weeks, supplemented by five other trials that evaluated semaglutide against different diabetes medications over a longer span of 30 to 56 weeks, some of which operated under an open-label design [20, 72].

Furthermore, additional evidence was obtained from large trials, including the SUSTAIN 6 trial (NCT01720446), which involved a separate cohort of 3,297 individuals at high cardiovascular risk [1]. This trial, conducted across 20 countries over 104 weeks, specifically monitored significant cardiovascular events, including heart attacks and strokes, revealing that semaglutide not only facilitated glycaemic control but also significantly lowered cardiovascular risks compared to placebo [1]. The aggregated data from both pivotal and supplementary studies reinforced the therapeutic potential of semaglutide in enhancing health outcomes for individuals with type 2 diabetes.

The journey of semaglutide from its clinical beginnings to FDA approval illustrates a methodical process bolstered by extensive biomedical research, underscoring its significance as a diabetes treatment option that transcends glycaemic management to address cardiovascular health as well.

Expansion to Cardiovascular Risk Reduction

In March 2024, the FDA expanded the indications for semaglutide, marketed as Wegovy, to include the reduction of cardiovascular risks for adults with established cardiovascular disease who are either overweight or obese. This decision was based on results from the placebo-controlled, double-blind SELECT trial, which involved over 17,600 participants globally. The trial aimed to assess the impact of semaglutide on major cardiovascular events while also providing standard care interventions for conditions such as hypertension and hyperlipidemia, along with lifestyle counselling [75, 76].

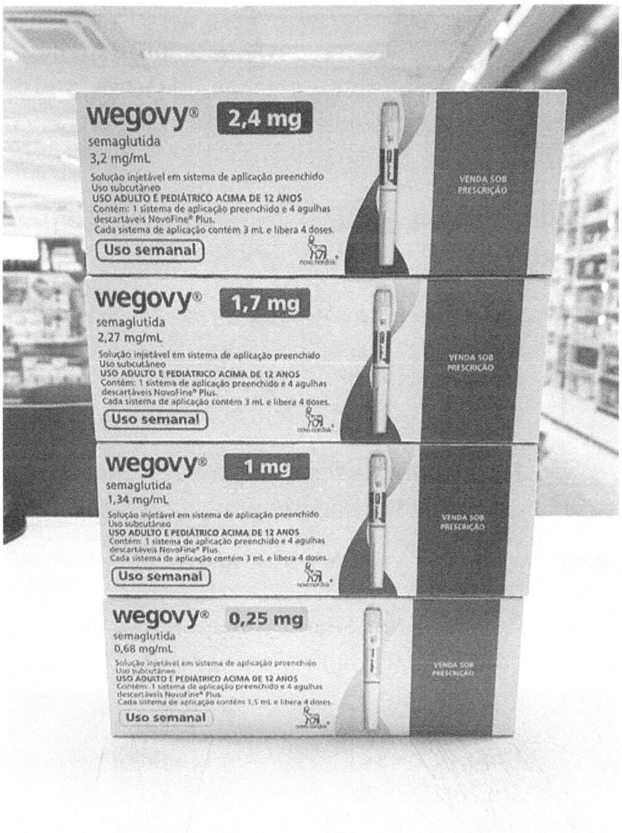

Figure 4: Photo of four different doses of Wegovy. Nelson R. de Lima Filho, CC BY 4.0, via Wikimedia Commons.

The pivotal findings of the SELECT trial were noteworthy; they revealed that 6.5% of individuals in the semaglutide cohort experienced a major cardiovascular event, compared to 8% in the placebo group. This statistic indicates a significant 20% reduction in the incidence of major adverse cardiovascular events (MACE), such as cardiovascular death, nonfatal myocardial infarction, and nonfatal stroke [75, 77]. These findings affirm semaglutide's unique status as the first anti-obesity medication that not only fosters significant weight loss — in some cases by up to 17% [76] — but also provides verified cardiovascular protection for those without diabetes, thereby demonstrating substantial therapeutic promise [1].

The implications of semaglutide's expanded approval are substantial, given that cardiovascular disease remains a leading cause of morbidity and mortality among individuals with obesity [18, 32]. Research has indicated that GLP-1 receptor agonists, including semaglutide, produce cardiovascular benefits beyond weight loss alone, highlighting their role in modulating metabolic factors that contribute to cardiovascular risk [78, 79]. The SELECT trial builds on this foundation, corroborating earlier findings that indicated a favourable cardiovascular safety profile for semaglutide in conjunction with lifestyle interventions and pharmacological therapy for obesity [71, 77].

The FDA's recent endorsement signifies a pivotal advancement in managing cardiovascular risk among overweight and obese adults, reaffirming semaglutide's role as a dual contributor to both weight management and cardiovascular health, thus reshaping clinical approaches to obesity treatment intertwined with cardiovascular care [1, 79].

Timeline of Semaglutide: Discovery, Development, and Clinical Milestones

1970s – Early Hormone Research

- Jens Juul Holst and Joel Habener begin studying gut hormones related to digestion and duodenal ulcer disease.
- Their work focuses on hormones released during eating and their effects on the pancreas.

1988 – Discovery of GLP-1's Potency

- Holst and Habener identify the strong insulin-stimulating effects of GLP-1 (glucagon-like peptide-1) using pig pancreas experiments.
- This discovery lays the foundation for the entire GLP-1–based drug class.

1993 – GLP-1 Tested in Humans

- Michael Nauck infuses GLP-1 into people with type 2 diabetes.

- GLP-1 normalises blood glucose by increasing insulin and suppressing glucagon—but natural GLP-1 breaks down too quickly for therapeutic use.

Late 1990s – Development of First GLP-1 Therapies

- Novo Nordisk begins targeted research on GLP-1–based drugs.
- 1998: A Novo Nordisk team led by Lotte Bjerre Knudsen develops liraglutide, the first long-acting GLP-1 receptor agonist used clinically.

Early 2000s – Next-Generation Molecule Created

- Novo Nordisk researchers Jesper Lau, Thomas Kruse, and Paw Bloch design and develop semaglutide, engineered to last a full week in the body.

2008 – First Semaglutide Clinical Trial

- A phase II trial begins evaluating semaglutide as a once-weekly treatment for type 2 diabetes.

2016–2017 – Large Phase III Trials Completed

- Semaglutide is tested in seven multi-country trials involving over 4,000 participants with type 2 diabetes.
- Trials run across 33 countries, comparing semaglutide with placebo and other diabetes medications.

December 2017 – FDA Approval for Type 2 Diabetes

- Semaglutide (brand name Ozempic) is approved in the United States for improving glycaemic control in adults with type 2 diabetes.

2019 – Oral Semaglutide Approved

- Rybelsus, the first-ever oral GLP-1 medication, receives FDA approval.

2021 – Semaglutide Approved for Obesity

- After highly successful STEP trials, Wegovy is approved for chronic weight management.
- A major phase III obesity trial shows an average 14.9% body-weight reduction at 68 weeks.

2021 – Major Scientific Recognition

- The Warren Alpert Foundation Prize is awarded to Holst, Habener, and Drucker for foundational incretin research leading to semaglutide and similar therapies.

2022 – Anti-Obesity Breakthrough Recognition

- Reviews identify semaglutide as one of the most effective weight-loss medications to date, second only to bariatric surgery.

2023 – One of the Most Prescribed Drugs in the U.S.

- Semaglutide becomes the 19th most commonly prescribed medication in the United States, with over 25 million prescriptions issued.

March 2024 – Cardiovascular Indication Approved

- The FDA approves Wegovy for reducing the risk of cardiovascular death, heart attack, and stroke in overweight or obese adults with established heart disease.
- Approval is based on a multinational trial of 17,600 participants, showing significant reductions in major cardiovascular events.

Why Semaglutide Stands Out Among GLP-1 Medications

Semaglutide has emerged as a leading therapy among GLP-1 receptor agonists, primarily due to its distinct therapeutic attributes that underscore its effectiveness, convenience of administration, and comprehensive clinical benefits.

1. Exceptional Effectiveness for Both Diabetes and Weight Loss

Clinical trials, such as the SUSTAIN and STEP studies, have demonstrated that semaglutide significantly outperforms other GLP-1 receptor agonists like exenatide, dulaglutide, and liraglutide in terms of HbA1c reduction and body weight loss [80, 81]. Notably, semaglutide has been shown to facilitate weight loss exceeding 10–15% of baseline body weight, comparable to surgical weight loss interventions [82, 83]. This positions semaglutide as a formidable option in the management of both type 2 diabetes and obesity, integrating effective glycaemic control with substantial weight loss outcomes that enhance patient adherence and overall health management [84].

2. Once-Weekly Dosing and Long Half-Life

A significant advantage of semaglutide is its pharmacokinetic profile that allows for once-weekly dosing due to its extended half-life of about seven days [81, 85]. This infrequent dosing not only enhances patient adherence compared to medications requiring daily administration but also minimizes fluctuations in therapeutic effects, thereby delivering consistent blood glucose control and appetite regulation [86, 87]. Real-world evidence supports the efficacy of semaglutide in maintaining treatment persistence compared to other GLP-1 receptor agonists [81, 86].

3. Only GLP-1 Available as Both Injection and Tablet

Semaglutide uniquely offers flexibility as it is the sole GLP-1 receptor agonist available in both injectable and oral formulations. This dual delivery system increases accessibility for patients, particularly those apprehensive about injections [81, 88]. The oral formulation, branded as Rybelsus, expands treatment reach for individuals who prefer pills over injections, thereby accommodating diverse patient preferences and potentially improving adherence [81, 88].

4. Superior Appetite Regulation and Weight-Control Mechanisms

Semaglutide distinctly activates pathways in the hypothalamus that are responsible for promoting satiety. This pronounced effect leads to enhanced appetite suppression and behavioural adjustments toward lower caloric intake, as evidenced by studies [80, 89]. While other GLP-1 agonists also provide appetite regulation, the depths of activation and resultant weight management with semaglutide are suggested to be superior, contributing to its overall efficacy and appeal in therapeutic settings [18, 82].

5. Robust Evidence for Cardiovascular Risk Reduction

Semaglutide stands out by providing substantial cardiovascular benefits, an aspect not commonly shared by other diabetes medications. The SUSTAIN 6 trial demonstrated a significant reduction in cardiovascular events among individuals using semaglutide, including reductions in heart attacks and strokes [50]. Furthermore, the SELECT trial indicated cardiovascular risk attenuation among non-diabetic obese patients, showcasing semaglutide's broad applicability beyond merely controlling diabetes [90, 91].

6. Strong Global Safety Profile and Widespread Clinical Adoption

With extensive investigation involving over 40,000 participants across diverse demographics, semaglutide is recognized for its favourable safety profile. Its tolerability and long-term effectiveness contribute to its rapid adoption in clinical practice worldwide, as it has been included in the World Health Organization's List of Essential Medicines [68, 85, 92]. This wide acceptance also reflects confidence in its benefits across varied patient populations [84, 93].

7. Benefits Beyond Glucose: Metabolic and Systemic Improvements

Beyond lowering blood glucose and promoting weight loss, semaglutide has demonstrated improvements in cardiovascular health markers, including reductions in blood pressure and favourable lipid profiles [20, 91, 93]. The comprehensive benefits of semaglutide for managing broader metabolic syndrome components emphasize its role as a multifunctional therapeutic agent, particularly for those primarily affected by obesity rather than diabetes [68, 87].

8. Next-Generation Molecular Design

The structural modifications in semaglutide enhance its stability and prolong its action, allowing for sustained therapeutic effects. These innovations result in improved durability compared to older GLP-1 therapies [18, 84]. Such advancements contribute to semaglutide's predictable pharmacological profile, which is essential for effective diabetes management and weight control [20, 94].

Semaglutide stands out in the GLP-1 medication class because of its unique combination of high efficacy, excellent adherence via convenient dosing schedules, and comprehensive metabolic benefits. As an innovative therapy, it plays a pivotal role in modern metabolic medicine, showcasing the potential for improved patient outcomes through its robust clinical evidence and practical administration strategies.

Brand Names: Ozempic, Wegovy, Rybelsus

Semaglutide is marketed worldwide under several brand names, each designed for specific medical purposes, dosages, and routes of administration. Although all three products contain the same active ingredient, they are not interchangeable, as they differ in their approved uses, formulations, and dose strengths.

Ozempic® – Injectable Semaglutide for Type 2 Diabetes

Ozempic is a once-weekly injectable form of semaglutide approved primarily for the treatment of type 2 diabetes. Its main role is to help individuals improve their glycaemic control—that is, to manage and stabilise blood-sugar levels.

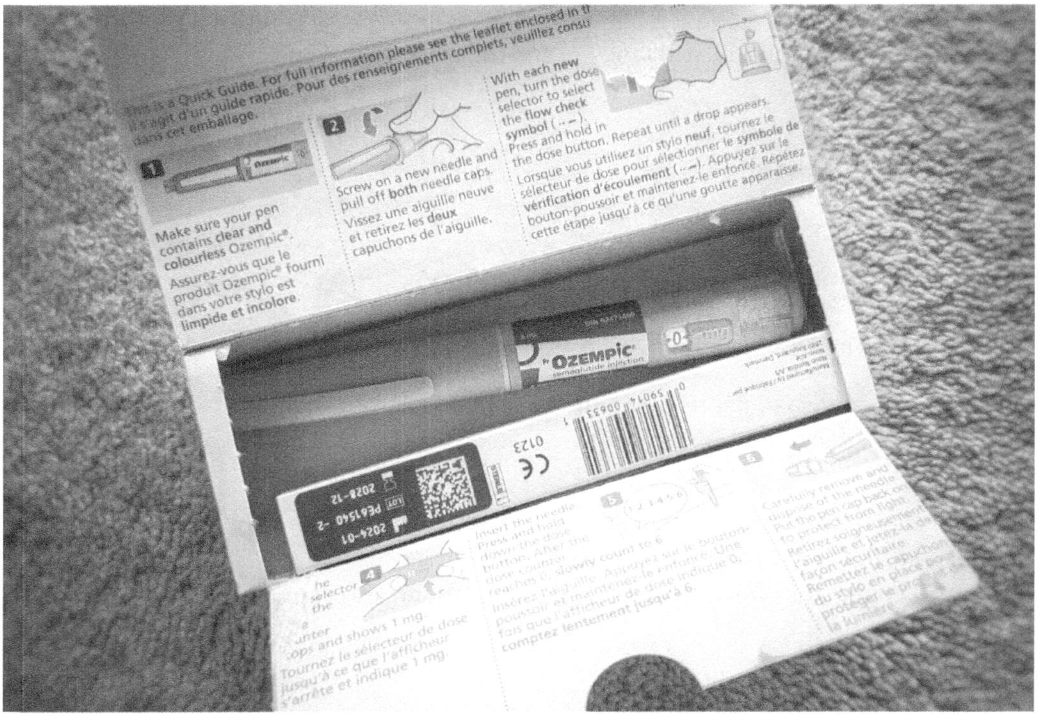

Figure 5: Ozempic Pen. Dennis Sylvester Hurd, CC0 1.0 Universal, via Flickr.

Key Features:

- **Route:** Subcutaneous injection (once weekly)
- **Approved Use:** Type 2 diabetes management
- **Secondary Benefits:** Weight loss and cardiovascular risk reduction in people with diabetes
- **Typical Doses:** 0.25 mg (starter), 0.5 mg, 1 mg, 2 mg

Ozempic helps lower HbA1c levels, reduces post-meal glucose spikes, and often results in modest to significant weight loss. Although it is widely used off-label for weight management, it is not approved specifically for obesity without diabetes, which is why Wegovy was later developed.

Wegovy® – Injectable Semaglutide for Obesity and Weight Management

Wegovy is a higher-dose, once-weekly injectable form of semaglutide specifically approved for chronic weight management in adults and adolescents with obesity, or adults who are overweight with weight-related health conditions. It is also approved for reducing the risk of major cardiovascular events in people with obesity and heart disease.

Key Features:

- **Route:** Subcutaneous injection (once weekly)
- **Approved Use:**
    - Obesity treatment
    - Weight management
    - Cardiovascular risk reduction in overweight/obese adults with heart disease
- **Typical Doses:** Rising titration up to 2.4 mg, a significantly higher dose than Ozempic

Wegovy's clinical trials (the STEP trials) demonstrated substantial weight loss—often 12–16% of initial body weight, much greater than any previous weight-loss medication. Because of this effectiveness, Wegovy has become a major therapy for obesity medicine.

Rybelsus® – Oral Semaglutide for Type 2 Diabetes

Rybelsus is the first and only oral tablet form of semaglutide and one of the first oral peptide medications ever approved. It is used exclusively for type 2 diabetes management.

Key Features:

- **Route:** Oral tablet (once daily)
- **Approved Use:** Type 2 diabetes
- **Typical Doses:** 3 mg (starter), 7 mg, 14 mg

The oral formulation creates a more accessible option for individuals who prefer not to use injections. However, its bioavailability is very low (1–2%), requiring strict instructions such as taking it on an empty stomach with a small amount of water and waiting at least 30 minutes before eating.

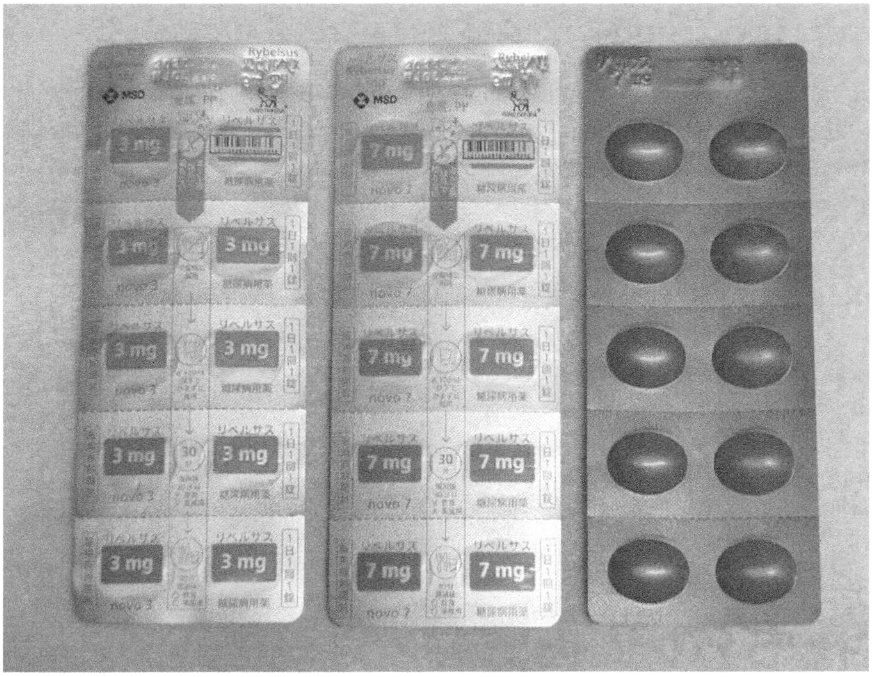

Figure 6: Rybelsus 3mg 7mg. Windshear, CC BY-SA 4.0, via Wikimedia Commons.

Table 2: Brand Comparison Summary.

Brand Name	Use	Route	Typical Dose	Key Benefit
Ozempic	Type 2 diabetes	Weekly injection	0.25–2 mg	Glucose control + weight loss
Wegovy	Obesity & CV risk reduction	Weekly injection	Up to 2.4 mg	Highest weight-loss efficacy
Rybelsus	Type 2 diabetes	Daily tablet	3–14 mg	First-ever oral GLP-1 option

Although all three brand names contain semaglutide, each serves a different role in modern metabolic medicine. Ozempic targets diabetes control, Wegovy is designed for high-efficacy weight reduction and cardiovascular protection, and Rybelsus provides a needle-free option for diabetes management. Together, they cover a broad spectrum of therapeutic needs, making semaglutide one of the most versatile and widely used medications of its class.

Oral Vs Injectable Forms

Semaglutide is distinctive among glucagon-like peptide-1 (GLP-1) receptor agonists due to its availability in both injectable and oral formulations: a once-weekly subcutaneous injection and a once-daily oral tablet. Despite both forms containing the same active ingredient, they differ in their pharmacokinetics, patient experience, and overall clinical outcomes, which may significantly impact dosing schedules and adherence.

The injectable formulations, marketed as Ozempic and Wegovy, are delivered subcutaneously, allowing semaglutide to enter the bloodstream efficiently. The bioavailability of the injectable form is approximately 89%, which results in stable drug levels and effective glycaemic control [42, 66]. Conversely, the oral formulation, sold as Rybelsus, must withstand the gastrointestinal environment, leading to a markedly lower absorption rate of only about 1-2% due to degradation in the gastrointestinal tract [58, 95]. This challenge is mitigated by the inclusion of sodium N-(8-2-hydroxybenzoyl amino) caprylate (SNAC), an absorption enhancer that protects semaglutide from degradation and facilitates its penetration through the gastric lining [58, 96].

Delivered Subcutaneously
Delivered subcutaneously means that the medication is injected *under the skin*, into the fatty tissue layer between the skin and the muscle. This method is commonly used for medicines that need slow, steady absorption into the bloodstream. Semaglutide injections (Ozempic and Wegovy) are given this way using a small needle, usually in the abdomen, thigh, or upper arm.

Mitigated by the Inclusion of Sodium N-(8-[2-hydroxybenzoyl]amino) Caprylate (SNAC)
This phrase means that a problem is reduced or helped by adding a substance called SNAC to the medication.
SNAC is an absorption enhancer included in the oral form of semaglutide (Rybelsus).
Normally, peptide drugs like semaglutide are destroyed in the stomach and absorbed very poorly. SNAC protects the drug in the stomach and helps it pass through the stomach lining into the bloodstream.
SNAC allows the semaglutide tablet to work even though the digestive system would normally break it down.

Dosing frequency and administration convenience vary significantly between these formulations. Weekly injections are favoured for their convenience and reduced burden of daily medication [97]. The subcutaneous delivery method uses user-friendly pre-filled pens with minimal discomfort for most patients, and no significant food-related restrictions apply prior to injection [42, 66]. In contrast, the oral formulation requires compliance with specific intake guidelines: it must be taken on an empty stomach with limited water, followed by a waiting period before consuming food or other medications to maximize absorption [98].

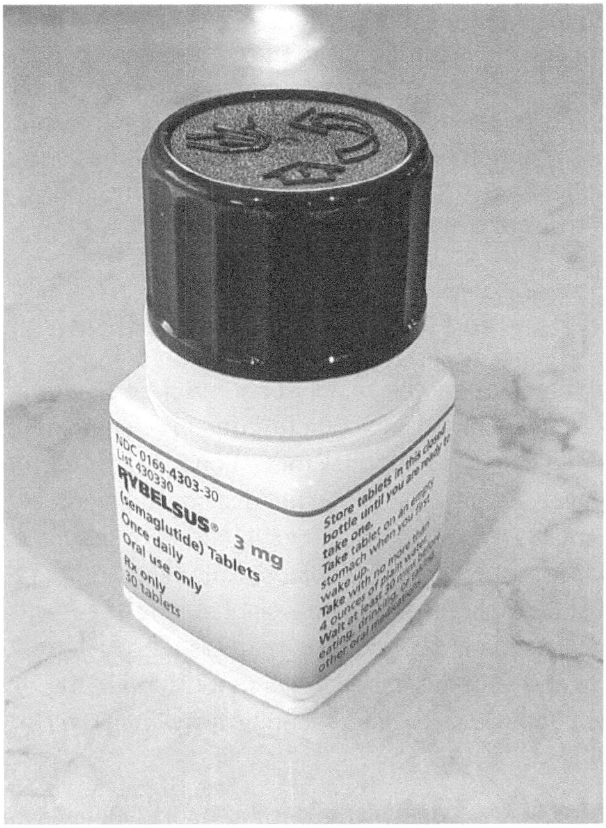

Figure 7: Rybelsus 3mg bottle. Grendelkhan, CC BY-SA 4.0, via Wikimedia Commons.

Clinical efficacy also diverges between the two forms. Studies report that the injectable semaglutide formulations generally provide more considerable reductions in HbA1c levels and weight loss compared to the oral version. For instance, injectable dosages have demonstrated reductions in HbA1c ranging from 1.5% to 1.8%, while oral semaglutide achieves reductions of about 1.0% to 1.4% in clinical trials [99, 100]. The injectable formulation typically produces stronger clinical outcomes due to the higher effective doses available, making it a better choice for patients seeking significant weight management and glycaemic control [99].

Both formulations share a similar side effect profile, including gastrointestinal disturbances such as nausea and vomiting. However, the injectable version may lead to more pronounced symptoms during dose adjustments due to the higher doses administered [62, 101]. Patient choice between formulations may depend on individual preferences; some may opt for the weekly injection for convenience and efficacy, while others might prefer the oral daily regimen to avoid needles, especially those new to GLP-1 therapies [96, 102].

Semaglutide's injectable form is characterized by higher potency, more consistent absorption, and the convenience of once-weekly dosing, making it a robust choice for managing type 2 diabetes and obesity. In contrast, the oral formulation presents a significant advancement in peptide therapeutic delivery as a needle-free alternative but necessitates adherence to stricter absorption conditions and is generally associated with lower overall efficacy.

How Widespread Its Use Has Become in Medicine and Media

Since its introduction, semaglutide has rapidly become a cornerstone in modern metabolic medicine, noted for its effectiveness in multiple domains, including blood sugar reduction, significant weight loss, and cardiovascular risk mitigation [32, 71, 103, 104]. Originally approved for the management of type 2 diabetes, semaglutide is now being widely prescribed for obesity management and metabolic syndrome, as well as in efforts to reduce cardiovascular risk. The compelling data surrounding semaglutide's efficacy is reflected in the STEP trials, which have established it as a robust therapeutic option for weight management, showing sustained weight loss and favourable changes in cardiometabolic markers [71, 105, 106]. By 2023, semaglutide achieved prominence as the 19th most prescribed medication in the United States, with more than 25 million prescriptions issued, underscoring its widespread adoption within clinical practice [107, 108].

Globally, semaglutide has been included in major treatment guidelines for diabetes and obesity, and it was added to the World Health Organization's List of Essential Medicines—a designation that emphasizes its centrality in global health initiatives [107, 109]. This guideline inclusion positions semaglutide not just as a treatment option but as a pivotal tool in managing chronic diseases that pose significant public health challenges. Its rapid integration into clinical pathways reflects the acknowledgment of obesity as a chronic disease [105, 107].

Culturally, semaglutide has transcended clinical limbs, generating substantial media and public interest due to its pronounced weight-loss effects. The STEP trials highlighted the dramatic outcomes resulting from semaglutide treatment, prompting discussions across various platforms, including television, news articles, and social media [110]. Terms like "Ozempic," "Wegovy," and "Ozempic face" have entered the public lexicon as the discussion of semaglutide encompasses lifestyle, wellness, and popular culture. This media visibility has consequently led to policy discussions addressing issues of access, ethical considerations regarding off-label use, and societal implications pertaining to body image and health equity [111, 112].

Ozempic Face
"Ozempic face" is an informal term used in media and social discussions to describe a change in facial appearance that some people notice after significant weight loss while using semaglutide (Ozempic or Wegovy). When a person loses weight quickly, especially in the face, it can lead to a thinner, more hollow, or sagging facial look. This is caused

by fat loss in the cheeks, jawline, and under the skin, which may make lines or wrinkles more visible.

The term does not refer to a medical condition and is not a side effect of the medication itself. Instead, it is simply the natural result of rapid or dramatic weight loss, regardless of the method used. Similar facial changes can occur with dieting, bariatric surgery, or illness. Some individuals may choose cosmetic treatments to restore fullness, while others experience gradual improvement as their weight stabilizes.

However, this rapid uptake also presents challenges such as supply shortages and the potential for off-label prescriptions that may complicate treatment paradigms [107, 113]. The emergence of discussions surrounding "Ozempic face" and concerns regarding the cosmetic use of the drug highlight the need for ongoing dialogue about the ethical ramifications of using semaglutide beyond its intended medical purposes [111]The conversation has evolved to encompass not only the pharmaceutical innovation itself but also the broader implications of weight management medications and their role in shaping societal views on health and wellness [32, 111, 112].

Semaglutide stands at the intersection of clinical practice, public health policy, and media culture. Its effectiveness as a treatment for obesity and metabolic disorders, combined with its enormous popularity in media, signifies a transformation in the approach to chronic diseases, shaping both medical treatment and public discourse.

Chapter 2

How Semaglutide Works in the Body

Semaglutide's clinical impact can only be fully understood by examining the biology it harnesses. Although widely known as a medication for type 2 diabetes and obesity, semaglutide works by amplifying a natural hormonal system that the body already uses to regulate appetite, digestion, and blood glucose. This system—centred around the incretin hormone GLP-1—coordinates signals between the gut, pancreas, brain, liver, and cardiovascular system, ensuring metabolic stability after eating. When this system becomes impaired, as it often does in diabetes and obesity, metabolic control begins to break down. Semaglutide's therapeutic effects arise from restoring and enhancing these pathways.

The chapter begins with the physiology of GLP-1 and the incretin system, outlining the key hormonal responses that occur immediately after food enters the digestive tract. These early processes start in specialised intestinal L-cells, which sense nutrients and release GLP-1 to help regulate insulin, glucagon, gastric emptying, and appetite. Understanding the role of L-cells and the rapid degradation of natural GLP-1 provides the foundation for appreciating why artificial GLP-1 receptor agonists—like semaglutide—were developed and how they differ from the body's short-lived hormone.

From there, the chapter explores how GLP-1 influences multiple organs. In the pancreas, it enhances glucose-dependent insulin secretion and suppresses glucagon. In the brain, it activates appetite-regulating neural pathways that reduce hunger and promote satiety. In the stomach, it slows gastric emptying to smooth post-meal glucose spikes. These physiological actions explain the powerful glucose-lowering, appetite-suppressing, and weight-reducing effects seen with semaglutide therapy.

The chapter then transitions into semaglutide's mechanism of action, demonstrating how this long-acting GLP-1 analogue engages the same pathways as natural GLP-1, but with far greater stability and duration. Because semaglutide resists enzymatic breakdown and binds strongly to albumin, it provides continuous receptor activation throughout the week—producing steadier metabolic control than older, shorter-acting GLP-1 medications. This extended action underpins improvements not only in glucose regulation but also in cardiovascular risk factors, inflammation, and liver metabolism.

Finally, the chapter contextualises semaglutide among other GLP-1 receptor agonists, detailing the structural, pharmacokinetic, and clinical advancements that make it one of the most effective therapies in modern metabolic medicine. Together, these sections build a comprehensive understanding of how semaglutide interacts with the body on molecular, cellular, and systemic levels, setting the stage for deeper exploration of its therapeutic applications in diabetes, obesity, and cardiometabolic disease.

Physiology of GLP-1 and the Incretin System

The incretin system is a key hormonal pathway that helps the body regulate blood glucose levels after eating. Its actions begin in the gut but influence multiple organs, including the pancreas, liver, stomach, and brain. Among the incretin hormones, glucagon-like peptide-1 (GLP-1) plays the most significant role in glucose homeostasis, appetite regulation, and metabolic health.

Incretins are a group of hormones produced in the gastrointestinal tract in response to food intake. The two major incretin hormones are:

- GLP-1 (Glucagon-Like Peptide-1)
- GIP (Glucose-Dependent Insulinotropic Polypeptide)

Their primary function is to enhance the body's insulin response to glucose. This is why the same amount of glucose produces a much stronger insulin release when consumed orally compared to being given intravenously—a phenomenon known as the incretin effect.

GLP-1 is produced in the L-cells of the small intestine, particularly the distal ileum and colon. When nutrients such as carbohydrates, fats, and proteins enter the digestive tract, these cells release GLP-1 into the bloodstream. It then travels throughout the body and acts on various organs involved in metabolic control.

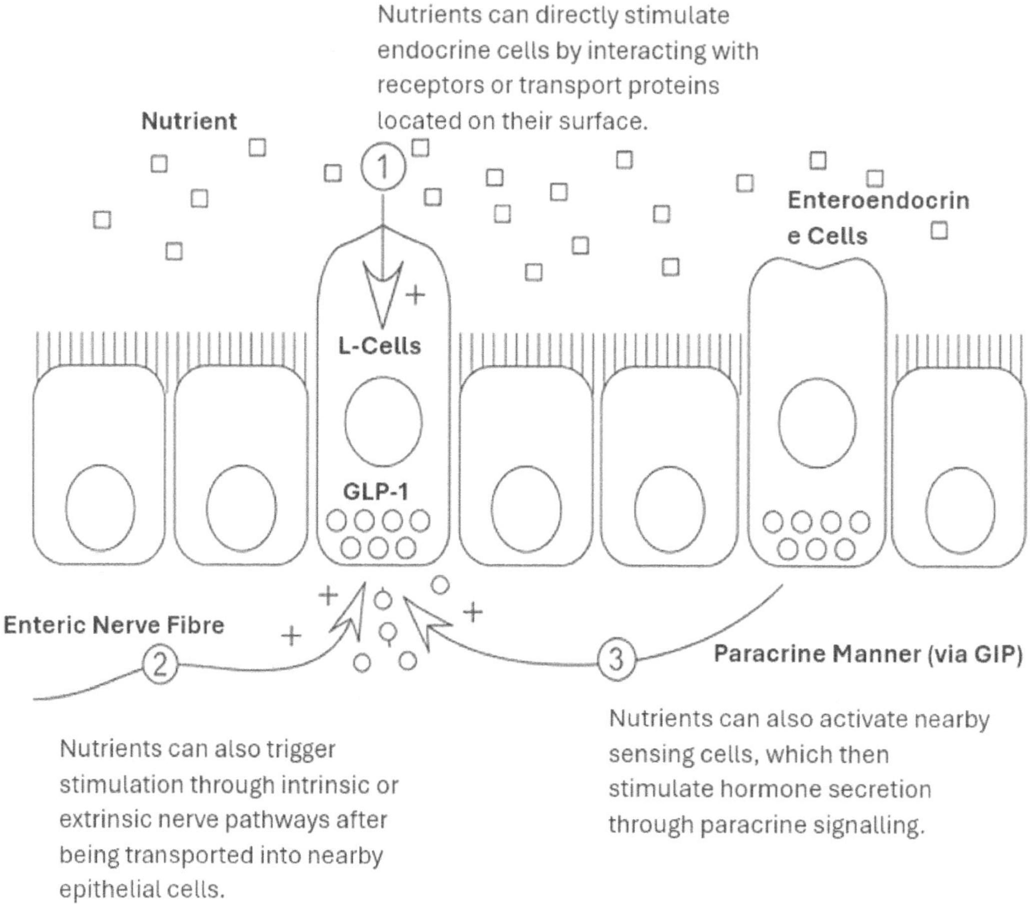

Figure 8: Nutrient sensing by enteroendocrine cells.

L-cells, specialized hormone-producing cells primarily located in the distal small intestine (ileum) and large intestine (colon), play a crucial role in metabolic regulation through the incretin system. They respond to the presence of nutrients by releasing hormones such as glucagon-like peptide-1 (GLP-1) and peptide YY (PYY), which are vital for regulating blood glucose levels, appetite, digestion, and overall metabolic balance. The positioning of L-cells in the gastrointestinal tract enables them to respond effectively to partially digested food and nutrient release. Various nutrients, including carbohydrates, proteins, fats, and dietary fibre, act as triggers for their activation, supported by evidence that indicates L-cells possess specific receptors and transporters facilitating nutrient sensing [114-116].

The secretion mechanisms of GLP-1 and PYY from L-cells significantly contribute to appetite management and digestive processes. For instance, GLP-1 enhances insulin secretion during hyperglycaemia, inhibits glucagon release, and slows gastric emptying, thereby promoting satiety. PYY further aids in appetite reduction and digestive modulation post-meal [116, 117]. These actions underscore the central role of L-cells not only in normal metabolic processes but also in the pharmacological effects of GLP-1-based therapies, such as semaglutide, which mimics GLP-1's actions, prolonging its effects against conditions such as type 2 diabetes and obesity [118, 119].

Research indicates that while L-cells are sensitive to nutrient stimuli, their responsiveness can diminish in individuals with type 2 diabetes or obesity. Studies show that GLP-1 secretion may be impaired in these populations, leading to reduced insulin responsiveness and heightened glucose levels post-meal [120, 121]. Therefore, medications like semaglutide serve a dual purpose: they enhance GLP-1 effects and help restore metabolic balance by compensating for the reduced activity of this hormone observed in these individuals [119, 122].

Moreover, GLP-1 is rapidly degraded by the enzyme dipeptidyl peptidase-4 (DPP-4), limiting its physiological effectiveness to a matter of minutes. Modern GLP-1 receptor agonists, such as semaglutide, have been engineered to resist this degradation, allowing for prolonged beneficial effects on glycaemic control and appetite regulation [123, 124].

L-cells are pivotal in nutrient sensing and hormonal regulation within the gut. Their hormones, primarily GLP-1 and PYY, are essential for managing blood sugar levels, appetite, and digestive processes. Due to their significance in metabolic functions and the context of developing therapies for diabetes and obesity, a deeper understanding of L-cell biology and GLP-1 signalling pathways presents invaluable opportunities to advance treatment strategies in metabolic diseases.

How GLP-1 Works in the Body

GLP-1 acts on specific receptors found in multiple tissues. Its effects are beneficial in the management of blood glucose and appetite:

1. Pancreas: Enhances Insulin, Reduces Glucagon

GLP-1 stimulates the beta cells of the pancreas to release insulin in a glucose-dependent manner—meaning insulin is only increased when blood sugar is high. This makes GLP-1 therapies much safer than some older diabetes medications because they carry a low risk of hypoglycaemia.

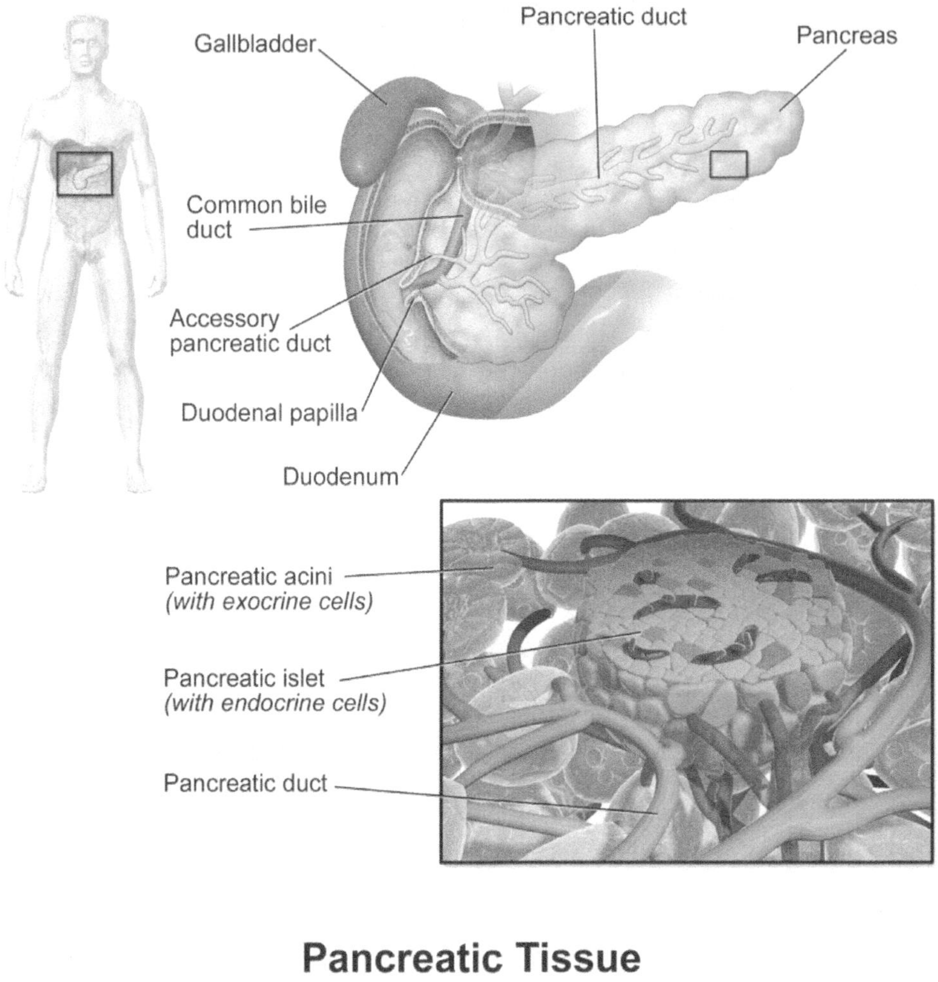

Figure 9: Structure of pancreas, revealing the Islet of Langerhans. "Medical gallery of Blausen Medical 2014". WikiJournal of Medicine 1 (2). DOI:10.15347/wjm/2014.010. ISSN 2002-4436., CC BY 3.0, via Wikimedia Commons.

At the same time, GLP-1 suppresses glucagon release from the pancreas's alpha cells. Glucagon raises blood glucose by stimulating the liver to release stored sugar. By reducing glucagon, GLP-1 helps prevent excessive glucose output after meals.

Alpha Cells
Alpha cells are specialised cells found in the islets of Langerhans in the pancreas. Their main function is to produce and release glucagon, a hormone that raises blood glucose levels. Glucagon is released when blood sugar is low, such as between meals or during fasting. It signals the liver to break down stored glycogen into glucose and release it into

> the bloodstream. Alpha cells work in balance with beta cells to help maintain stable blood sugar levels throughout the day.
>
> **Beta Cells**
> Beta cells are the most abundant cells in the islets of Langerhans in the pancreas. They are responsible for producing and releasing insulin, the hormone that lowers blood glucose levels. Insulin allows glucose to enter the body's cells, where it can be used for energy or stored for later use. Beta cells respond directly to rising blood sugar after eating. In type 2 diabetes, beta cells may become impaired, unable to produce enough insulin, or may be affected by insulin resistance in the body's tissues.

2. Stomach: Slows Gastric Emptying

GLP-1 slows the speed at which food leaves the stomach. This lowers post-meal glucose spikes by allowing glucose to enter the bloodstream more gradually. It also contributes to prolonged feelings of fullness.

3. Brain: Reduces Appetite and Increases Satiety

GLP-1 receptors in the hypothalamus help regulate hunger and fullness. GLP-1 intensifies "satiety" signals and decreases hunger signals, leading to reduced food intake. This mechanism is one reason why GLP-1–based medications, including semaglutide, are effective for weight loss.

4. Liver: Indirect Glucose Control

Although GLP-1 does not act directly on the liver, its effects on insulin and glucagon help regulate hepatic glucose production, contributing to overall glycaemic control.

Rapid Breakdown of Natural GLP-1

One limitation of natural GLP-1 is its extremely short half-life—around 1–2 minutes. It is rapidly degraded by the enzymes DPP-4 (dipeptidyl peptidase-4) and neutral endopeptidase. This rapid breakdown makes natural GLP-1 unsuitable as a medication without modification.

Modern GLP-1 receptor agonists like semaglutide are engineered to resist this breakdown and remain active in the body for much longer.

Importance of the Incretin System in Diabetes

In people with type 2 diabetes, the incretin effect is significantly reduced. This contributes to:

- insufficient insulin release
- inappropriate glucagon secretion
- higher post-meal blood glucose levels

By mimicking or enhancing incretin activity, GLP-1–based therapies help restore these metabolic pathways. Semaglutide, as a long-acting GLP-1 receptor agonist, effectively compensates for reduced endogenous GLP-1 function.

> The physiology of GLP-1 and the incretin system is central to understanding how the body manages blood glucose after eating. GLP-1 enhances insulin release, suppresses glucagon, slows digestion, and reduces appetite—making it a highly effective therapeutic target. Semaglutide builds on these natural pathways by providing a longer-acting, more potent version of GLP-1 that improves metabolic function in people with diabetes, obesity, and cardiovascular risk.

Mechanism of Action

Pancreatic Effects (Insulin ↑, Glucagon ↓)

One of the most important actions of semaglutide is its direct effect on the pancreas, where it helps regulate blood glucose through two coordinated hormonal changes: an increase in insulin release and a decrease in glucagon secretion. These effects are critical for maintaining healthy blood sugar levels, especially after eating.

Semaglutide activates GLP-1 receptors on the beta cells of the pancreas. Beta cells are responsible for producing insulin, the hormone that lowers blood glucose by allowing cells to take up and use glucose for energy. When semaglutide stimulates these receptors, it enhances insulin release—but only when blood glucose levels are elevated. This is known as glucose-dependent insulin secretion, and it is a key safety feature of GLP-1–based medications, as it greatly reduces the risk of hypoglycaemia. In essence, semaglutide helps beta cells respond more effectively to meals, improving post-meal glucose control.

At the same time, semaglutide reduces the activity of alpha cells in the pancreas. Alpha cells produce glucagon, a hormone that raises blood glucose by signalling the liver to release stored glucose into the bloodstream. In people with type 2 diabetes, glucagon levels can remain inappropriately high, contributing to elevated fasting and post-meal blood sugar. By suppressing glucagon secretion when glucose levels are high, semaglutide prevents excess glucose release from the liver and helps keep blood sugar within a healthier range.

Together, these two coordinated actions—increasing insulin and decreasing glucagon when glucose is high—allow semaglutide to stabilise blood sugar levels more effectively than many older diabetes medications. They also mimic the natural actions of GLP-1 released by intestinal L-cells after a meal, making semaglutide a powerful therapeutic extension of the body's own physiological mechanisms.

Effects on Appetite Regulation Through the Hypothalamus

Getting to Know Semaglutide and Other GLP-1–Based Medications

Semaglutide exerts powerful effects on appetite and food intake by acting on specific regions of the hypothalamus, the part of the brain responsible for controlling hunger, satiety, and energy balance. These central effects are a major reason why semaglutide produces significant and sustained weight loss in people using the medication.

After semaglutide enters the bloodstream, it crosses the blood–brain barrier and binds to GLP-1 receptors located in several appetite-regulating centres of the hypothalamus. Two key areas involved are the arcuate nucleus (ARC) and the paraventricular nucleus (PVN). The arcuate nucleus contains two important groups of neurons:

- POMC/CART neurons, which promote satiety and reduce food intake
- NPY/AgRP neurons, which stimulate hunger and increase appetite

Semaglutide enhances the activity of the satiety-promoting POMC/CART neurons while suppressing the hunger-generating NPY/AgRP neurons. This dual action shifts the balance toward reduced caloric intake, decreased cravings, and earlier onset of fullness during meals.

Arcuate Nucleus (ARC)
The arcuate nucleus is a key region of the hypothalamus located near the base of the brain. It contains specialised groups of neurons that regulate hunger, satiety, and energy balance. Because it receives signals from hormones such as GLP-1, insulin, ghrelin, and leptin, the arcuate nucleus acts as a central "control hub" for appetite regulation and metabolic homeostasis.

Paraventricular Nucleus (PVN)
The paraventricular nucleus is another important structure within the hypothalamus involved in regulating appetite, stress responses, metabolism, and hormone release. It integrates signals from appetite-regulating neurons in the arcuate nucleus and helps determine whether the body should increase or decrease food intake.

POMC/CART Neurons
POMC/CART neurons are appetite-suppressing neurons located in the arcuate nucleus.

- POMC stands for *pro-opiomelanocortin*, a precursor molecule that breaks down into peptides that reduce food intake.
- CART stands for *cocaine- and amphetamine-regulated transcript*, another satiety-promoting peptide.

When activated, POMC/CART neurons send signals that increase satiety, decrease hunger, and reduce eating behaviour. GLP-1 agonists like semaglutide stimulate these neurons.

NPY/AgRP Neurons
NPY/AgRP neurons are appetite-stimulating ("hunger") neurons also located in the arcuate nucleus.

- NPY stands for *neuropeptide Y*, which strongly increases hunger.

- AgRP stands for *agouti-related peptide*, which promotes feeding and blocks satiety signals.

When activated, these neurons increase hunger, trigger food-seeking behaviour, and promote weight gain. Semaglutide reduces their activity, helping decrease appetite.

Vagus Nerve

The vagus nerve is the longest cranial nerve and a major communication pathway between the gut and the brain. It carries information about stomach stretch, nutrient content, and fullness to brain regions involved in appetite regulation. By transmitting "I am full" signals from the digestive system, the vagus nerve plays a crucial role in regulating hunger and meal size.

Nucleus Accumbens

The nucleus accumbens is a structure located in the brain's reward system. It processes motivation, pleasure, and reinforcement, including the rewarding aspects of eating. It influences cravings and the desire to consume high-calorie, palatable foods. Semaglutide affects this region by reducing reward-driven eating and improving control over food choices.

In addition to these direct effects, semaglutide also strengthens communication between the gut and the brain. Signals from the gastrointestinal tract—especially those related to stomach fullness and nutrient presence—are transmitted to the hypothalamus through the vagus nerve. Semaglutide amplifies these signals, reinforcing the body's natural satiety response after eating. This means people feel satisfied sooner and remain full for longer periods, leading to a sustained reduction in food consumption.

Semaglutide's impact on appetite is further supported by its ability to influence reward pathways in the brain. These pathways, which involve regions such as the nucleus accumbens, help regulate motivation to eat and cravings for high-calorie or highly palatable foods. By modulating these circuits, semaglutide can reduce emotional or reward-driven eating and shift preferences toward healthier, lower-calorie foods.

The combined effect of these mechanisms is a profound reduction in appetite and caloric intake, which—when maintained over time—results in clinically significant weight loss. Unlike traditional appetite suppressants, semaglutide works by enhancing the body's *natural* satiety signals rather than forcing a state of reduced hunger. This contributes to more sustainable weight management and better adherence to treatment.

Gastric Emptying

One of the important ways semaglutide helps regulate blood sugar and support weight loss is by slowing gastric emptying, the rate at which food leaves the stomach and enters the small intestine. This effect is part of the natural action of the hormone GLP-1, which semaglutide mimics.

After a meal, semaglutide activates GLP-1 receptors located on nerves in the stomach wall, particularly those connected to the vagus nerve, which communicates digestive information to the brain. This activation sends signals that reduce stomach muscle contractions and delay the movement of food into the small intestine. As a result, nutrients—especially glucose—enter the bloodstream more slowly and steadily. This prevents the rapid spikes in blood sugar that often occur after eating, providing smoother post-meal glucose control.

Slowing gastric emptying also contributes to increased satiety, or prolonged feelings of fullness. When food stays in the stomach longer, stretch receptors remain activated, sending "fullness" signals to the brain. This reduces meal size, decreases hunger between meals, and supports overall calorie reduction. These effects are an important reason why semaglutide produces significant and sustained weight loss in many individuals.

The impact on gastric emptying is strongest during the early phases of treatment and gradually lessens over time as the body adapts. Even though the effect becomes less pronounced, it continues to play a supportive role alongside semaglutide's central appetite-regulating actions in the brain.

In summary, semaglutide slows gastric emptying by reducing stomach contractions and delaying the movement of food into the intestine. This leads to smoother blood-sugar control, reduced appetite, smaller meal sizes, and longer-lasting satiety—key components of its therapeutic benefits in diabetes and obesity.

Cardiometabolic Improvements

Semaglutide, a glucagon-like peptide-1 (GLP-1) receptor agonist, is increasingly recognized for its diverse cardiometabolic benefits beyond its primary function of glycaemic control in individuals with type 2 diabetes. Evidence from multiple studies indicates that semaglutide leads to significant improvements in cardiovascular risk profiles, enhances metabolic health, and reduces inflammatory markers, contributing to cardiometabolic improvements across varied populations.

One of the foremost mechanisms by which semaglutide achieves these effects is through substantial weight loss. As demonstrated in the SUSTAIN-6 trial, semaglutide significantly reduces body weight, a critical factor in mitigating cardiovascular strain, improving blood pressure, and enhancing insulin sensitivity [18, 79]. Excess visceral fat is known to promote a pro-inflammatory state and contribute to metabolic dysfunction. Studies indicate that semaglutide achieves weight loss by decreasing appetite and prolonging gastric emptying, which, in turn, fosters improved blood glucose management and lipid profiles [72, 125]. Notably, reduced body weight correlates strongly with enhanced cardiometabolic outcomes, emphasizing semaglutide's role as an effective therapy aimed at combating obesity-related complications [126].

In addition to its weight-loss effects, semaglutide directly impacts cardiovascular function. GLP-1 receptors are present in vascular tissues; thus, their activation by semaglutide leads to improved endothelial function and vasodilation, resulting in reduced blood pressure and enhanced blood flow [9, 18]. Clinical trials confirm that semaglutide administration leads to significant reductions in both systolic and diastolic blood pressure, even among individuals without diabetes, thus extending its benefits to a broader population [18, 127]. Furthermore, the effects on lipid profiles include decreases in low-density lipoprotein (LDL) cholesterol and triglycerides, while promoting increases in high-density lipoprotein (HDL) cholesterol, further reducing cardiovascular risks associated with atherosclerosis [72, 128].

Another crucial aspect of semaglutide's cardiometabolic improvement lies in its anti-inflammatory effects. Chronic low-grade inflammation, commonly associated with obesity and type 2 diabetes, exacerbates cardiovascular risks. GLP-1 receptor activation has demonstrated a potential to reduce pro-inflammatory cytokines, thereby improving vascular health and decreasing the risk of cardiac events [129, 130]. Notably, semaglutide has been shown to decrease epicardial fat inflammation, suggesting a dual benefit for both cardiovascular and metabolic health [52, 126].

Moreover, the results of the SELECT trial underscore semaglutide's significance in reducing major adverse cardiovascular events (MACE), including heart attacks, strokes, and cardiovascular-related mortality, indicating its profound impact on overall cardiovascular safety [79, 131]. These findings align with the current understanding that effective management of diabetes, obesity, and cardiovascular disease requires a multifaceted approach, which semaglutide effectively addresses through its various mechanisms of action.

Semaglutide presents a potent option for improving cardiometabolic health through interconnected pathways of weight management, cardiovascular function, lipid control, and inflammation reduction. Its comprehensive benefits make it a critical intervention for individuals facing the intersection of diabetes, obesity, and cardiovascular disease.

Differences Between Semaglutide and Older GLP-1 Agonists

Semaglutide represents a significant advancement in the class of GLP-1 receptor agonists (GLP-1 RAs) compared to older formulations such as liraglutide, exenatide, dulaglutide, and lixisenatide. This analysis will discuss key differences between semaglutide and its predecessors, focusing on molecular structure, half-life, potency, weight loss outcomes, availability of oral formulations, cardiovascular benefits, gastrointestinal tolerability, and the supporting clinical evidence.

1. Structural Modifications and Molecular Design

Semaglutide's advanced design includes amino acid substitutions that provide resistance against enzymatic degradation, a long fatty-acid side chain that enhances binding to albumin, and improved receptor-binding affinity. Prior GLP-1 agents such as exenatide and liraglutide lack these modifications, which leads to their rapid inactivation within the body [72, 132]. Semaglutide's structural innovations result in a greatly extended half-life, contributing to its enhanced physiological responses, including prolonged activity and more potent effects on glycaemic control and appetite regulation [18, 20, 85].

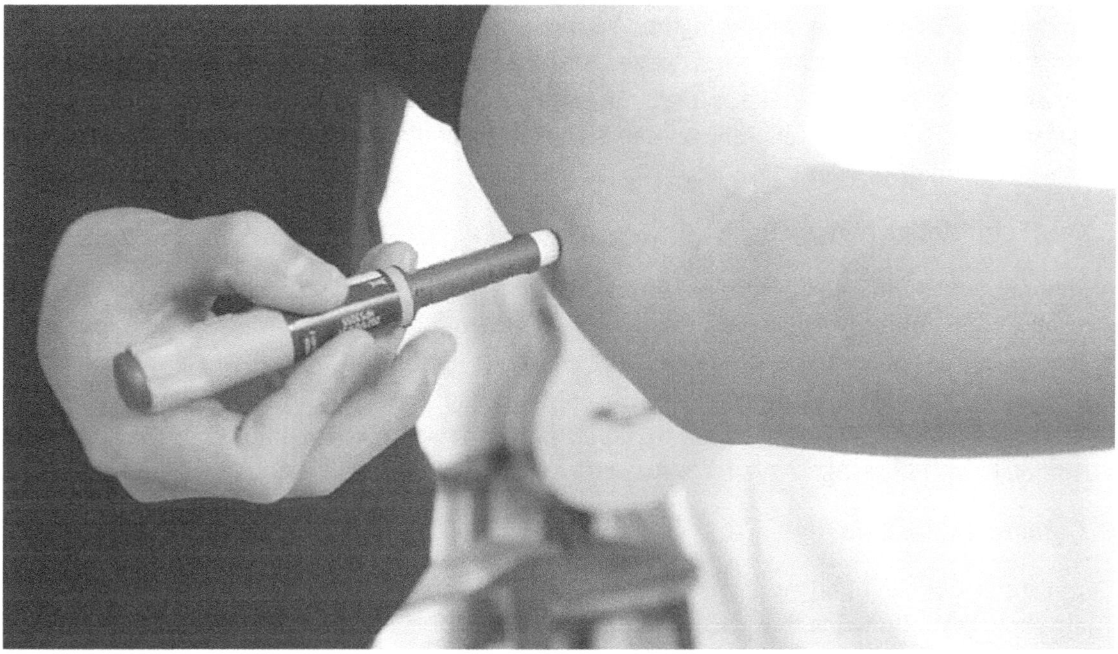

Figure 10: Saxenda Injection (Liraglutide) injected on arm. 무난러, CC BY 3.0, via Wikimedia Commons.

2. Duration of Action (Half-Life and Dosing Frequency)

The pharmacokinetics of semaglutide allow for once-weekly dosing (Ozempic, Wegovy for injections) or daily oral administration (Rybelsus), significantly optimizing convenience and adherence for patients compared to older agents like exenatide and liraglutide, which require more frequent dosing—up to daily injections [85, 133, 134]. Semaglutide's half-life of approximately seven days contrasts sharply with liraglutide's 13 hours and exenatide's 2–4 hours, thereby offering greater stability in blood levels [133, 135]. This longer duration not only enhances patient compliance but also contributes to better overall therapeutic outcomes [18, 85].

3. Potency and Receptor Affinity

Clinical data demonstrates that semaglutide exhibits significantly higher potency and receptor-binding affinity compared to older GLP-1 agonists, such as liraglutide and dulaglutide [72, 136].

This increased potency translates into superior glucose-lowering capabilities and appetite suppression, with semaglutide leading to weight loss results that are comparable to bariatric surgery [85, 136]. Older GLP-1 RAs typically yield modest weight losses, whereas semaglutide can facilitate body weight reductions of 12–16% in trials, thereby presenting a highly effective option for both diabetes management and obesity treatment [133, 136, 137].

4. Weight Loss Effects

The weight loss effects of semaglutide are particularly noteworthy, as evidenced by substantial clinical trial findings that show marked weight reductions in comparison to older GLP-1 formulations. For instance, while liraglutide 3 mg leads to weight losses of approximately 5–8%, semaglutide 2.4 mg has achieved losses of around 12–16% [20, 136]. The physiological mechanisms underlying these effects in semaglutide are thought to include stronger engagement with appetite-regulating areas in the brain, leading to diminished cravings, reduced hunger, and earlier feelings of fullness [20, 72].

5. Oral Formulation Availability

Another critical differentiation is that semaglutide is available in an oral formulation (Rybelsus), a novel offering among GLP-1 RAs. The other GLP-1 agents require injections, which can be a barrier for many patients due to needle aversion or discomfort [85, 134]. Semaglutide achieves oral viability through a combination with SNAC (sodium N-(8)-trans-hexadecenoate), an absorption enhancer, enabling it to withstand the harsh gastric environment and be effectively absorbed [134, 135, 138].

6. Cardiovascular Benefits

Semaglutide has exhibited more profound cardiovascular benefits compared to older GLP-1 RAs. Trials show that it reduces the risk of major adverse cardiovascular events (MACE) significantly and demonstrates efficacy even in non-diabetic populations [18, 137, 139]. Comparatively, while liraglutide and dulaglutide also provide cardiovascular advantages, semaglutide's effects are noted to be broader and more significant, reflecting improved outcomes in blood pressure, lipid levels, and inflammatory markers [132, 135, 139].

7. Gastrointestinal Tolerability and Dosing Strategy

Although gastrointestinal side effects are common among all GLP-1 RAs due to their mechanism of action—specifically delayed gastric emptying—semaglutide's milder side-effects profile at optimal dosages may be attributed to its titration strategies and dosing flexibility [20, 72, 85]. The structured titration schedules employed for semaglutide can enhance patient tolerability, ultimately fostering adherence over time compared to the more rigid dosing requirements of previous agents [135, 139].

8. Clinical Evidence Base

Moreover, semaglutide has the most extensive clinical trial framework validating its efficacy and safety. Its pivotal trials—including SUSTAIN, PIONEER, and SELECT—encompass diverse populations and a wealth of data that highlight its effectiveness across diabetes, obesity, and cardiovascular risk [85, 130, 133, 140]. This extensive evidence foundation surpasses that of older GLP-1 RA formulations, which, although robust, do not encompass the same breadth of evidence [20, 137].

> The advancements embodied in semaglutide over older GLP-1 receptor agonists present a compelling case for its use as a preferred agent in the management of type 2 diabetes and obesity. Its structural innovations, prolonged duration of action, superior potency, effective weight loss outcomes, oral formulation availability, enhanced cardiovascular benefits, and a robust clinical trial portfolio distinguish it significantly from its predecessors.

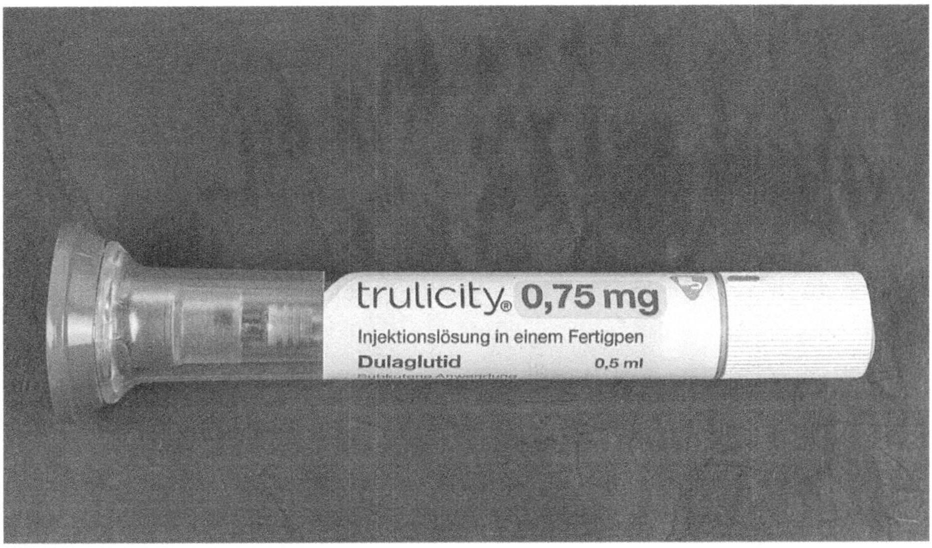

Figure 11: Autoinjector with Trulicity (0.75mg) by Lilly (Dulaglutid). Raimond Spekking, CC BY-SA 4.0, via Wikimedia Commons.

Table 3: Comparison Table: Semaglutide vs. Older GLP-1 Receptor Agonists.

Feature / Characteristic	Semaglutide (Ozempic, Wegovy, Rybelsus)	Older GLP-1 Agonists (Exenatide, Liraglutide, Dulaglutide, Lixisenatide)
Year Introduced	2017–2021	2005–2014
Molecular Design	Highly modified GLP-1 analogue with long fatty-acid side chain for albumin binding and prolonged stability	Less extensive modification; more susceptible to enzymatic breakdown

Feature / Characteristic	Semaglutide (Ozempic, Wegovy, Rybelsus)	Older GLP-1 Agonists (Exenatide, Liraglutide, Dulaglutide, Lixisenatide)
Half-Life	~7 days	Exenatide: 2–4 hours; Lixisenatide: 2–3 hours; Liraglutide: 13 hours; Dulaglutide: ~5 days
Dosing Frequency	*Injectable:* Once weekly *Oral:* Once daily	Exenatide: Twice daily or once weekly Lixisenatide: Once daily Liraglutide: Once daily Dulaglutide: Once weekly
Available Forms	Injectable and oral tablet (Rybelsus)	Injectable only
Bioavailability	Injectable: ~89% Oral: 1–2% (with SNAC enhancer)	High for injectables; no oral formulation possible
Potency / Receptor Affinity	Very high; stronger receptor binding	Moderate; weaker binding and shorter receptor activation
Glucose Lowering	Strong and consistent; excellent HbA1c reductions	Effective but generally less potent than semaglutide
Weight-Loss Effect	Substantial (10–16%+ body weight), depending on dose	Liraglutide: 5–8% Exenatide/Dulaglutide: smaller weight reductions
Appetite Suppression	Strong central effects on hypothalamic appetite pathways	Moderate appetite effects; less impact on hedonic (reward) eating
Cardiovascular Benefits	Proven MACE reduction in both diabetics and non-diabetics (SELECT trial)	Cardiovascular benefit shown for some agents (e.g., liraglutide, dulaglutide), but not as strong or broad
Gastric Emptying	Moderate slowing (most pronounced early in therapy)	Variable; strong early effect for short-acting agents
GI Side Effects	Similar class effects; stronger early due to potency but mitigated by slow titration	Common; more frequent with shorter-acting agents

Feature / Characteristic	Semaglutide (Ozempic, Wegovy, Rybelsus)	Older GLP-1 Agonists (Exenatide, Liraglutide, Dulaglutide, Lixisenatide)
Clinical Trial Programs	Extensive: SUSTAIN, PIONEER, STEP, SELECT	Earlier, smaller programs depending on drug (e.g., LEADER for liraglutide)
Use in Obesity	Approved (Wegovy) with large trials supporting weight management	Liraglutide 3 mg approved; others primarily diabetes-focused
Use in Cardiovascular Risk Reduction	FDA-approved for reducing cardiovascular death, MI, and stroke	Liraglutide and dulaglutide have cardioprotective evidence but not as broad
Overall Clinical Impact	Considered next-generation, high-efficacy GLP-1 RA	Effective but less potent; foundational earlier therapies

Why Low-Dose Sustained Action Works

Semaglutide is engineered to deliver small, steady levels of GLP-1 receptor activation over a long period, rather than short bursts of high concentration. This design is one of the main reasons it is more effective than many older GLP-1 agonists and produces significant benefits in both diabetes and obesity treatment. Low-dose sustained action aligns closely with how the body naturally regulates appetite, blood glucose, and metabolic pathways.

One of the key advantages of sustained action is the stability of hormone signalling. GLP-1 is a hormone the body normally releases in short pulses after eating, but it is rapidly broken down within minutes. Semaglutide's long half-life allows it to remain active for an entire week, maintaining a consistent level of GLP-1 receptor engagement. This avoids the fluctuations seen with shorter-acting drugs, which can lead to inconsistent glucose control, unstable appetite signals, and varying side-effect intensity. With semaglutide, the steady receptor activation results in more predictable physiological responses and a smoother therapeutic effect throughout the day.

Stability of Hormone Signalling

Stability of hormone signalling refers to the body receiving a steady, consistent level of hormonal activation over time, rather than rapid spikes and drops. When hormone levels remain stable, the biological systems they regulate—such as appetite, blood glucose, digestion, and metabolism—can function smoothly and predictably.

In the context of GLP-1–based medications like semaglutide, stable hormone signalling means that the drug activates GLP-1 receptors at a low but continuous level throughout the day (or week), avoiding sudden surges that may cause side effects or inconsistent physiological responses. This stable activation improves tolerability, enhances therapeutic effects, and closely mimics the body's natural patterns of hormone regulation.

A sustained low dose also improves tolerability, especially in the gastrointestinal system. Sudden spikes in GLP-1 activity can overstimulate gut receptors, causing nausea, vomiting, and abdominal discomfort. By keeping hormone levels stable rather than peaking sharply, semaglutide reduces the likelihood of acute side effects. Slow titration schedules further help the body adapt gradually to the drug, improving long-term adherence and patient comfort.

Slow Titration Schedules

Slow titration schedules refer to the gradual increase of a medication's dose over time, rather than starting immediately at the full therapeutic dose. This step-by-step approach allows the body to adjust to the drug's effects, helping to reduce side effects, improve tolerability, and increase the likelihood that patients can remain on the treatment long-term.

For GLP-1 medications like semaglutide, slow titration schedules are especially important because sudden high doses can cause gastrointestinal symptoms such as nausea or vomiting. By starting low and increasing the dose every few weeks, the digestive system and the brain's appetite-centre receptors adapt gradually, making treatment safer and more comfortable.

Another important reason low-dose sustained action works is its influence on the central appetite-regulation system. The brain regions involved in hunger and satiety—particularly the arcuate nucleus of the hypothalamus—respond best to continuous, gentle modulation rather than short, intense bursts. Semaglutide's constant presence supports ongoing suppression of hunger-stimulating neurons (NPY/AgRP) and enhances activity in satiety-promoting neurons (POMC/CART). This leads to a persistent reduction in appetite and cravings throughout the week, supporting consistent calorie reduction and long-term weight loss.

The same principle applies to glucose metabolism. Beta cells in the pancreas respond naturally to glucose levels, releasing insulin as needed. By providing stable GLP-1 receptor activation, semaglutide enhances this glucose-dependent insulin response without forcing excessive insulin release. At the same time, it steadily suppresses glucagon secretion when glucose is high, preventing sharp rises in blood sugar. This balance is far more physiologic and safer than medications that push insulin production regardless of glucose levels.

Finally, sustained action supports long-term cardiometabolic improvements. Gradual, consistent weight loss reduces inflammation, improves lipid profiles, and lowers blood pressure. Stable glycaemic control prevents glucose swings that damage blood vessels. Over time, these steady improvements combine to significantly reduce the risk of major adverse cardiovascular events.

Low-dose sustained action works because it mirrors natural hormonal rhythms, maintains steady receptor activation, enhances tolerability, stabilises appetite and glucose-regulation pathways, and supports long-term cardiometabolic health. This pharmacological design is a major reason why semaglutide has become one of the most effective GLP-1 therapies available today.

Pathways

Semaglutide, a GLP-1 receptor agonist, has emerged as a multifaceted therapeutic agent with significant implications for the treatment of type 2 diabetes, obesity, and cardiometabolic diseases. Its effects are underpinned by complex interactions across various physiological systems, including the pancreas, gastrointestinal tract, central nervous system, liver, adipose tissue, and cardiovascular system. At the heart of these actions is the activation of GLP-1 receptors, which are critical in regulating appetite, glucose homeostasis, and other metabolic functions.

The activation of GLP-1 receptors situated on pancreatic beta cells is one of the primary mechanisms by which semaglutide exerts its therapeutic effects. By facilitating glucose-dependent insulin secretion and suppressing glucagon release, semaglutide helps to modulate both fasting and postprandial blood glucose levels, effectively promoting glycaemic control [79, 125]. Furthermore, this action in the pancreas is complemented by its effects on reducing glucagon secretion, which assists in limiting hepatic glucose production—a phenomenon critical in the pathophysiology of diabetes [28, 125].

Moreover, semaglutide's impact extends beyond glucose regulation; it also includes significant neurobiological alterations. Upon crossing the blood-brain barrier, semaglutide activates GLP-1 receptors in areas of the hypothalamus involved in appetite control. This leads to a dual action where neuronal pathways enhance satiety through the activation of pro-opiomelanocortin (POMC) neurons while inhibiting hunger signals through the suppression of neuropeptide Y (NPY) and agouti-related peptide (AgRP) neurons [28, 141]. Thus, semaglutide leads to notable decreases in food cravings and caloric intake, aiding in weight management [141, 142].

In the gastrointestinal tract, semaglutide plays a crucial role by decelerating gastric emptying, acting on GLP-1 receptors located in the stomach [141, 143]. This leads to delayed nutrient absorption, which contributes to the prevention of rapid postprandial glucose spikes and prolongs the sensation of fullness after meals. Although the initial effects on gastric emptying may diminish over time, they are critical for achieving glycaemic control during the early stages of therapy [28, 143].

The hepatic effects of semaglutide are noteworthy, although they occur indirectly. By enhancing insulin sensitivity and reducing glucagon levels, semaglutide facilitates a decrease in hepatic glucose output, showing significant improvements for conditions such as metabolic-associated steatosis [28, 79, 125]. The weight reductions associated with semaglutide therapy further contribute to liver fat reduction, enhancing metabolic health markers in patients with obesity and diabetes [28, 141].

Cardiovascular outcomes associated with semaglutide treatment are also impressive. Data indicates that GLP-1 receptor activation can lead to favourable modifications in cardiovascular risk factors, including reductions in blood pressure and improvements in lipid profiles [144, 145]. These cardiovascular benefits stem not only from systemic metabolic changes but also from direct effects on vascular tissues where GLP-1 receptors mediate anti-inflammatory and vasodilatory effects [28, 141]. Improved endothelial function, reduction in visceral fat, and decreased levels of inflammatory markers collectively contribute to diminished cardiovascular risks associated with diabetes and obesity [144, 146].

Lastly, at a molecular level, semaglutide is a synthetic analogue of GLP-1, designed for enhanced stability and prolonged activity within the bloodstream. This modification includes amino acid substitutions and a fatty-acid side chain that allows for significant binding to serum albumin, thereby extending its half-life to approximately seven days [79, 125]. This pharmacokinetic profile ensures sustained receptor activation and minimizes the fluctuations in hormone levels that are often seen with shorter-acting GLP-1 agonists, improving patient adherence and long-term management of metabolic conditions [147].

Chapter 3

Approved Uses and Medical Indications

Building on the scientific foundations established in the earlier chapters, the clinical significance of semaglutide becomes clearer when its physiological actions are connected to real-world medical outcomes. Chapter 1 introduced semaglutide as a long-acting GLP-1 receptor agonist designed to amplify the body's natural incretin system. Chapter 2 expanded this understanding by examining how semaglutide acts across multiple organ systems—pancreatic hormone regulation, appetite and satiety signalling, gastrointestinal motility, hepatic metabolism, cardiovascular pathways, and long-term energy balance. Together, these chapters highlight why semaglutide has emerged as one of the most effective therapeutic tools in modern metabolic medicine.

Chapter 3 now shifts from the underlying biology to the *clinical applications* of semaglutide—how its mechanisms translate into approved uses, medical indications, and tangible patient benefits. Semaglutide's influence on insulin secretion, glucagon suppression, gastric emptying, appetite regulation, cardiovascular function, and systemic inflammation forms the basis for its broad therapeutic potential. These physiological effects underpin its approved roles in managing type 2 diabetes, chronic weight disorders, and cardiovascular risk reduction, as well as its emerging applications in conditions such as MASLD/MASH, PCOS, and prediabetes.

This chapter examines these indications in detail, beginning with semaglutide's established role in the treatment of type 2 diabetes—where it has helped redefine standards of glycaemic control and cardiometabolic protection. It then explores its evidence-based use in chronic weight management, a landmark advancement that positions semaglutide at the forefront of modern obesity care. The chapter further discusses its expanding recognition in cardiovascular medicine and reviews emerging research in related metabolic conditions. Finally, it considers how global regulatory environments shape access, usage, and health-system integration.

By linking semaglutide's biological pathways with its clinical applications, this chapter provides a comprehensive overview of how a single medication can address multiple interconnected metabolic diseases—reflecting a paradigm shift in the treatment of diabetes, obesity, and cardiometabolic health.

Treatment of Type 2 Diabetes (T2DM)

Semaglutide has established itself as a significant therapeutic option in the management of Type 2 Diabetes Mellitus (T2DM). Its mechanism of action is complex, addressing several core defects of the disease, including impaired insulin secretion, elevated glucagon levels, slowed glucose uptake, and dysfunctional appetite and weight regulation, thereby enhancing overall glycaemic control and offering ancillary benefits such as weight reduction and cardiovascular risk mitigation [52, 148].

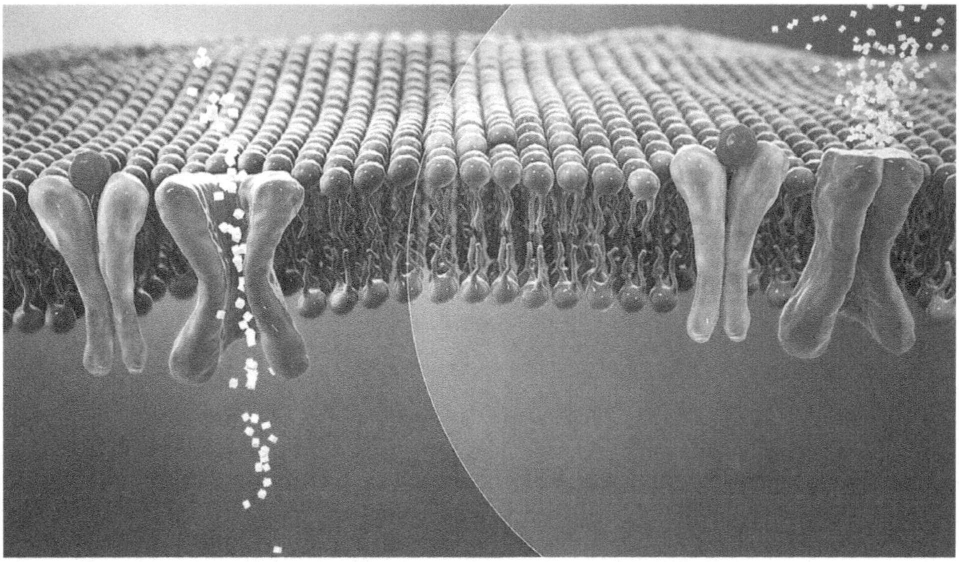

Figure 12: Mechanism of normal Blood Sugar (white crystals) absorption (Left) Vs. insulin resistance in Type 2 Diabetes (Right). Manu5, CC BY-SA 4.0, via Wikimedia Commons.

As a glucagon-like peptide-1 (GLP-1) receptor agonist, semaglutide operates through various pathways. It stimulates insulin secretion from pancreatic beta cells when glucose levels are elevated, suppresses glucagon secretion from alpha cells, and slows gastric emptying. These actions together contribute to lower post-prandial glucose spikes and enhanced insulin sensitivity [46, 149]. Clinical evidence supports the substantial efficacy of semaglutide, with trials demonstrating reductions in the glycated haemoglobin (HbA1c) level by 1.0 to 1.5 percentage points, allowing many patients to reach target glycaemic goals when used alongside metformin or other oral agents [52, 150].

Lower Post-Prandial Glucose Spikes
Post-prandial glucose spikes are sharp increases in blood sugar that occur after eating, especially meals high in carbohydrates.
Lowering post-prandial glucose spikes means reducing the size and speed of these rises, leading to smoother blood-glucose levels and better metabolic control. Medications like semaglutide slow digestion

and improve insulin response, which helps prevent these rapid jumps in blood sugar.

Enhanced Insulin Sensitivity
Insulin sensitivity describes how effectively the body's cells respond to insulin.
Enhanced insulin sensitivity means cells are more responsive, allowing glucose to enter them more easily. This lowers blood sugar levels and reduces the workload on the pancreas. Improved insulin sensitivity is a major benefit of weight loss, exercise, and some diabetes medications.

Glycated Haemoglobin (HbA1c)
HbA1c is a blood test that measures the percentage of haemoglobin (a protein in red blood cells) that has glucose attached to it. It reflects the average blood-glucose level over the past 2–3 months.
Higher HbA1c levels indicate poorer glycaemic control. It is the primary marker used to diagnose diabetes and monitor the effectiveness of treatment.

Metformin or Other Oral Agents
Metformin is the most commonly prescribed first-line medication for Type 2 Diabetes. It lowers blood sugar by reducing liver glucose production and improving insulin sensitivity.
Other oral agents refer to additional diabetes medications taken by mouth, such as:

- SGLT2 inhibitors
- DPP-4 inhibitors
- Sulfonylureas
- Thiazolidinediones

These drugs work through different mechanisms and may be combined with semaglutide to improve overall glycaemic control.

Moreover, weight management remains a critical issue in T2DM, as obesity exacerbates insulin resistance and compromises glucose regulation. Semaglutide's appetite-suppressing effects facilitate significant weight loss, often exceeding 5-10%, especially when administered at therapeutic doses (0.5–1 mg weekly) [68, 151]. The SUSTAIN trials highlighted the weight-loss capabilities of semaglutide, reinforcing its status as a standout treatment among previous glucose-lowering medications [68].

Additionally, cardiovascular risks associated with T2DM are notable, with many patients facing heightened vulnerability to major adverse cardiovascular events (MACE). Notably, semaglutide has been shown to reduce the risk of MACE, including heart attacks and strokes, notably illustrated in the landmark SUSTAIN-6 trial, which reported improvements in blood pressure, reductions in LDL cholesterol, decreased inflammation, and enhanced vascular function [52,

152, 153]. These cardiovascular benefits position semaglutide as a superior choice over traditional diabetes medications, which often neglect such systemic outcomes.

In its formulation, semaglutide is available as both an injectable option (Ozempic), which is administered weekly, and as an oral tablet (Rybelsus), which is taken daily. While both formulations contain the same active ingredient, their paths of delivery differ significantly; the injectable formulation is typically favoured in clinical practice for its enhanced potency and more pronounced effects on glycaemic control and weight loss [46, 150].

Semaglutide can be prescribed either as monotherapy for patients not tolerating metformin or in combination with various agents, providing flexibility in treatment regimens. Unlike older medications like sulfonylureas or insulin, semaglutide has a minimal risk of hypoglycaemia due to its glucose-dependent mechanism of action [68, 102]. Typically, it is indicated for adults with T2DM who require better glycaemic control, face challenges with obesity or excessive weight, or have an elevated cardiovascular risk [52, 151]. However, it is contraindicated in Type 1 Diabetes and diabetic ketoacidosis.

Semaglutide has become a cornerstone in modern T2DM management due to its ability to improve glycaemic control, promote weight reduction, and lower cardiovascular risk. Its broad efficacy and safety profile, demonstrated through extensive clinical trials, reaffirm its critical role in addressing the multifaceted challenges posed by T2DM.

Weight Management in Obesity and Overweight with Comorbidities

Semaglutide, marketed under the brand name Wegovy, has been approved in numerous countries for chronic weight management in adults classified as obese or overweight, specifically those presenting with weight-related medical conditions. This medication is administered at higher doses (up to 2.4 mg weekly) and is designed to support weight loss and long-term weight maintenance efforts. The approval of semaglutide for these applications is anchored in robust evidence from large-scale clinical trials—most notably the STEP (Semaglutide Treatment Effect in People with Obesity) trials—which demonstrate significant and sustained reductions in body weight and appetite, alongside notable improvements in obesity-related health risks [32, 84, 154].

Eligibility for treatment with semaglutide is determined based on specific criteria. Adults must have a body mass index (BMI) of 30 kg/m^2 or higher, which fulfills the clinical definition of obesity. Moreover, it is indicated for individuals with a BMI of 27 kg/m^2 or more who also have at least one weight-associated comorbidity, such as type 2 diabetes, hypertension, cardiovascular diseases, obstructive sleep apnoea, and dyslipidaemia [154, 155]. These specific eligibility criteria ensure that treatment is targeted at individuals whose excess weight significantly contributes to their health risks, thus maximizing the clinical benefits of semaglutide therapy [156, 157].

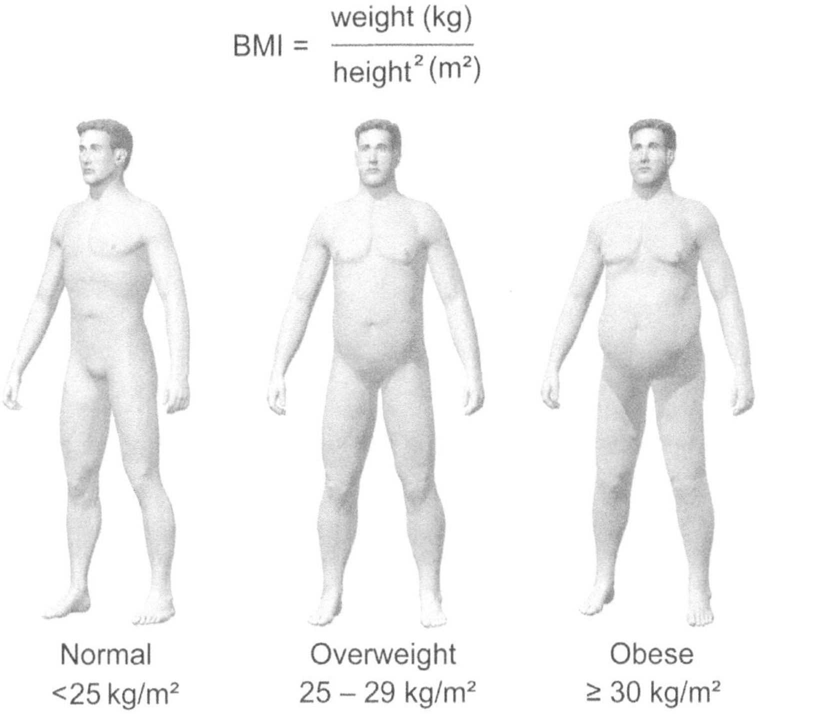

Figure 13: Obesity and BMI. BruceBlaus, CC BY-SA 4.0, via Wikimedia Commons.

> **Overweight**
> Overweight refers to a body weight that is above what is considered healthy for a given height. It is typically defined using the Body Mass Index (BMI), where a BMI of 25.0 to 29.9 kg/m^2 falls within the overweight range. People who are overweight may have a higher risk of developing conditions such as high blood pressure, type 2 diabetes, and heart disease, especially if excess weight is carried around the abdomen.
>
> **Obese**
> Obese describes a level of excess body fat that is high enough to pose significant health risks. It is generally defined as having a BMI of 30 kg/m^2 or higher. Obesity is associated with increased risk of serious conditions such as type 2 diabetes, cardiovascular disease, stroke, sleep apnoea, fatty liver disease, and certain cancers. Obesity is recognised as a chronic medical condition that often requires long-term management.

The mechanism through which semaglutide exerts its weight-reducing effects is primarily via appetite regulation. By activating GLP-1 (glucagon-like peptide-1) receptors in the hypothalamus—central to appetite control—semaglutide effectively reduces hunger and enhances feelings of fullness. It also delays gastric emptying, diminishes cravings, and alters reward-driven eating behaviours [88, 158]. Consequently, these actions facilitate a consistent reduction in caloric intake, which is a crucial component of effective long-term weight management [84, 156].

The efficacy of semaglutide as a therapeutic agent for obesity has positioned it as one of the most effective medications for weight management approved to date. During the STEP trials, participants receiving weekly doses of 2.4 mg experienced average weight reductions of approximately 15% of their initial body weight, with some individuals achieving losses of around 20% or more [32, 159]. These outcomes are substantially greater than those typically observed with lifestyle interventions alone and rival the success rates seen with certain bariatric surgical procedures, yet with significantly less risk involved [154, 158].

In addition to inducing weight loss, semaglutide provides substantial improvements in various obesity-related health conditions. Clinical studies indicate enhancements in blood glucose levels, insulin sensitivity, and significant reductions in blood pressure and fats, such as LDL cholesterol and triglycerides. Furthermore, it has been shown to decrease liver fat and inflammation while also improving symptoms associated with obstructive sleep apnoea [157-159]. These multifaceted benefits illustrate the integrative nature of obesity in affecting metabolic, cardiovascular, and musculoskeletal health [156, 157].

It's also critical to note that semaglutide has been approved for adults who are classified as overweight but not obese, provided they present with one or more weight-related comorbidities. Even moderate excess weight is associated with escalated risks of type 2 diabetes, cardiovascular diseases, and other metabolic disorders [154, 160]. Therefore, semaglutide promotes medically significant weight loss, which can decelerate disease progression and enhance overall health outcomes [88, 156].

Obesity is a chronic, relapsing condition that necessitates long-term management strategies rather than short-term dieting approaches. Semaglutide is aimed at long-term use to help sustain weight loss by continually supporting appetite control and mitigating overeating triggers. This ongoing therapy is best utilized in conjunction with lifestyle modifications, including nutritional counselling and increased physical activity, to enhance effectiveness [156, 157, 161]. Regulatory agencies also recommend the inclusion of reduced-calorie diets and physical activities alongside semaglutide to optimize weight management efforts [32, 84].

While generally well tolerated, semaglutide may produce gastrointestinal side effects such as nausea, vomiting, and diarrhea, particularly during the initial phase of dose escalation [118]. Typically, these effects are mild to moderate and can often be mitigated through gradual dose increases. Notably, semaglutide is not intended for individuals seeking weight loss for purely cosmetic reasons and is contraindicated for those with a normal BMI [154, 160].

> Semaglutide (Wegovy) represents a significant advancement in the pharmacological landscape for chronic weight management in individuals classified as obese or overweight, especially those with associated medical conditions. Its strong efficacy in achieving notably sustained body weight reductions through appetite suppression and other physiological mechanisms sets a new precedent for the long-term medical management of obesity as a chronic disease [32, 154, 159].

Cardiovascular Risk Reduction

Semaglutide has gained approval in multiple countries, including the United States and within the European Union, primarily for its role in managing type 2 diabetes and reducing the incidence of major adverse cardiovascular events (MACE). MACE encompasses cardiovascular death, non-fatal heart attacks, and non-fatal strokes, reflecting a growing recognition of the relationship between obesity, type 2 diabetes, and cardiovascular disease. Research underscores how semaglutide not only improves metabolic conditions but also addresses key pathological processes contributing to cardiovascular risk, including inflammation and vascular damage [1, 79].

The significant cardiovascular benefits of semaglutide were highlighted in the landmark SUSTAIN-6 trial. This pivotal study demonstrated a reduction in MACE when comparing semaglutide treatment to placebo among participants with type 2 diabetes who were already receiving standard care for blood pressure and glucose management [1, 79]. Subsequent meta-analyses have reaffirmed these findings, indicating that semaglutide is associated with decreased cardiovascular events [11, 162]. The SELECT trial further expanded the applicability of semaglutide by establishing its effectiveness in reducing cardiovascular events even among individuals without diabetes who are overweight or have pre-existing cardiovascular conditions [163]. These trials collectively suggest that GLP-1 therapies like semaglutide may play a broader role in cardiology that extends beyond glucose control [164].

Mechanistically, the cardiovascular risk reduction associated with semaglutide can be attributed to several interrelated factors. A principal factor is the drug's capacity to induce significant weight loss, particularly targeting visceral fat, which is closely linked to systemic inflammation, insulin resistance, and endothelial dysfunction [6, 79]. Studies have shown that effective weight management via semaglutide contributes to lowering blood pressure and improving lipid profiles, evidenced by reductions in both LDL cholesterol and triglycerides, critical markers of cardiovascular health [72, 165]. Such improvements promote the stabilization of arterial plaque and enhance overall vascular health.

Moreover, semaglutide appears to exert anti-inflammatory effects, with relevant studies indicating a reduction in inflammatory markers often exacerbated by obesity and metabolic syndrome [6, 166]. Enhanced endothelial function and reduced vascular stiffness observed in patients receiving semaglutide suggest beneficial changes in vascular health, further supporting the assertion that semaglutide positively impacts the circulatory system and cardiac workload [167]. Stability in glycaemic control afforded by semaglutide is particularly important in individuals with type 2 diabetes, as it helps protect blood vessels against oxidative stress—an important factor in diabetic vascular complications [168, 169].

The multifaceted benefits associated with semaglutide—ranging from significant weight loss, improved inflammatory and cardiometabolic markers, to enhanced glycaemic control—contribute to observed reductions in the incidence of MACE. This evidence underscores the complex interlink between obesity, diabetes, and cardiovascular health, positioning semaglutide as a critical asset in contemporary cardiometabolic management practices [1, 170].

Emerging Evidence: NAFLD/NASH, PCOS, Prediabetes

Although semaglutide is primarily approved for type 2 diabetes and chronic weight management, a rapidly growing body of research suggests promising roles in other metabolic conditions—especially non-alcoholic fatty liver disease (NAFLD)/non-alcoholic steatohepatitis (NASH), now often termed MASLD/MASH, polycystic ovary syndrome (PCOS), and prediabetes. These indications are at various stages of investigation and, in many jurisdictions, remain off-label or emerging uses, but the data provide important insight into semaglutide's broader metabolic impact.

NAFLD / NASH / MASLD / MASH

Metabolic dysfunction-associated steatotic liver disease (MASLD) and metabolic dysfunction-associated steatohepatitis (MASH), previously classified under the broader umbrella of non-alcoholic fatty liver disease (NAFLD) and non-alcoholic steatohepatitis (NASH), respectively, reflect a significant paradigm shift that underscores their intricate connection with obesity, insulin resistance, and other metabolic risk factors [171-173]. MASLD embodies a spectrum of hepatic conditions characterized by steatosis and can progress to steatohepatitis, indicating the progression of liver inflammation and injury. The clinical implications of these conditions are profound, as the excessive accumulation of fat within the liver can lead to more severe outcomes, including fibrosis, cirrhosis, and potentially liver-related morbidity and mortality [174, 175]. This evolution in nomenclature aims to enhance awareness and understanding of the pathophysiological processes driving these diseases, promoting better diagnostic and therapeutic strategies [176, 177].

NAFLD – Non-Alcoholic Fatty Liver Disease
Definition: NAFLD is a condition in which excess fat accumulates in the liver of people who drink little or no alcohol. It represents the earliest stage of metabolic liver disease.
How it emerges: NAFLD develops when the liver receives more fat than it can process or export. This typically occurs in people with:

- obesity

- insulin resistance
- type 2 diabetes
- high triglycerides
- metabolic syndrome

Over time, fat builds up within liver cells (hepatic steatosis), which can progress to inflammation and more serious liver injury if metabolic stress continues.

NASH – Non-Alcoholic Steatohepatitis
Definition: NASH is the more severe form of NAFLD. It occurs when fat accumulation in the liver is accompanied by inflammation, liver-cell injury (ballooning), and varying degrees of fibrosis.
How it emerges: NASH develops when the metabolic stress that caused fatty liver also triggers:

- oxidative stress
- chronic inflammation
- hepatocyte injury
- activation of scar-forming cells

If untreated, NASH can lead to significant scar tissue (fibrosis), cirrhosis, liver failure, or liver cancer.

MASLD – Metabolic Dysfunction–Associated Steatotic Liver Disease
Definition: MASLD is the updated medical term replacing NAFLD. It emphasises that steatotic (fatty) liver disease is strongly linked to metabolic dysfunction, not just fat accumulation.
How it emerges: MASLD develops when liver fat is present *in combination with* at least one metabolic risk factor, such as:

- overweight or obesity
- insulin resistance or type 2 diabetes
- hypertension
- dyslipidaemia
- elevated waist circumference

This terminology reflects the role of metabolic drivers—rather than alcohol—in disease development.

MASH – Metabolic Dysfunction–Associated Steatohepatitis
Definition: MASH is the updated term for NASH. It describes steatotic liver disease with inflammation, hepatocyte injury, and scarring, occurring in the context of metabolic dysfunction.
How it emerges: MASH develops when MASLD progresses due to ongoing metabolic stress. The liver moves beyond simple fat storage to:

- chronic inflammation
- liver-cell damage
- collagen deposition and fibrosis

Without intervention, MASH can progress to advanced fibrosis, cirrhosis, portal hypertension, and hepatocellular carcinoma.

How These Conditions Progress Along a Spectrum

These four terms represent a continuum of metabolic liver disease:

1. **MASLD / NAFLD** → liver fat accumulation (steatosis)
2. **MASH / NASH** → inflammation and cell injury
3. **Fibrosis** → scar tissue formation
4. **Cirrhosis** → advanced scarring and liver dysfunction
5. **End-stage disease** → liver failure or liver cancer

Progression is driven primarily by:

- obesity (especially visceral fat)
- insulin resistance
- chronic inflammation
- sedentary lifestyle
- high-fat/high-sugar diets

Because semaglutide improves these metabolic drivers—especially weight and insulin resistance—it is considered a promising therapy in MASLD/MASH.

Semaglutide has emerged as a promising therapeutic agent for the treatment of MASLD and MASH. Its mechanisms of action, including substantial weight loss, improved insulin sensitivity, and reduced inflammation, specifically address the underlying metabolic dysfunction associated with these liver diseases [172, 173, 178]. Clinical trials have provided robust evidence supporting the efficacy of semaglutide. A pivotal phase 2 study demonstrated a remarkable 59% resolution rate of NASH in patients treated with a daily dose of 0.4 mg of semaglutide, in stark contrast to 17% in the placebo group [179, 180]. Moreover, subsequent trials utilizing a once-weekly 2.4 mg dose have shown beneficial effects on liver fat content, markers of liver injury, and metabolic parameters in patients with advanced disease, underscoring semaglutide's potential as a transformative therapy [179, 181].

Despite these promising findings, it is crucial to note that while semaglutide significantly improves steatosis and inflammation, its effects on reversing fibrosis appear less consistent [171, 175]. Systematic reviews and meta-analyses converge on the conclusion that semaglutide offers significant benefits for steatosis and steatohepatitis, though substantial fibrosis regression remains challenging and may necessitate extended treatment durations [177, 182]. Moreover, ongoing large-scale studies, such as the ESSENCE phase 3 trial, aim to further elucidate semaglutide's impacts on liver histology and associated metabolic markers in multiple cohorts, thereby solidifying its role in clinical practice for MASLD and MASH [173, 176].

The reclassification of NAFLD and NASH to MASLD and MASH aligns with mounting evidence highlighting their association with metabolic dysfunction. The emergence of semaglutide as a substantial therapeutic option offers hope for enhanced management of these liver diseases. However, while current data support the notion that semaglutide improves liver health, the complexities surrounding fibrosis regression and long-term outcomes warrant further investigation to fully assess its efficacy and optimal usage in clinical settings [181, 182].

Polycystic Ovary Syndrome (PCOS)

Polycystic ovary syndrome (PCOS) is a prevalent endocrine and metabolic disorder characterized by a triad of features: oligo- or anovulation, elevated androgen levels, and polycystic ovarian morphology visible through ultrasound [183-185]. The condition is closely associated with obesity, insulin resistance, and dyslipidaemia, resulting in increased cardiometabolic risks [186, 187]. Importantly, obesity has been identified as a significant contributor to the reproductive and metabolic dysfunctions that accompany PCOS [187, 188]. Recent evidence suggests the efficacy of GLP-1 receptor agonists, such as semaglutide, in ameliorating these symptoms. The therapeutic potential of semaglutide is underscored by its ability to enhance weight loss, improve insulin sensitivity, and mitigate some androgen-related features, making it a focal point in recent research aimed at managing PCOS-related complications [189, 190].

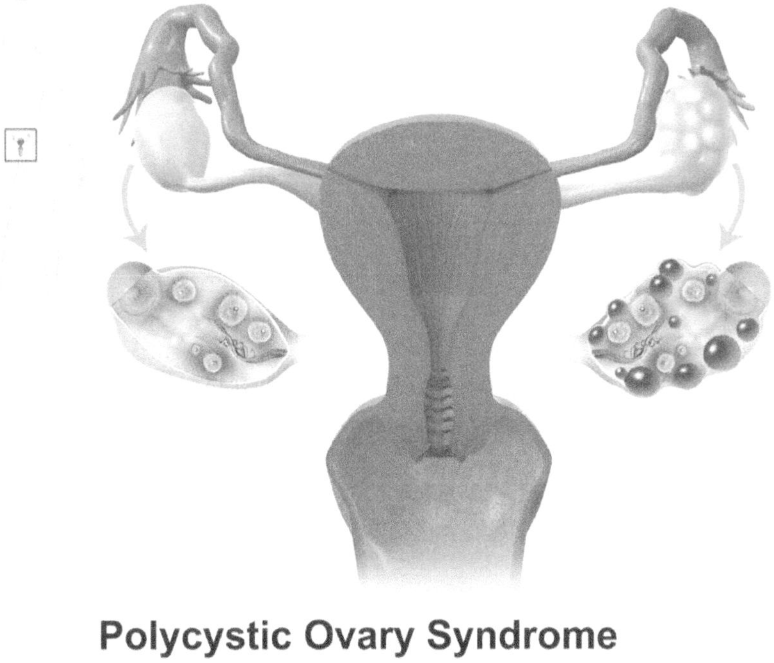

Figure 14: A medical illustration depicting PCOS. BruceBlaus, CC BY-SA 4.0, via Wikimedia Commons.

Research demonstrates that semaglutide can lead to marked improvements in various metabolic parameters in women with PCOS. A systematic review consolidating findings on GLP-1 receptor agonists revealed substantial benefits over standard therapies, including reductions in body weight, body mass index (BMI), and insulin resistance levels, alongside improvements in reproductive and metabolic markers [190, 191]. Additionally, studies on the combined use of metformin and semaglutide have indicated superior outcomes compared to metformin alone, including notable decreases in weight, waist circumference, and inflammatory markers. Such findings highlight the compound's potential not only for weight management but also for enhancing menstrual regularity and restoring ovulatory function in affected women [185, 192].

Emerging evidence also reveals implications of semaglutide in younger populations. Observational studies show that adolescent and young adult females with PCOS may experience significant weight loss when treated with GLP-1 receptor agonists compared to dietary counselling alone. This suggests that semaglutide may provide widespread benefits across different age demographics, influencing both weight and metabolic regulation in this subset of patients [193, 194]. Furthermore, experimental studies indicate that semaglutide might impact neurological responses to food cues, promoting healthier eating behaviours and appetite control strategies vital for managing obesity in women with PCOS [186, 195].

Nevertheless, limitations persist within the research landscape. Most studies are characterized by small sample sizes and varied methodologies, creating challenges in generalizing the findings [188, 196]. Long-term effects of semaglutide use regarding reproductive outcomes—such as fertility rates and live birth outcomes—remain inadequately defined, particularly as its application for PCOS is often off-label and primarily focused on metabolic risk reduction rather than reproductive enhancement [185, 187]. As further research unfolds, it will be crucial to delineate the long-term safety and efficacy of semaglutide and its role in comprehensive PCOS management strategies.

Growing evidence supports the beneficial role of GLP-1 receptor agonists like semaglutide in managing the metabolic and reproductive sequelae of PCOS. These agents offer promising avenues for treatment, particularly for women struggling with obesity and associated insulin resistance while also influencing eating behaviours, suggesting a multifaceted approach to managing this complex condition.

Prediabetes

Prediabetes represents a significant metabolic state characterized by elevated blood glucose levels, indicating a critical transitional phase prior to the onset of type 2 diabetes mellitus (T2DM). Individuals classified as having prediabetes exhibit impaired fasting glucose (IFG) and/or impaired glucose tolerance (IGT), conditions associated with a heightened risk of progressing to T2DM and other cardiovascular diseases [197, 198]. The progression from prediabetes to diabetes is particularly pronounced among individuals with obesity, especially those accumulating visceral fat, which has been identified as a major contributor to insulin resistance [199]. Data suggest that lifestyle interventions aimed at weight reduction can significantly mitigate these risks; however, pharmacological interventions such as the administration of GLP-

1 receptor agonists like semaglutide have gained attention for their efficacy in reversing the prediabetic state [200].

Semaglutide, a GLP-1 receptor agonist, has demonstrated notable effectiveness in the management of obesity and insulin sensitivity in prediabetic populations. Clinical trials such as the STEP program have indicated that once-weekly semaglutide not only facilitates significant weight loss but also leads to considerable improvements in glycaemic control, resulting in a high percentage of individuals returning to normoglycemia [200]. For example, in studies from the STEP program, those on semaglutide had much higher rates of reverting from prediabetes to normal glycaemic status compared to placebo [200]. Additionally, other clinical datasets have illustrated that the weight loss achieved with semaglutide correlates strongly with improvements in HbA1c and fasting plasma glucose levels, signifying its potential role as a preventative measure against T2DM [200, 201].

The implications of these findings are substantial within clinical practice, especially for individuals with both prediabetes and obesity. Semaglutide not only aids in achieving sustained weight loss but also enhances metabolic profiles, decreasing HbA1c and improving postprandial glucose regulation [200-202]. Despite these benefits, regulatory approval for its use specifically in diabetes prevention remains limited, as current prescriptions primarily target obesity management [79]. Nevertheless, the data support the use of semaglutide as an adjunct to lifestyle interventions for improving glycaemic control and possibly delaying the transition from prediabetes to T2DM [200, 203].

Prediabetes is a critical risk factor for developing T2DM, predominantly influenced by obesity and insulin resistance. Semaglutide has emerged as a promising therapeutic option to facilitate weight loss and improve insulin sensitivity, thereby offering a strategic approach to prevent diabetes progression. Continued research into long-term outcomes and regulatory approvals will be essential to validate semaglutide's role in diabetes prevention.

Overall Summary

Across conditions such as NAFLD/MASLD/MASH, PCOS, and prediabetes, semaglutide's emerging therapeutic roles reflect a shared underlying pattern. The medication consistently promotes significant weight loss, enhances insulin sensitivity, improves glycaemic control, and reduces inflammation and ectopic fat deposition. Because these metabolic disturbances are central drivers across many related disorders, semaglutide's ability to target these mechanisms leads to broad improvements in conditions that share overlapping pathophysiology.

Despite these promising findings, several important considerations remain. Regulatory approvals vary between countries and across specific conditions, meaning that semaglutide is formally indicated for some uses but not others. In particular, the evidence base for PCOS and prediabetes, while growing, is still evolving, and in many regions treatment of these conditions with semaglutide is considered off-label. As with all metabolic therapies, treatment decisions should be carefully individualised, taking into account patient-specific risks, comorbidities, and clinical goals, and must be made under the guidance of a qualified health professional.

Differences Between Regulatory Approvals In US, Australia, EU, UK, Asia

In the United States, semaglutide has received approval from the Food and Drug Administration (FDA) for multiple indications. It is available in various formulations, including the weekly injectable Ozempic and the daily oral version Rybelsus, both specifically indicated for the management of type 2 diabetes [66]. Furthermore, the FDA has approved Wegovy, a higher-dose formulation of semaglutide, for chronic weight management, influenced by extensive clinical trial programs, including the STEP and SELECT studies that evaluate its effectiveness and safety [105, 163, 204]. The FDA has also expanded the indications for semaglutide to include cardiovascular risk reduction for adults with obesity and established cardiovascular disease, reflecting the medication's robust evidence base in addressing obesity and its related comorbidities within the U.S. population [205].

In contrast, Australia's Therapeutic Goods Administration (TGA) has approved semaglutide formulations for diabetes and obesity management; however, the implementation has been notably more conservative. Factors such as supply chain issues and the phased introduction of Wegovy have hindered widespread access, leading to a gap between regulatory approval and practical availability [206]. Additionally, the Pharmaceutical Benefits Scheme (PBS) dictates subsidization, which can restrict access despite TGA approvals, further complicating the situation for Australian patients [207].

Within the European Union, the European Medicines Agency (EMA) has generally aligned with U.S. approvals in permitting semaglutide for type 2 diabetes and obesity [208]. However, disparities exist in reimbursement decisions and eligibility for different population segments across member states. For instance, while Germany may have quicker uptake of new medications, countries like Greece may enforce stricter eligibility criteria, thus impacting accessibility [208].

The United Kingdom's Medicines and Healthcare Products Regulatory Agency (MHRA), operating independently post-Brexit, has mirrored trends seen in U.S. and EU approvals, allowing semaglutide for type 2 diabetes and weight management [71]. However, access remains contingent on the National Institute for Health and Care Excellence (NICE), which evaluates cost-effectiveness and establishes guidelines that can impose restrictions, such as BMI cut-offs for Wegovy [71, 206].

Globally, Asia presents a mixed landscape for semaglutide approvals. Japan's PMDA and South Korea have approved the medication primarily for diabetes management, with more rigorous criteria for weight-management approvals reflecting regional regulatory caution [208]. Countries like Singapore have aligned closely with U.S. and EU trends, while China has approached semaglutide approvals more slowly, requiring local clinical data to support effective use [71, 208].

These international discrepancies in semaglutide's approval and usage highlight the influence of local healthcare priorities, regulatory processes, and economic models. Understanding these differences is essential for clinicians and patients as they navigate the complexities of treatment options and the potential for off-label usage, particularly in regions where semaglutide's utilization might not be comprehensively approved yet [163, 204, 206].

Table 4: Comparison Table: Semaglutide Regulatory Approvals Across Global Regions.

Region / Regulator	Brands Approved	Approved Indications	Cardiovascular Risk Reduction Approval	Notable Regional Considerations
United States (FDA)	Ozempic (weekly injection) Rybelsus (oral) Wegovy (weekly injection)	- Type 2 diabetes (Ozempic, Rybelsus) - Chronic weight management for obesity/overweight with comorbidities (Wegovy)	**Approved** (2024): For adults with obesity/overweight and established cardiovascular disease	Broadest and earliest approvals; strong national focus on obesity treatment; indications informed by large U.S.-based trials (STEP, SELECT)
Australia (TGA)	Ozempic Rybelsus Wegovy (approved but staged rollout)	- Type 2 diabetes (Ozempic, Rybelsus) - Chronic weight management (Wegovy)	**Not yet aligned with U.S. timing**; cardiovascular indication pending independent review	Access strongly influenced by PBS subsidy decisions; slower rollout of Wegovy; conservative approach to obesity medications
European Union (EMA)	Ozempic Rybelsus Wegovy	- Type 2 diabetes (Ozempic, Rybelsus) - Chronic weight management (Wegovy)	**Approved**: For adults with overweight/obesity and cardiovascular disease	Harmonised approval across member states, but reimbursement varies by country
United Kingdom (MHRA)	Ozempic Rybelsus Wegovy	- Type 2 diabetes (Ozempic, Rybelsus) - Chronic weight management (Wegovy)	**Under evaluation / aligned with EMA direction**	NICE guidelines determine access within the NHS; weight management use limited to specific BMI

Region / Regulator	Brands Approved	Approved Indications	Cardiovascular Risk Reduction Approval	Notable Regional Considerations
				thresholds and clinical conditions
Japan (PMDA)	Ozempic Rybelsus Wegovy (recent approval with strict criteria)	- Type 2 diabetes (Ozempic, Rybelsus) - Limited obesity indication (Wegovy)	**Not widely approved**; cardiovascular indication lagging	Historically cautious with obesity drugs; stricter safety standards; frequently requires local clinical data
South Korea	Ozempic Wegovy	- Type 2 diabetes (Ozempic) - Obesity treatment (Wegovy)	**Not widely approved**	Rapid uptake of Wegovy due to high demand; regulatory pathway similar to Western standards
Singapore	Ozempic Rybelsus Wegovy	- Type 2 diabetes (Ozempic, Rybelsus) - Obesity treatment (Wegovy)	**Emerging alignment with U.S./EU decisions**	Closely follows U.S./EU regulatory trends; fast adoption of new metabolic therapies
China	Ozempic	- Type 2 diabetes (Ozempic)	**Not approved**; obesity indications pending	More cautious and data-intensive regulatory process; slower approval of weight-management therapies; oral and obesity indications lag behind

Limitations and Contraindications

Far Reaching Potential

A large, real-world evaluation involving 2.4 million participants has provided one of the most comprehensive assessments to date of the risks and benefits associated with glucagon-like peptide-1 receptor agonists (GLP-1RAs), including semaglutide. These medications are already well established as effective treatments for type 2 diabetes and obesity, but the new findings indicate that their impact may extend far beyond glucose control and weight management. Using extensive data from the United States Department of Veterans Affairs, researchers investigated 175 different health outcomes in 215,970 people prescribed GLP-1RAs as part of routine diabetes care [209]. The outcomes of these patients were compared with multiple cohorts receiving other commonly used diabetes medications, including sulfonylureas, DPP-4 inhibitors, and SGLT2 inhibitors [209].

Sulfonylureas
Definition: Sulfonylureas are a class of oral medications used to treat type 2 diabetes by stimulating the pancreas to release more insulin. They bind to sulfonylurea receptors (SUR1) on pancreatic beta cells, causing insulin secretion *regardless of blood glucose level*.
Key features:

- Increase endogenous insulin production
- Effective at lowering blood glucose
- Risk of hypoglycaemia due to glucose-independent action
- Common examples: glipizide, glyburide (glibenclamide), glimepiride

Role: Older, widely used drugs but less favoured today due to hypoglycaemia and weight gain.

DPP-4 Inhibitors (Dipeptidyl Peptidase-4 Inhibitors)
Definition: DPP-4 inhibitors are oral type 2 diabetes medications that block the enzyme DPP-4, which normally breaks down incretin hormones (including GLP-1 and GIP). By inhibiting DPP-4, these drugs increase the levels and duration of natural incretins.
Physiological effects:

- Enhance glucose-dependent insulin secretion
- Suppress glucagon when glucose is high
- Modest improvements in HbA1c
- Low risk of hypoglycaemia

Common examples: sitagliptin, saxagliptin, linagliptin, alogliptin
Role: Considered weight-neutral and safe but less potent than GLP-1 receptor agonists.

SGLT2 Inhibitors (Sodium–Glucose Cotransporter-2 Inhibitors)
Definition: SGLT2 inhibitors are oral medications that lower blood glucose by blocking the SGLT2 transporter in the proximal renal tubules of the kidneys. This reduces glucose reabsorption and increases urinary glucose excretion ("glycosuria").
Physiological effects:

- Lower blood glucose *independently of insulin*
- Promote mild weight loss and blood-pressure reduction
- Improve cardiovascular and renal outcomes

Common examples: empagliflozin, dapagliflozin, canagliflozin, ertugliflozin
Role: Highly valued in modern diabetes management for heart- and kidney-protective benefits.

The results revealed a complex profile of both benefits and risks. GLP-1RA use was associated with *reduced risk in 42 health outcomes*, many of which extend beyond traditional metabolic effects. Participants taking these medications had significantly lower risks of several neurological, psychiatric, infectious, respiratory, and cardiometabolic conditions [209]. Notably, lower rates were seen in substance use disorders, psychotic disorders, seizures, and neurocognitive diseases such as Alzheimer's disease and dementia. These findings suggest potential neuroprotective benefits that are still not fully understood [209]. The medications were also linked with fewer respiratory illnesses, fewer coagulation problems, and a reduced risk of major cardiovascular conditions including deep vein thrombosis, pulmonary embolism, stroke, cardiac arrest, heart failure, and myocardial infarction. Taken together, these effects indicate that GLP-1RAs may offer broad, systemic improvements in health, likely related to their ability to reduce inflammation, improve metabolic function, and influence organ systems far beyond the pancreas [209].

However, the study also identified *increased risks in 19 health outcomes*, most of which relate to gastrointestinal or autonomic side effects already recognised in clinical practice. Patients using GLP-1RAs had higher rates of nausea, vomiting, abdominal pain, gastritis, and diverticulitis—consistent with the well-known gastrointestinal intolerance associated with this class [209]. Additional risks included hypotension, syncope (fainting), and arthritis. These adverse effects emphasise the need for careful monitoring, slow dose titration, and appropriate patient selection. The findings also come amid other recent reports suggesting a possible increased risk of suicidal ideation in individuals with anxiety or depression who take semaglutide, though this remains an area of active investigation and conflicting evidence [209].

Australian clinicians and researchers have offered perspectives on the implications of this major U.S. study. Obesity and bariatric medicine specialist Dr Georgia Rigas welcomed the findings, describing them as an important step forward that highlights the "far-reaching potential" of GLP-1Ras [209]. She noted that the benefits appear to extend well beyond blood sugar and body weight, touching on cardiovascular, respiratory, and neurological health. Dr Rigas emphasised that the side-effect profile observed in the study is consistent with what clinicians already recognise, which may give further confidence in the use of GLP-1 therapies in appropriate patients [209]. At the same time, she acknowledged that these medications have become extremely popular in Australia—particularly semaglutide as Ozempic—driven in part by social media interest in weight loss. This has resulted in prolonged shortages, off-label demand, and the emergence (and subsequent banning) of unregulated replica versions. With formal availability of weight-loss-specific versions such as Wegovy and Mounjaro expanding, regulatory authorities continue to closely monitor safety, supply, and prescribing patterns.

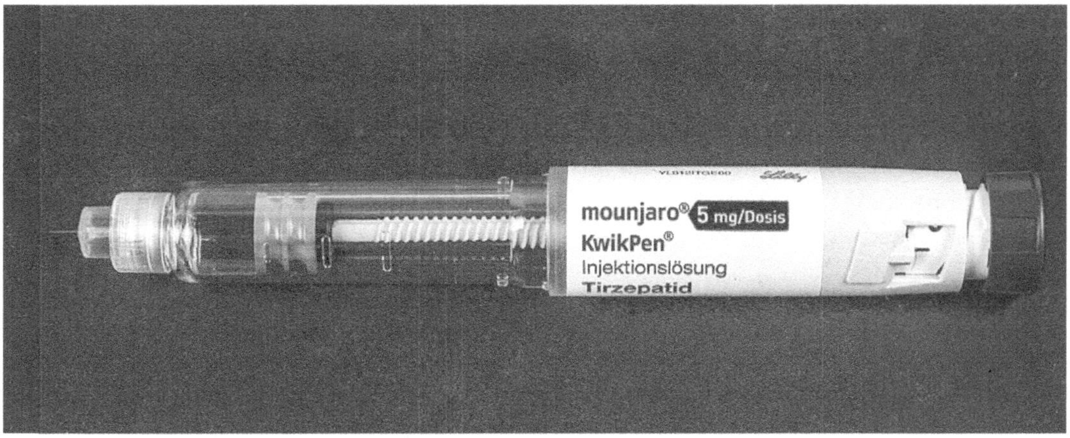

Figure 15: Lilly Mounjaro KwikPen Tirzepatid 5 mg per dose rate. Raimond Spekking, CC BY-SA 4.0, via Wikimedia Commons.

Public health expert Professor Tony Blakely from the University of Melbourne also commented on the study, highlighting how it adds to the expanding understanding of GLP-1RAs as potentially transformative agents in metabolic and cardiovascular medicine. He noted that while the results are promising, they apply primarily to people with diabetes—the population included in the study. For people without diabetes who use GLP-1 drugs mainly for weight loss, the effects may not be identical, as diabetes-related inflammation and metabolic dysfunction could partly explain the wide-ranging benefits seen in the research. This distinction underscores the need for further targeted studies in non-diabetic populations using GLP-1 medications for obesity alone [209].

The authors of the study concluded that their findings offer important insights into both the positive and negative health effects of GLP-1RAs and may help guide clinical decisions and future research priorities [209]. However, they emphasised that the study population—composed largely of older, white male veterans—limits the generalisability of the results. More diverse research cohorts are needed to determine whether these wide-ranging benefits and risks apply across different ages, genders, and ethnic groups. Despite these limitations, the study represents a major contribution to understanding the broader systemic effects of semaglutide and related therapies, reinforcing their growing role in modern metabolic, cardiovascular, and preventive medicine [209].

Limitations and Contraindications of Semaglutide

Semaglutide represents a significant therapy for type 2 diabetes, obesity, and cardiometabolic risk reduction; however, its use is subject to specific clinical limitations due to contraindications and patient-specific risk factors. Understanding these factors is vital for effective and safe prescribing.

1. Absolute Contraindications

Absolute contraindications are critical in determining when semaglutide should not be prescribed. A significant concern surrounding semaglutide is its association with an increased risk of medullary thyroid carcinoma (MTC), as highlighted by studies indicating that rodent models have shown a heightened risk of thyroid C-cell tumours [210]. Semaglutide is thus contraindicated in individuals with a personal or family history of MTC or with genetic predispositions such as Multiple Endocrine Neoplasia type 2 (MEN2) [210]. Additionally, known hypersensitivity to semaglutide or its components represents a critical reason for abstaining from this medication [210].

2. Relative Contraindications / Situations Requiring Caution

Relative contraindications necessitate close monitoring and careful assessment rather than an outright prohibition of therapy. Pregnancy and breastfeeding present notable challenges. Animal studies have suggested potential foetal harm, prompting recommendations for discontinuation at least two months prior to conception due to the drug's long half-life [32]. Furthermore, the safety of semaglutide during breastfeeding remains uncertain, typically leading to avoidance in lactating mothers [211].

History of pancreatitis is another area of caution. While a causal relationship between GLP-1 receptor agonists, including semaglutide, and pancreatitis exists, the risk is notably reported among those with a history of acute pancreatitis or gallstone-related pancreatitis [133]. Patients with severe gastrointestinal disorders should also be administered semaglutide cautiously, as the drug's mechanism—slowing gastric emptying—can exacerbate symptoms in conditions like gastroparesis or gastric outlet obstruction [212].

The impact of semaglutide on diabetic retinopathy is particularly concerning; clinical trials have documented a transient worsening of retinopathy upon rapid glucose control improvements, which requires careful monitoring in at-risk populations [130, 213]. Lastly, patients with significant renal impairment need to be managed vigilantly, especially during episodes of gastrointestinal distress that could precipitate acute kidney injury due to dehydration [60].

3. Known Limitations of Semaglutide

Despite its advantages, semaglutide presents limitations, particularly in tolerability concerning gastrointestinal side effects (e.g., nausea and vomiting), which are evidently dose-dependent and the most reported during therapy escalation [161]. Moreover, the potential for weight regain after cessation of semaglutide usage underscores the necessity for ongoing management of obesity as a chronic condition; long-term dependency on therapy reflects the broader nature of obesity treatment [32, 133].

Cost and access issues further complicate its prescription in practice; the high price of semaglutide and variability in insurance coverage can restrict patient availability to this therapy [205]. Additionally, the necessity for a prolonged titration period—where dosages gradually increase over several weeks to minimize side effects—affects timely access to effective treatment [32, 133].

4. Limitations in Specific Populations

Certain populations, such as the elderly or adolescents, present unique challenges when prescribing semaglutide. Older adults may be more susceptible to complications like dehydration and muscle loss during weight management, necessitating individualized dosing [96]. For adolescents, the long-term effects of semaglutide on growth and bone density during puberty remain under exploration, thereby invoking caution when considering therapy in younger populations [96]. Furthermore, semaglutide is not approved for type 1 diabetes management, primarily due to the risk of ketoacidosis when insulin dosing is improperly adjusted [32].

5. Limitations Related to Mechanism of Action

The pharmacodynamics of semaglutide also present limitations. Over time, patients can develop a tolerance to the effects of GLP-1 receptor agonists, leading to diminished efficacy [133]. Additionally, while semaglutide showcases efficacy in treating early-stage non-alcoholic fatty liver disease, its limitations become evident regarding advanced liver fibrosis and cirrhosis, which merits further investigation [210].

Table 5: Contraindications and Conditions Requiring Caution for Semaglutide.

Category	Condition	Level of Concern	Why It Matters	Clinical Guidance
Absolute Contraindications	**Personal or family history of Medullary Thyroid Carcinoma (MTC)**	**Do NOT use**	Based on rodent studies showing C-cell tumours; human relevance uncertain but risk cannot be excluded.	Avoid semaglutide entirely; choose alternative therapy.
	Multiple Endocrine Neoplasia type 2 (MEN2)	**Do NOT use**	Strong association with thyroid C-cell hyperplasia and malignancy.	Contraindicated in all formulations.
	Serious hypersensitivity to semaglutide or excipients	**Do NOT use**	Risk of anaphylaxis or severe allergic reactions.	Permanently discontinue if reaction occurs.
Pregnancy and Lactation	**Pregnancy**	**Avoid use**	Potential foetal harm; weight loss unsafe in pregnancy; long half-life means prolonged exposure.	Stop ≥2 months before planned conception.

Category	Condition	Level of Concern	Why It Matters	Clinical Guidance
	Breastfeeding	**Avoid use**	Limited data on drug passage into breast milk.	Use alternative therapy until breastfeeding ends.
Use with Caution	**History of pancreatitis**	**Caution**	GLP-1 RAs associated with pancreatitis; causality unclear.	Avoid if previous episodes were severe; monitor symptoms.
	Severe gastrointestinal disease (e.g., gastroparesis)	**Caution**	Semaglutide slows gastric emptying, may worsen motility disorders.	Prefer alternative treatment in severe cases.
	Diabetic retinopathy (especially proliferative)	**Caution**	Rapid glucose lowering linked with transient worsening of retinopathy.	Start slowly; ophthalmology follow-up recommended.
	Renal impairment during dehydration	**Caution**	Severe vomiting/diarrhoea may cause acute kidney injury.	Monitor renal function; ensure adequate hydration.
	Gallbladder disease (gallstones, cholecystitis)	**Caution**	Rapid weight loss increases gallstone risk.	Monitor for biliary symptoms.
	History of mental health conditions (e.g., depression, suicidal ideation)	**Caution**	Some reports of mood changes and rare suicidal ideation.	Assess psychiatric history; monitor mood throughout treatment.
	Elderly or frail patients	**Caution**	Risk of dehydration, excessive weight loss, sarcopenia.	Consider lower dose or closer monitoring.
Populations Not Approved	**Type 1 diabetes**	**Not approved**	Semaglutide does not replace insulin; risk of ketoacidosis if insulin reduced.	Do not use as monotherapy or insulin substitute.

Category	Condition	Level of Concern	Why It Matters	Clinical Guidance
	Children <12 years (for obesity) and <18 years (for diabetes)	**Not approved (except Wegovy 12–17 yrs in some regions)**	Limited long-term safety data.	Follow regional approvals strictly.

Semaglutide is a powerful therapeutic option for diabetes and obesity management, but its clinical application is confined by numerous absolute and relative contraindications, along with several inherent limitations that necessitate thorough evaluation and monitoring. Understanding these parameters is essential for appropriate clinical decision-making.

Chapter 4

Forms, Dosing, and Administration

Chapters 2 and 3 established a comprehensive understanding of semaglutide's mechanisms of action, clinical effects, and approved therapeutic uses across type 2 diabetes, obesity, cardiovascular risk reduction, and emerging metabolic indications. These earlier chapters highlighted how semaglutide interacts with multiple physiological systems—pancreatic, gastrointestinal, hepatic, neurological, and cardiovascular—and why its ability to activate GLP-1 receptors throughout the body leads to widespread metabolic benefits. Together, these insights form the scientific foundation required for understanding how the medication should be administered in real-world clinical practice.

This chapter builds on that foundation by turning from *what semaglutide does* to *how semaglutide is used*. Forms, dosing schedules, and administration strategies are central to the drug's safe and effective use, particularly because semaglutide's potency, long half-life, and gastrointestinal effects require thoughtful titration and precise patient instructions. This chapter explains the practical differences between injectable and oral formulations, outlines the rationale behind dose-escalation schedules, and explores the essential principles governing timing, missed doses, switching formulations, and long-term treatment adherence.

Where previous chapters examined the pharmacology and clinical outcomes, this chapter focuses on the key practical questions such as:

- How should injectable versus oral semaglutide be administered for maximum efficacy?
- Why do both formulations require slow, structured dose escalation?
- What adjustments are needed when transitioning between brands or delivery routes?
- How do storage, handling, and proper injection technique impact safety and effectiveness?

By detailing these considerations, Chapter 4 provides essential guidance for clinicians, educators, and patients. It translates semaglutide's pharmacological complexity into practical steps that support safe initiation, optimal titration, and long-term therapeutic success—ensuring the powerful benefits described in earlier chapters can be achieved consistently in everyday clinical care.

Overview of Injectable (Subcutaneous) Formulations

Injectable semaglutide has emerged as a clinically established formulation of this glucagon-like peptide-1 receptor agonist (GLP-1 RA). Administered as a once-weekly subcutaneous injection, it harnesses semaglutide's long half-life to provide a stable pharmacokinetic profile characterized by predictable absorption and high bioavailability, which is estimated at approximately 89% [214, 215]. Designed for self-administration, semaglutide is marketed under two primary brand names: Ozempic for the management of type 2 diabetes and Wegovy for chronic weight management [71].

The route of administration for semaglutide, specifically subcutaneous injection, is pivotal for its therapeutic efficacy. Approved injection sites include the abdomen, thigh, and upper arm, allowing for consistent absorption [66]. Each injection utilizes a pre-filled, multi-dose pen injector, simplifying the administration process for patients who may lack prior injection experience. This design facilitates ease of dosing, with Ozempic allowing for variable dosing and Wegovy using fixed-dose increments [71].

Route of Administration

Injectable semaglutide is administered subcutaneously, meaning the medication is injected into the fatty tissue just beneath the skin. Approved injection sites include:

- the abdomen
- the front of the thigh
- the upper arm

These areas provide consistent absorption and are suitable for self-injection.

One of the significant advantages of semaglutide's injectable formulation is its once-weekly dosing schedule. This scheduling is supported by its half-life, which helps maintain stable blood concentration levels with a single injection [216]. Patients are typically instructed to administer their dose on the same day each week, although they have flexibility in adjusting the dosing day, provided a minimum of 48 hours has elapsed since the last injection [217]. Gradual titration of the initial dosage is recommended to minimize gastrointestinal side effects; Ozempic starts at 0.25 mg weekly, advancing to 2 mg based on glycaemic needs, while Wegovy commences at 0.25 mg and can reach a maintenance dose of 2.4 mg [66, 71].

Dosing Frequency

One of the main advantages of injectable semaglutide is once-weekly dosing. Thanks to its extended half-life (~7 days) and albumin-binding properties, the medication maintains stable blood levels with a single injection every seven days. Patients are advised to inject on the same day each week, with flexibility to change the day if needed (as long as at least 48 hours have passed since the previous dose).

Dose Strengths and Titration

Injectable semaglutide is titrated gradually to improve tolerability and minimise gastrointestinal side effects.

Ozempic (Type 2 Diabetes):

- Starts at 0.25 mg weekly (non-therapeutic introduction dose)
- Increased to 0.5 mg
- May be escalated to 1 mg or 2 mg weekly depending on glycaemic targets

Wegovy (Weight Management):

- Begins at 0.25 mg and increases stepwise through 0.5 mg, 1.0 mg, and 1.7 mg
- Reaches the therapeutic maintenance dose of **2.4 mg weekly**

The slow escalation is essential because it allows the gastrointestinal system and appetite pathways to adjust to the drug's effects.

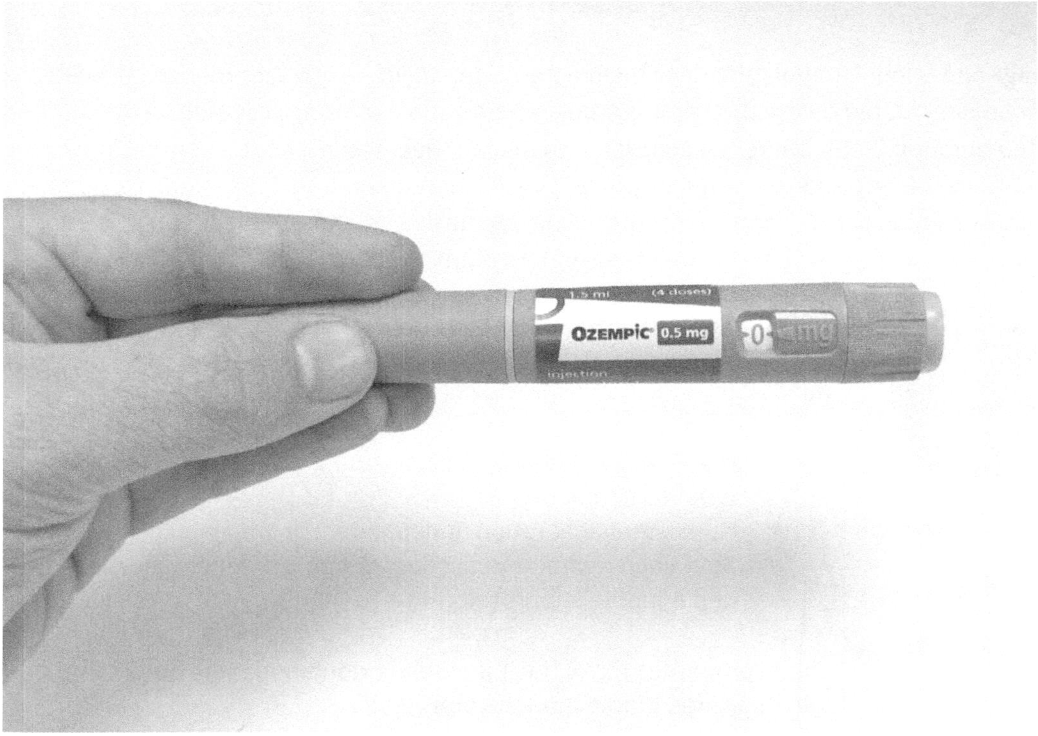

Figure 16: Ozempic Injector Pen. Chemist4U, CC BY-SA 2.0, via Flickr.

The injectable form offers several pharmacokinetic advantages. Importantly, its absorption is unaffected by food intake, fostering sustained activation of GLP-1 receptors, which are crucial for regulating glucose levels and appetite [215]. Beyond efficacy in glycaemic control, semaglutide demonstrably supports weight loss, making it a dual-purpose agent for populations with type 2 diabetes and those seeking to manage obesity [71]. The clinical evidence obtained from various trials showcases semaglutide as facilitating significant weight reduction while presenting a favourable safety profile comparable to other GLP-1 RAs [66].

Delivery Device

Injectable formulations come in pre-filled, multi-dose pen injectors designed for ease of use. The pens:

- require no vial preparation
- use ultra-thin, disposable needles
- allow dose selection in some versions (Ozempic)
- deliver fixed-dose increments in others (Wegovy)

This design supports independent administration and is well suited for individuals without prior injection experience.

Storage and administration practices for injectable semaglutide are user-friendly; pre-filled pens must be refrigerated before their first use but can be stored at room temperature thereafter for a limited duration [215]. Users are instructed to discard needles after each use, emphasizing the importance of not sharing pens to prevent cross-contamination [88]. Most patients report minimal injection site discomfort due to the fine needle design, thereby facilitating the integration of semaglutide into their healthcare management plans [66, 71].

Pharmacokinetic Advantages

Injectable semaglutide provides:

- High bioavailability (~89%), ensuring the majority of the dose reaches circulation
- Consistent absorption, independent of food intake
- Sustained receptor activation, supporting steady glucose control and appetite suppression

These properties make the injectable formulation more potent and clinically predictable than the oral version.

Storage and Handling

Injectable semaglutide pens must be stored:

- refrigerated before first use
- at room temperature after opening (for a limited time depending on product guidelines)

Needles are replaced after each injection, and pens must never be shared.

Suitability and Patient Considerations

Injectable semaglutide is appropriate for:

- individuals comfortable with self-injection
- patients needing strong glycaemic control
- those with significant obesity who require higher doses for weight management

Because the injection is weekly and the needle is very small, most users report minimal discomfort and find the regimen easier than expected.

In summary, injectable semaglutide represents a significant advancement in the treatment of type 2 diabetes and obesity, characterized by efficacy, user-friendly administration, and a stable pharmacokinetic profile that supports sustained therapeutic benefits.

Overview of Oral Semaglutide (Rybelsus)

Oral semaglutide, marketed under the brand name Rybelsus, is the first oral formulation of a glucagon-like peptide-1 (GLP-1) receptor agonist. This innovation in peptide-based therapy marks a significant advancement since traditional peptides have historically struggled with stability in the gastrointestinal tract and effective absorption. Rybelsus incorporates a unique formulation strategy that allows for once-daily tablet administration, thus facilitating the management of type 2 diabetes mellitus (T2DM) in ways that injectable forms of semaglutide do not. Although Rybelsus and injectable semaglutide contain the same active ingredient, their pharmacokinetics, dosing, and administration requirements differ significantly [42, 151, 218].

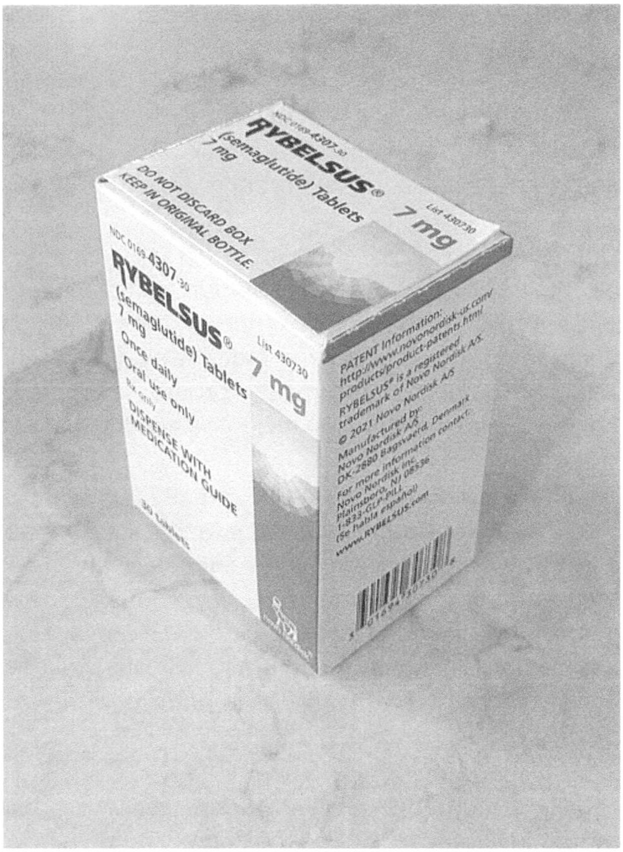

Figure 17: Box of Rybelsus (semaglutide) 7mg. Grendelkhan, CC BY-SA 4.0, via Wikimedia Commons.

The design of Rybelsus aims to deliver semaglutide through the stomach rather than directly into the bloodstream. Peptides are generally prone to degradation by gastric acid and digestive enzymes, which limits their oral bioavailability. Rybelsus addresses this issue by using an absorption enhancer known as sodium N-(8-2-hydroxybenzoylamino)caprylate (SNAC). This enhancer temporarily increases the local gastric pH, protecting semaglutide from degradation and allowing it to pass through the gastric lining into the bloodstream. Despite this enhancement, the oral bioavailability of semaglutide is low, approximating 1-2% of the dose compared to the nearly complete bioavailability of its injectable counterpart. Nevertheless, the doses utilized in clinical settings can still lead to significant improvements in glycaemic control for patients with T2DM [42, 45, 58, 219].

Sodium N-(8-[2-hydroxybenzoyl]amino)caprylate (SNAC)

Sodium N-(8-[2-hydroxybenzoyl]amino)caprylate (SNAC) is a specialised absorption enhancer used in the oral formulation of semaglutide (Rybelsus). Its purpose is to overcome one of the major challenges in drug delivery: peptides are normally destroyed by stomach acid and digestive enzymes and cannot easily cross the gastrointestinal lining. By temporarily altering the stomach's local environment, SNAC protects semaglutide and allows enough of the peptide to be absorbed into the bloodstream for therapeutic effect. Without this compound, oral semaglutide would not be possible.

Chemically, SNAC is a small, non-therapeutic molecule classified as a permeation enhancer. It is the sodium salt of a modified fatty acid linked to a benzoyl amino group, a structure that enables it to interact with both lipids and proteins. These interactions allow SNAC to momentarily modulate some of the stomach's protective barriers, creating the right conditions for semaglutide to survive and be absorbed.

Peptide drugs like semaglutide normally cannot be taken orally because the stomach environment is highly acidic, digestive enzymes rapidly break down proteins, and large molecules cannot easily pass through the gastric mucosa. Under these conditions, virtually all ingested semaglutide would be degraded before reaching the bloodstream. SNAC solves this problem by creating a local "microenvironment" around the dissolving tablet, preserving the peptide long enough for absorption to occur.

SNAC works through several complementary mechanisms. First, it temporarily raises the pH in the immediate vicinity of the tablet, reducing acid-mediated degradation of semaglutide and creating a more neutral zone where the peptide remains stable. This effect is tightly localised and does not significantly alter the overall stomach pH. Second, SNAC reduces the activity of digestive enzymes that would otherwise break down semaglutide, and it also interacts directly with the peptide to further stabilise it. Third and most importantly, SNAC increases the permeability of the stomach lining by briefly enhancing membrane fluidity in the gastric epithelial cells. This allows semaglutide to cross the gastric wall through the cells themselves—a unique mechanism, since most peptides are absorbed in the small intestine rather than the stomach.

These actions are carefully controlled. SNAC's effects are short-lived, disappear once the tablet passes from the stomach, and remain confined to a small local area. The compound does not damage the stomach lining and is considered non-toxic, having undergone extensive safety testing. Its use in Rybelsus represents a major advance in oral peptide delivery.

By enabling semaglutide to survive the stomach and enter the bloodstream, SNAC makes the world's first oral GLP-1 receptor agonist possible. Even with SNAC, only about 1–2% of a dose reaches circulation, but because semaglutide is highly potent and long-acting, this small fraction is sufficient for clinical benefit. In contrast, the injectable version has a bioavailability of around 89%.

Because oral absorption is limited, any interference can significantly reduce how much semaglutide enters the bloodstream. This is why strict administration rules are required for Rybelsus: it must be taken on an empty stomach, with no more than 120 mL of water, and followed by at least 30 minutes without food, drink, or other medications. These conditions ensure SNAC can create the optimal environment for absorption.

The administration of oral semaglutide requires specific timing and dietary restrictions to optimize absorption. Patients are instructed to take the medication once daily on an empty stomach, with no more than 120 mL of plain water, and to avoid ingesting food or drinks for at least 30 minutes afterward. These conditions are essential to reduce interference from gastric contents and to allow for optimal uptake of the limited amount of semaglutide that can be absorbed. While these requirements may complicate the regimen compared to the simplicity of a weekly injection, many patients prefer the oral form, which helps alleviate the aversion to needles common among individuals with T2DM [60, 101, 219].

The dosing regimen for Rybelsus is designed to promote tolerance through a gradual escalation approach. Treatment typically begins at a lower dose of 3 mg for the first 30 days, allowing the body to adjust to the medication. After this initial period, the dose is increased to 7 mg daily, a dosage associated with significant glucose-lowering effects in many individuals. If further glycaemic control is desired, the dose can be raised to the maximum approved level of 14 mg daily. Importantly, while the oral version of semaglutide is not specifically approved for weight management, some patients do experience modest weight loss as a secondary benefit [60, 101, 220].

From a pharmacological standpoint, oral semaglutide offers advantages, particularly for individuals who prefer non-injectable therapies or those reluctant to initiate treatment with injectable GLP-1 receptor agonists. However, due to its lower bioavailability, the oral formulation generally provides less potency compared to injectable forms, particularly in terms of weight loss outcomes. Nonetheless, Rybelsus is an important option for enhancing glycaemic control within a comprehensive diabetes management plan that may include dietary modifications, physical activity, and other pharmacological agents [95, 220].

Rybelsus expands the accessibility of GLP-1-based therapies and offers an effective alternative for patients seeking a needle-free option for diabetes medication. While the strict adherence to administration guidelines and daily intake may introduce some complexity, the ability to provide meaningful glycaemic control through an oral route represents a significant advancement in diabetes treatment strategies [42, 219, 220].

Dose-Escalation Schedules and Rationale

The rationale for using dose-escalation schedules when prescribing semaglutide, whether for type 2 diabetes or chronic weight management, is grounded in both physiological safety and therapeutic efficacy. Semaglutide operates as a glucagon-like peptide-1 (GLP-1) receptor agonist, impacting several systems within the body including appetite regulation, glucose metabolism, and gastrointestinal function. This multifaceted mechanism necessitates a careful approach to drug administration to mitigate adverse effects and enhance treatment adherence [88, 154, 221].

Physiological Rationale for Dose Escalation

The initiation of treatment typically begins with a low dose that is gradually increased over several weeks. This gradual titration allows the body to acclimatize to semaglutide's effects, which can induce gastrointestinal issues such as nausea, vomiting, and diarrhea [32, 88, 221]. Clinical evidence suggests that the majority of gastrointestinal adverse events (AEs) occur during the initial escalation phase, highlighting the importance of allowing patients' gastrointestinal systems to adjust to the medication [221, 222]. Research indicates that when semaglutide is administered without this careful titration, patients experience a higher incidence and severity of these AEs, which can lead to treatment discontinuation [223, 224].

Semaglutide's action on the central nervous system to suppress appetite underscores the need for a controlled dosing schedule. A swift reduction in appetite may prompt acute side effects, including dizziness or dehydration, as the body struggles to adapt to new dietary intakes [32, 225]. By incrementally increasing the dose, clinicians can facilitate a smoother recalibration of the body's appetite-regulating pathways, minimizing the risk of abrupt adverse reactions [222, 226].

Therapeutic Efficacy and Patient Management

The dose-escalation process also contributes to improved patient adherence to treatment. High dropout rates, often influenced by the initial experience of severe side effects, can be mitigated through gradual titration, as patients report a relatively smoother transition through early treatment stages [88, 227]. The importance of maintaining a manageable side-effect profile cannot be overstated, particularly in managing obesity, where long-term treatment commitment is required for sustained weight loss [154, 228, 229].

Additionally, pharmacokinetic considerations play a significant role in the rationale for slow dose escalation. Semaglutide is characterized by a long half-life, approximately seven days, requiring careful monitoring and dose adjustments to avoid rapid drug accumulation, which could lead to severe AEs [230, 231].

Animal models and clinical studies have provided insights into the pharmacodynamics of semaglutide, demonstrating that gradual escalation improves tolerability and therapeutic outcomes [225, 230, 232]. For example, titration protocols that involve smaller increments and a lower starting dose show enhanced gastrointestinal tolerability versus more aggressive escalation schemes [88, 224, 231]. These findings support the practice of a systematic dose adjustment strategy to leverage semaglutide's efficacy while safeguarding patient comfort throughout the treatment continuum [88, 154, 231].

> The rationale behind the gradual dose-escalation schedule for semaglutide is fundamentally tied to its complex physiological actions and is purposefully designed to optimize therapeutic outcomes while minimizing side effects. This patient-centred approach enhances overall treatment adherence and therapeutic effectiveness, ultimately leading to improved long-term outcomes in both glycaemic control and weight management.

Why the First Dose Is Not Therapeutic

The initial starting dose of semaglutide—such as the 0.25 mg weekly injectable dose or the 3 mg daily oral dose—is deliberately set at a level too low to produce meaningful GLP-1 receptor activity. These early doses are not intended to deliver therapeutic benefits. Instead, they function as "acclimation doses" that help the body adjust gradually to the medication. At this stage, the goal is to reduce the likelihood of nausea, prepare the gastrointestinal system for the drug's effects, and allow appetite-regulation and glucose-regulation pathways to adapt without being overwhelmed. Only after the dose is increased stepwise do patients reach levels that provide full therapeutic impact.

Acclimation doses are low, introductory doses of a medication that are intentionally below the therapeutic range. Their purpose is not to produce full clinical effects, but to allow the body to gradually adjust to the drug. Acclimation doses help reduce early side effects, improve tolerability, and prepare metabolic, gastrointestinal, or neurological pathways for higher, effective doses that will follow during dose escalation.

Typical Dose-Escalation Schedules

Wegovy (2.4 mg weekly for weight management)

Usually increased in 4-week intervals:

1. **0.25 mg weekly**
2. **0.5 mg weekly**
3. **1.0 mg weekly**
4. **1.7 mg weekly**
5. **2.4 mg weekly** (maintenance)

Ozempic (for type 2 diabetes)

Common schedule:

1. **0.25 mg weekly**
2. **0.5 mg weekly**
3. **1.0 mg weekly** (or **2.0 mg** for select patients)

The initial 0.25 mg dose is not therapeutic—it is simply to allow the body to adapt.

Rybelsus (oral semaglutide)

1. **3 mg daily** (starter dose; not therapeutic)
2. **7 mg daily** (therapeutic for many)
3. **14 mg daily** (max dose)

Dose-escalation schedules are essential for safe and effective semaglutide therapy. They:

- minimise gastrointestinal symptoms
- allow appetite and metabolic pathways to adapt

- prevent premature discontinuation
- support stable long-term use
- ensure controlled pharmacokinetics

This structured, gradual approach is a key reason semaglutide is well tolerated and successful in both diabetes and obesity treatment.

Storage, Handling, Pen Devices, Injection Technique

Semaglutide is supplied in pre-filled, multi-dose pen injectors designed for safe, accurate, and convenient self-administration. Proper storage, handling, and injection technique are essential to maintain medication potency, ensure consistent dosing, and minimise injection-related discomfort. This section outlines best practices for using injectable semaglutide, applicable to both Ozempic and Wegovy.

Storage Requirements

Proper storage protocols for semaglutide are critical for maintaining the medication's stability, efficacy, and safety. Before the pen is first opened, it must be stored in a refrigerator at temperatures between 2°C and 8°C (36°F to 46°F). Freezing semaglutide is particularly detrimental as it can damage the medication, requiring the disposal of any pen that has been frozen. The importance of refrigeration prior to opening is underscored by the need to protect the medication from light, which can also compromise its integrity [233, 234].

Once opened, the storage requirements for semaglutide become more flexible. Patients can either keep it refrigerated or at room temperature, provided that the temperature does not exceed 30°C (86°F). Different formulations of semaglutide have specific guidelines regarding their room temperature stability: Ozempic can be stored at room temperature for up to 56 days, while Wegovy's stability at room temperature is limited to 28 days [234]. It is crucial to avoid exposure to direct heat or sunlight during this time, and the pen should be recapped after each use to protect not only the contents but also the needle interface. There are significant risks associated with using semaglutide past its expiration date, as this could lead to reduced effectiveness or safety concerns. If the solution appears discoloured, cloudy, or contains visible particles, the pen must be discarded to prevent adverse health effects [233].

Furthermore, general safety measures, such as keeping the medication out of the reach of children, are vital to prevent accidental overdoses or mishandling. These precautions are consistent across various studies that examine the pharmacological treatment of conditions related to semaglutide [233, 234].

Correct storage ensures semaglutide remains stable, effective, and safe.

Before First Use

- Pens must be stored in the refrigerator at 2°C to 8°C (36°F to 46°F).
- They should not be frozen. A pen that has been frozen must be disposed of.
- Store the pen in its original carton to protect it from light.

After First Use

- Once opened, the pen can be stored in:
    - the refrigerator, or
    - room temperature (up to 30°C / 86°F) for a limited period depending on the product:
        - Ozempic: up to 56 days
        - Wegovy: up to 28 days
- Avoid exposing the pen to heat or direct sunlight.
- Always recap the pen after each injection to protect the medication and needle interface.

General Storage Considerations

- Never use the pen past its expiration date.
- If the solution appears cloudy, discoloured, or contains particles, the pen must not be used.
- Pens should be kept out of reach of children.

Handling Guidelines

Safe handling of semaglutide pens is essential for maintaining accurate dosing and reducing the risk of infection. Proper technique not only ensures that each injection delivers the intended amount of medication but also protects users from avoidable complications such as contamination or accidental needle injuries.

A new, sterile, disposable needle must be used for every injection. Reusing needles increases the risk of infection, blunts the needle tip, and can affect dose delivery. After completing the injection, the needle should be removed immediately. This helps prevent medication leakage, reduces the amount of air that can enter the pen, minimises contamination, and lowers the chance of accidental needle sticks.

Pen safety is another critical consideration. Semaglutide pens must never be shared, even if a new needle is attached. Sharing pens poses a serious risk because bloodborne pathogens can be transmitted through microscopic traces of blood that may remain inside the pen device. Each pen is intended for use by one individual only.

Before each injection, patients should carry out a quick safety check. They should confirm that they are using the correct medication and dose, ensuring they have selected the right pen strength. The solution inside the pen should be examined carefully; it must appear clear and colourless. A new needle should then be attached securely. In some cases, the pen may need to be primed—Ozempic pens, for example, require priming only before the very first use of a new pen. These steps help ensure safe handling and consistent, accurate dosing every time the medication is administered.

Pen Devices

Semaglutide pens are specifically designed to make treatment simple, consistent, and accessible for users, including those with little or no prior experience with injections. Their thoughtful design allows patients to administer their medication safely at home without needing to handle vials, syringes, or complex preparation steps.

One of the key features of semaglutide pens is their pre-filled, multi-dose design, which eliminates the need to draw medication from a vial. Ozempic pens use a "dial-a-dose" mechanism that allows patients to select different dose increments, making it easy to adjust doses gradually during titration or according to clinical needs. In contrast, Wegovy pens deliver fixed single-dose strengths, with each pen containing only one dose level. This feature reduces user error during stepwise dose increases for weight-management therapy, as each stage uses a different pen.

The pens also use ultra-thin needles—typically 32 to 34 gauge—which are designed to minimise discomfort and require only a shallow insertion into the subcutaneous tissue. This enhances comfort and helps encourage long-term adherence to weekly injections.

Needle Gauge

Needle gauge refers to the thickness of the needle: the higher the gauge number, the thinner the needle. A 32–34 gauge needle is among the thinnest available for medical injections and is significantly narrower than standard insulin needles or typical blood-draw needles.

Because these needles are extremely fine, they cause very little sensation when they pass through the skin. This is particularly important for semaglutide, as it is intended for regular weekly self-injection, often by people with no prior experience using injectable medications. The thinness of the needle also allows for a shallow, subcutaneous injection into the fatty layer just under the skin, rather than a deeper intramuscular injection, further reducing discomfort.

Overall, the use of 32–34 gauge needles helps improve user confidence, reduces injection anxiety, and increases long-term adherence to semaglutide therapy.

User-centred design elements make the pens even easier to use. Audible clicks confirm dose selection and injection progress, helping users feel confident that the dose has been delivered correctly. Clear dose windows allow visual confirmation of the selected dose, and the pens' ergonomic shape provides a comfortable, stable grip. These combined features support a reliable and user-friendly injection experience.

Injection Technique

Proper injection technique is critical for the effective and safe delivery of semaglutide, a glucagon-like peptide-1 receptor agonist prescribed for type 2 diabetes and weight management. Achieving consistent absorption and minimizing complications hinge on using correct methodologies. Studies indicate that improper injection techniques can lead to suboptimal glycaemic control, increased pain, and potential complications such as lipohypertrophy, where the local fat tissue reacts adversely to repeated injections in the same spot [235, 236] . Thus, adhering to recommended practices is essential in preventing such issues and enhancing patient comfort during administration.

Semaglutide is primarily injected subcutaneously in three approved anatomical locations: the abdomen (at least 5 cm away from the navel), the thigh, and the outer arm. It is advisable to rotate these injection sites weekly to prevent tissue irritation and complications [71, 237]. The need for site rotation is further supported by research indicating that consistent use of the same site can lead to tenderness and detrimental changes in skin texture, such as those observed with lipodystrophy [236, 238]. This rotation strategy has been emphasized in the guidelines to mitigate these risks and promote healthy tissue maintenance [237].

The injection procedure involves a meticulous step-by-step approach that includes handwashing, site disinfection, attaching a sterile needle, conducting a flow check with a new pen, and ensuring proper angle and technique during injection. The correct angle for subcutaneous injections is typically a 90-degree insertion, with recommendations for individuals with minimal subcutaneous fat to pinch a fold of skin [239, 240]. Evidence suggests that the duration the needle remains in place post-injection contributes to complete dose delivery, advocating for tip withdrawal after a duration of six seconds to ensure all medication is released [241]. This element of procedure is particularly relevant to prevent both injection-related discomfort and potential complications related to pharmacokinetic absorption variances observed with subcutaneous versus intramuscular placements [242].

Patient comfort can also be enhanced through measures such as allowing the injection pen to reach room temperature before use, which has been shown to reduce sensations of pain during administration [239, 240]. A swift needle insertion technique can minimize discomfort, thereby improving the overall experience for the patient [236]. This holistic approach to injection technique—emphasizing both preparation and execution—encapsulates the necessary steps to ensure safe and reliable delivery of semaglutide while emphasizing the role of education on proper methods to empower patients in self-administration scenarios [236, 243].

Step-by-Step Injection Procedure

1. Wash hands and clean the injection site with an alcohol swab.

2. Attach a new needle and remove the caps.

3. Check the flow (only for a new Ozempic pen).

4. Select the prescribed dose using the dose selector.

5. Insert the needle into the skin at a 90-degree angle. A skin fold may be used for thin individuals.

6. Press and hold the dose button until the counter reaches zero.

7. Continue holding the needle in place for **6 seconds** to ensure full delivery.

8. Remove the needle, discard it in a sharps container, and recap the pen.

Disposal of Used Needles

Used needles must be placed in a designated sharps container.

They should never be discarded in household waste or recycling bins.

Many pharmacies offer:

- sharps containers,
- collection services, or
- community disposal programs.

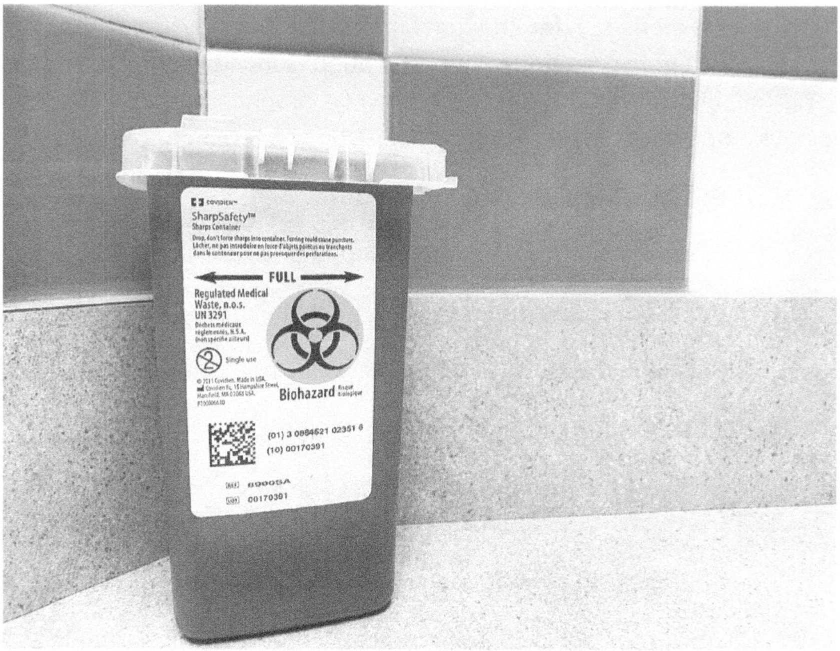

Figure 18: Example of a sharps disposal container. Tony Webster from Minneapolis, Minnesota, United States, CC BY 2.0, via Wikimedia Commons.

Injectable semaglutide requires careful attention to storage, handling, and injection technique to ensure safety, efficacy, and patient comfort. Pens must be refrigerated before first use, stored properly afterwards, and used with a new needle for every injection. The device design supports easy self-administration, and consistent injection technique—along with proper site rotation—ensures reliable delivery of the medication each week. Mastery of these practical aspects is a key component of successful long-term semaglutide therapy.

Timing Considerations, Missed Doses, Switching Formulations

Semaglutide's long half-life, weekly dosing schedule (for injectables), and strict administration rules (for the oral form) require careful attention to timing. Proper timing ensures stable drug levels, maximises therapeutic benefits, and reduces the risk of side effects. Understanding what to do if a dose is missed—and how to safely switch between injectable and oral formulations—is an important part of effective treatment.

Timing Considerations

The pharmacokinetics of injectable semaglutide allow for a once-weekly administration, as demonstrated by its long half-life of approximately one week, contributing to stable therapeutic levels between doses [244, 245]. Key considerations for administration include choosing a consistent weekly injection day, flexibility in the timing of injections with regard to meals, and maintaining adherence to the recommended spacing of doses according to the 48-hour rule to mitigate potential side effects [42, 245].

Key timing principles:

- **Choose a consistent weekly injection day.**
- Injections can be taken **at any time of day**, with or without food.
- The chosen day may be changed if necessary, as long as the timing respects the 48-hour rule for spacing doses.
- Because the medication accumulates gradually, maintaining a predictable weekly rhythm helps reduce side effects and keeps blood levels steady.

The long half-life of semaglutide allows for gradual accumulation in the body, fostering a predictable pharmacokinetic profile, which is crucial in optimizing its therapeutic effects and minimizing gastrointestinal side effects commonly associated with GLP-1 receptor agonists [136, 215]. Employing a systematic approach to administration, including maintaining a regular schedule, has been shown to enhance patient adherence and improve overall therapeutic outcomes, thereby enabling effective glucose control and weight management [136, 221].

In contrast, oral semaglutide, marketed as Rybelsus, presents a more complex administration protocol. Its absorption is significantly influenced by gastric contents, necessitating that it be taken first thing in the morning on an empty stomach, with only a small amount of water, and requiring a 30-minute window before consuming any food or additional medications [22, 246]. This stricter regimen reflects the lower bioavailability of oral semaglutide compared to its injectable counterpart, necessitating adherence to precise timing elements to ensure effective systemic absorption [45, 246].

Rybelsus must be taken:

- **first thing in the morning**, immediately after waking
- **on an empty stomach**
- with **no more than 120 mL (about half a cup) of water**
- followed by **at least 30 minutes with no food, drink, or other medications**

Research indicates that the pharmacokinetic properties of oral semaglutide are impacted by formulations designed to enhance its absorption, such as the inclusion of sodium N-(8-2-hydroxybenzoylamino)caprylate (SNAC), which interacts with the gastric environment to improve efficacy [42, 247]. This approach exemplifies the challenges faced with orally administered GLP-1 receptor agonists, where greater attention to dosing conditions is paramount in achieving desired therapeutic concentrations and consequently, better metabolic control for patients with type 2 diabetes [22, 248].

While both formulations of semaglutide provide valuable options for managing type 2 diabetes and obesity, their respective administration principles highlight crucial differences that healthcare providers and patients must navigate for optimized therapeutic outcomes. Injectable semaglutide's weekly regimen fosters adherence due to its simplicity, while oral semaglutide's regimen requires greater patient diligence but offers an alternative for those averse to injections.

Missed Doses

Semaglutide has gained attention for its long half-life, which provides flexibility in dosing regimens, particularly in cases where patients may miss their scheduled injections. Its pharmacokinetic properties demonstrate that the drug can maintain stable concentrations in the body, allowing for missed doses to be managed effectively without significant impact on therapeutic levels, though adherence to specific guidelines is crucial to avoid adverse effects and maintain the drug's efficacy [222, 249].

For subcutaneously administered semaglutide, if a patient misses a weekly dose, they may take it as soon as they remember, provided that at least 48 hours remain before the next scheduled dose. If the next dose is less than 48 hours away, the missed dose should be skipped, and patients must resume their regular dosing schedule instead of doubling up. This is to prevent excessive accumulation of the drug and an increased risk of gastrointestinal side effects, such as nausea [48, 215]. The terminal half-life of subcutaneous semaglutide is approximately one week, facilitating effective drug levels even when doses are missed [222, 249].

Oral semaglutide, marketed under the brand name Rybelsus, has a distinct approach to missed doses. If a daily dose is forgotten, patients are advised to skip it and continue with the next scheduled dose the following morning. This caution is due to the requirement for oral semaglutide to be taken on an empty stomach; failure to adhere to this can significantly affect absorption and lead to inconsistent drug levels, diminishing therapeutic efficacy [45, 250, 251]. Thus, it is essential to follow the recommendation of not taking additional tablets to compensate for a missed dose to avoid adverse side effects and ensure the treatment remains safe and effective [42, 252].

The pharmacokinetics of oral semaglutide indicates that meal timing significantly influences absorption. Studies have shown that absorption is greatly reduced after meals, emphasizing the importance of taking the medication in a fasting state for optimal drug absorption [249, 251]. The half-life of oral semaglutide allows for daily dosing, contributing to stable blood levels, even with variability in absorption due to factors such as gastrointestinal conditions [95]. Proper management of missed doses—whether via injection or oral route—is critical in maintaining steadiness in blood drug levels and safeguarding patients against potential side effects associated with improper dosing practices [42, 250].

> Semaglutide's long half-life indeed offers flexibility in dosing when injections or oral tablets are missed; however, strict adherence to specific dosing recommendations is paramount to avoid excessive drug accumulation and to ensure continued therapeutic benefits. The nuances in the administration guidelines for both the injectable and oral forms underscore the importance of understanding pharmacokinetics and the implications of missed doses [42, 222, 249, 250].

Switching Formulations

Transitioning between oral and injectable forms of semaglutide can arise due to various clinical considerations such as evolving treatment goals, tolerance to side effects, or a shift from managing diabetes to effectively treating obesity. Both formulations—oral semaglutide (Rybelsus) and the injectable forms (Ozempic/Wegovy)—contain the same active ingredient, semaglutide, which facilitates a generally straightforward switch. Nonetheless, it necessitates careful titration to maintain tolerability and minimize gastrointestinal side effects [245, 253].

When patients move from oral semaglutide to an injectable formulation, guidelines suggest that no washout period is typically required. However, regardless of previous oral dosing levels, the injectable version should start at the lowest dosage of 0.25 mg weekly. This initial cautious approach allows the gastrointestinal tract to acclimatize to the different absorption characteristics associated with the injectable form, thereby reducing the likelihood of nausea and other digestive issues [245, 254, 255]. A patient transitioning from 7 mg or 14 mg Rybelsus would therefore commence with 0.25 mg of Ozempic, adhering to a specified titration schedule thereafter [49].

Conversely, the reverse transition—from an injectable semaglutide formulation to oral semaglutide—mandates a cautious approach as well. Patients should initiate treatment with the acclimation dose of 3 mg Rybelsus, irrespective of the injectable dosage they were previously using. After maintaining this dose for 30 days, the treatment can be escalated to 7 mg, with the possibility of increasing to 14 mg if necessary for therapeutic benefit [245, 256]. The significant differences in delivery methods can prompt some patients to experience recurrent gastrointestinal symptoms during this transition, which illustrates the importance of careful titration [257].

The transition from one injectable formulation to another—between Ozempic and Wegovy—similarly requires careful dose adjustment. With Ozempic primarily indicated for type 2 diabetes and Wegovy specifically designed for weight management, the patient switching from Ozempic to Wegovy should restart at Wegovy's initial dose of 0.25 mg weekly and follow the established titration regimen for weight management [103, 258]. Similarly, shifting back from Wegovy to

Ozempic necessitates returning to a 0.25 mg weekly starting dose. Clinicians need to exercise sound clinical judgment during these transitions, particularly when moving patients between high maintenance doses, to ensure patient safety and minimize adverse effects [258, 259].

> Transitioning between different formulations of semaglutide needs to be guided by evidence-based practices. This ensures effective management of conditions and patient safety by carefully monitoring dose adjustments to mitigate side effects during the switching process.

Table 6: Switching Between Semaglutide Formulations.

Switch Type	Guidance / Principles	Example or Notes
Oral → Injectable (Rybelsus → Ozempic/Wegovy)	• No washout period usually required (same molecule). • Start at the lowest injectable dose (0.25 mg weekly), regardless of previous oral dose. • Allows re-acclimation and reduces gastrointestinal side effects.	From **7 mg or 14 mg Rybelsus → 0.25 mg Ozempic weekly**, then follow standard titration.
Injectable → Oral (Ozempic/Wegovy → Rybelsus)	• Start with **3 mg Rybelsus**, even if on a high injectable dose. • Increase to **7 mg after 30 days**. • Increase to **14 mg** only if needed. • Mild GI side effects may recur temporarily.	Begin oral therapy with **3 mg Rybelsus** → 7 mg → 14 mg (if needed).
Ozempic ↔ Wegovy (injectable → injectable)	• Both contain semaglutide but have different indications and dose strengths. • Switching **Ozempic → Wegovy** requires restarting at Wegovy's lowest dose (0.25 mg) and following weight-loss titration. • Switching **Wegovy → Ozempic** usually restarts at 0.25 mg weekly.	Ozempic → Wegovy: start at **0.25 mg weekly**, titrate upward. Wegovy → Ozempic: restart **0.25 mg weekly** for diabetes.

Semaglutide's long duration of action offers flexibility but requires careful attention to timing. Weekly injectable dosing benefits from consistent scheduling, while oral semaglutide has strict morning administration rules due to its unique absorption enhancer. Missed dose instructions prioritise safety and controlled drug levels, and switching between formulations or branded products requires re-titration to minimise side effects and maintain tolerability. Understanding these timing and transition principles is essential for achieving optimal therapeutic outcomes.

Example Charts/Tables for Dose-Titration

Semaglutide Dosing Table (Injectable and Oral)

The following dose-titration tables provide a clear visual framework for understanding how semaglutide therapy is initiated, increased, and maintained across its various formulations and approved indications. Because semaglutide must be introduced gradually to minimise side effects—particularly gastrointestinal discomfort—these tables distil complex prescribing instructions into an organised, step-by-step format. They transform detailed pharmacological guidance into an accessible reference that supports learning, clinical judgement, and patient comprehension.

These tables serve several important functions. First, they simplify the complexity of semaglutide dosing. Because dosing differs by formulation (injectable vs oral), brand (Ozempic, Wegovy, Rybelsus), indication (type 2 diabetes vs obesity), and therapeutic goals, the tables bring together this information in a structured way. This allows readers to quickly compare different titration pathways and understand the logic behind each escalation schedule.

Second, the tables support clinical decision-making. Health professionals can use them to plan appropriate titration timelines, anticipate dose increases, explain the concept of "acclimation doses," distinguish between introductory and therapeutic doses, and evaluate whether an injectable or oral option is better suited to a patient's needs. As a result, they function as practical tools for prescribing, monitoring, and adjusting treatment.

Third, the tables improve patient understanding and adherence. Many patients find multi-week titration schedules confusing or difficult to remember. Visual charts help them see how the dose changes over time, understand why gradual escalation is necessary, recognise when to expect therapeutic benefits, and feel more confident about their treatment plan. Clear expectations enhance adherence and reduce uncertainty or anxiety.

Fourth, the tables highlight key pharmacological differences between oral and injectable semaglutide. By outlining distinctions in dosing frequency, bioavailability, titration duration, and maintenance doses, they make it easier for readers to appreciate how each formulation behaves in the body and why individual treatment pathways differ.

Finally, the tables reinforce core pharmacotherapy concepts. The general principles of dose escalation—such as acclimation dosing, slow titration, the importance of tolerability, the rationale for higher maintenance doses, and the role of gradual dose increases in long-term success—are applicable not only to semaglutide but to many GLP-1 receptor agonists and long-acting metabolic therapies.

Table 7: Dose-Escalation Schedule for Semaglutide (Injectable: Ozempic & Wegovy).

Indication / Brand	Week	Dose	Purpose
Ozempic (Type 2 Diabetes)	Weeks 1–4	**0.25 mg weekly**	Acclimation dose (not therapeutic)
	Weeks 5–8	**0.5 mg weekly**	Initial therapeutic dose
	Week 9+	**1.0 mg weekly**	Standard therapeutic dose
	Optional escalation	**2.0 mg weekly**	For additional glycaemic control if needed
Wegovy (Obesity / Weight Management)	Weeks 1–4	**0.25 mg weekly**	Acclimation dose
	Weeks 5–8	**0.5 mg weekly**	Continued acclimation
	Weeks 9–12	**1.0 mg weekly**	Intermediate dose
	Weeks 13–16	**1.7 mg weekly**	Pre-maintenance dose
	Week 17+	**2.4 mg weekly**	Full maintenance dose for weight loss

Table 8: Dose-Escalation Schedule for Semaglutide (Oral: Rybelsus).

Week	Dose (Daily)	Purpose
Weeks 1–4	**3 mg**	Acclimation dose (not therapeutic)
Weeks 5–8	**7 mg**	Therapeutic dose for many patients
Week 9+	**14 mg**	Maximum dose; used if additional glucose lowering is needed

Table 9: Key Differences Between Injectable and Oral Dosing.

Feature	Injectable Semaglutide	Oral Semaglutide
Frequency	Once weekly	Once daily

Feature	Injectable Semaglutide	Oral Semaglutide
Bioavailability	~89%	~1–2%
Acclimation Dose	0.25 mg weekly	3 mg daily
Highest Therapeutic Dose	2.4 mg (Wegovy) or 2.0 mg (Ozempic)	14 mg
Titration Duration	8–16 weeks depending on indication	8 weeks

Table 10: General Principles of Dose Escalation.

Concept	Explanation
Acclimation dose	Allows the body to adjust; not intended for full therapeutic effect
Gradual titration	Reduces gastrointestinal side effects and improves tolerability
Higher maintenance dose	Required for significant weight loss or maximum glycaemic control
Slow escalation	Prevents early dropout and supports long-term adherence

Taken together, the tables communicate several key insights. The injectable dosing charts clearly show the full week-by-week escalation pathway and the distinction between introductory and therapeutic phases, including why Wegovy requires higher maintenance doses than Ozempic. The oral dosing table explains that the initial 3 mg tablet is not therapeutic and that meaningful clinical benefits begin at 7 mg, with 14 mg reserved for patients needing additional glycaemic improvement. Comparisons between oral and injectable formulations highlight differences in potency, bioavailability, and dosing schedules, helping readers understand why treatment pathways vary. Lastly, the table outlining general principles of dose escalation clarifies how gradual titration improves tolerability, supports metabolic stability, and enhances long-term treatment adherence.

Chapter 5

Clinical Benefits and Expected Outcomes

Following the foundational understanding of semaglutide's mechanisms of action, dosing strategies, pharmacology, and therapeutic principles explored in the previous chapter, this chapter shifts the focus from *how* semaglutide works to *what it achieves in real-world clinical practice*. Once patients reach therapeutic doses and maintain consistent treatment, semaglutide produces a broad spectrum of measurable metabolic, cardiovascular, and behavioural benefits that extend well beyond glucose lowering or appetite suppression alone.

Chapter 5 examines these outcomes in depth. It begins with a detailed overview of improvements in glycaemic control and HbA1c reduction, highlighting semaglutide's role as a leading therapy in diabetes management. Building on this, the chapter explores weight-loss outcomes, typical timeframes, patient variability, and realistic expectations based on both clinical trials and practical experience. Cardiovascular effects—including blood pressure, lipid changes, inflammation reduction, and landmark findings from major trials such as SUSTAIN, PIONEER, and SELECT—are presented to demonstrate semaglutide's evolving role as a cardiometabolic treatment, not just a glucose-lowering medication.

The chapter also reviews the medication's impact on liver health, particularly non-alcoholic fatty liver disease, and explains the metabolic and behavioural changes that underpin durable therapeutic benefits. Finally, it outlines the patient profiles most likely to respond well, enabling clinicians and readers to better understand who benefits most, why, and how to set personalised expectations.

Together, these discussions provide a comprehensive picture of semaglutide's clinical value, connecting physiological effects with meaningful health outcomes and preparing the reader for subsequent chapters on monitoring, long-term management, and optimisation of care.

Glycaemic Control and Hba1c Reduction

Semaglutide has emerged as one of the most effective medications for improving glycaemic control in individuals with type 2 diabetes. It operates through multiple biological pathways, which collectively enhance its therapeutic efficacy. Specifically, semaglutide increases insulin secretion, reduces glucagon release, slows gastric emptying, and increases feelings of satiety.

These mechanisms ensure more stable blood glucose levels throughout the day, leading to significant reductions in both fasting and post-prandial glucose levels and consistent improvements in HbA1c, the standard measure of long-term blood sugar control. Research indicates that semaglutide can lower HbA1c by an average of 1.0% to 1.8% in clinical settings, with some patients achieving decreases greater than 2.0% [52, 260, 261].

Glycated haemoglobin (HbA1c) is the most important marker used to assess long-term blood glucose control in people with diabetes. It reflects the amount of glucose that becomes attached to haemoglobin in red blood cells over their lifespan. Because these cells live for around 120 days, HbA1c provides an average of blood glucose levels over the previous 8–12 weeks, making it a strong predictor of complications such as eye, kidney, and nerve disease [262].

HbA1c matters because it correlates closely with the risk of diabetic complications, offers a long-term view of glucose control that daily finger-prick readings cannot provide, and requires no fasting or preparation. Since 2010, an HbA1c level of 6.5% or higher has been accepted as a diagnostic test for diabetes [262]. Despite its usefulness, HbA1c is not perfect and must always be interpreted within the broader clinical context.

HbA1c forms when glucose binds to haemoglobin A (HbA), the main adult haemoglobin. The degree of glycation depends on blood glucose levels and on how long red blood cells survive. Because only half of an HbA1c result reflects the previous 30 days, rapid improvements or deteriorations in glucose control may take several weeks to appear in the HbA1c value [262].

For diagnosing diabetes, HbA1c levels of 6.5% or above indicate diabetes, 5.7–6.4% indicate prediabetes, and levels below 5.7% are considered normal [262]. The test is convenient and stable, with less day-to-day variation than glucose tests, but it is more expensive, less sensitive in early disease, and can be inaccurate in certain medical conditions.

A range of factors can cause falsely low or falsely high HbA1c measurements. Conditions such as blood loss, pregnancy, renal failure, or haemolysis shorten red-blood-cell lifespan and may lower HbA1c [262]. In contrast, iron, B12 or folate deficiency, asplenia, severe hypertriglyceridaemia, or smoking can increase HbA1c. These limitations highlight the need to avoid interpreting HbA1c in isolation [262].

Clinical trials such as the DCCT and UKPDS demonstrated that lowering HbA1c reduces complications, though intensive control also increases the risk of hypoglycaemia. The Australian Diabetes Society recommends a general HbA1c target of 7.0% for most adults, more stringent targets for younger individuals with early disease, and relaxed targets for older adults or those with significant comorbidities. Targets must be individualised based on disease duration, life expectancy, comorbidities, and hypoglycaemia risk [262].

HbA1c results may be reported as a percentage (NGSP method) or in mmol/mol (IFCC method), and both are commonly displayed together in Australia. Point-of-care HbA1c devices now provide immediate results and are MBS-funded, but all methods have limitations and cannot capture daily glucose fluctuations [262].

Because HbA1c does not detect short-term variations, hypoglycaemia, or post-meal spikes, complementary monitoring tools are often required. Self-monitoring of blood glucose (SMBG) provides information about daily highs and lows, while continuous glucose monitoring (CGM) tracks glucose every few minutes and reveals patterns, trends, and time-in-range [262]. Fructosamine and glycated albumin offer shorter-term measures of glycaemic control and may be useful when HbA1c is unreliable, though they are not routine tests [262].

Different populations require different approaches. CGM is especially beneficial in type 1 diabetes to reduce hypoglycaemia risk. In renal failure, HbA1c may be inaccurate, making SMBG or CGM more reliable [262]. During pregnancy, HbA1c is not recommended for diagnosis, and glucose monitoring should rely on OGTT and SMBG or CGM. When HbA1c does not match glucose readings, technique, equipment accuracy, or laboratory variation must be reviewed [262].

Overall, HbA1c is a central tool in diabetes management but is only one part of the picture. It should be used alongside daily glucose data from SMBG or CGM, interpreted in context, and tailored to individual circumstances to guide safe and effective diabetes care.

Glycaemic control is pivotal for mitigating diabetes-related complications, such as neuropathy, nephropathy, retinopathy, cardiovascular diseases, and the risk of hospitalization due to glucose instability. The ability of semaglutide to reduce overall glucose variability leads to enhanced long-term metabolic health and lower risks of chronic complications [263, 264]. Indeed, maintaining an HbA1c level below 7.0% is recommended for most adults with type 2 diabetes to minimize these risks [263].

Mechanistically, semaglutide activates GLP-1 receptors present in various tissues, including the pancreas, stomach, and brain, to exert multiple beneficial effects. It promotes insulin secretion in a glucose-dependent manner, meaning it does so primarily during elevated glucose conditions, thereby limiting the potential for hypoglycaemia. Additionally, it inhibits glucagon release, leading to decreased endogenous glucose production, which is crucial for improving fasting blood glucose levels. Furthermore, it slows gastric emptying, which is critical for preventing rapid glucose spikes post-meal, and exerts appetite-reducing effects that support weight loss—a factor closely linked to improved insulin sensitivity and HbA1c reduction [52, 260].

Longitudinal studies, notably the Diabetes Control and Complications Trial (DCCT) and the United Kingdom Prospective Diabetes Study (UKPDS), highlight that for every 1% reduction in HbA1c, there is a corresponding decline of up to 35-40% in the risk of microvascular complications [265, 266]. Moreover, glycaemic improvements with semaglutide not only diminish microvascular risks but also mitigate macrovascular complications, thus effectively lowering rates of heart attacks, strokes, and cardiovascular mortality [11]. Clinical trials have demonstrated that patients using semaglutide experience better cardiovascular outcomes, underscoring its cardioprotective benefits independent of HbA1c reductions [77, 79].

In addition to its metabolic advantages, semaglutide offers notable benefits in stabilizing daily glucose levels. The medication actively reduces both fasting and postprandial glucose spikes, leading to less variability in blood glucose levels throughout the day. This stability can dramatically improve patients' quality of life, diminishing symptoms related to fluctuating glucose levels, such as fatigue, headaches, and cognitive difficulties [130, 267]. As glucose patterns stabilize, many patients report increased energy and improved mental clarity, which can enhance adherence to treatment regimens [268].

The therapeutic benefits of semaglutide extend to weight management, which is particularly significant given the high prevalence of obesity among individuals with T2D. Weight loss achieved through semaglutide administration leads to enhanced insulin sensitivity and a decrease in insulin resistance, which are vital for maintaining healthy glucose levels [67]. This dual action—lowering HbA1c and promoting weight loss—can result in many patients needing fewer diabetes medications, including insulin, thus mitigating the risk of hypoglycaemia, which is a common concern in diabetes management [67, 269].

Additionally, semaglutide's unique glucose-dependent mechanism minimizes the risk of hypoglycaemia, allowing for simpler and safer treatment regimens. This safety profile is especially beneficial for older adults, who are more susceptible to glucose-related complications [270, 271]. Expected outcomes with semaglutide prompt a significant shift in diabetes care paradigms, emphasizing the drug's role in managing not only glycaemic levels but overall patient health, leading to fewer hospitalizations and potentially reduced healthcare costs over time [272, 273].

Clinical trials, such as those conducted in the PIONEER program, have consistently demonstrated the effectiveness of semaglutide compared to other diabetes treatments. Oral semaglutide, for instance, has shown reductions in HbA1c similar to or superior to those achieved with established therapies like sitagliptin, confirming its utility in various patient populations [260, 274]. Notably, real-world data supports these findings, indicating that patients initiating treatment with semaglutide experience substantial reductions in HbA1c, particularly among those with higher baseline levels [261, 263].

Semaglutide significantly enhances glycaemic control through its multifaceted mechanisms of action, facilitating improvements in HbA1c and reducing the risks of diabetes-related complications. The evidence from both clinical trials and real-world studies underscores its role as a cornerstone in modern diabetes therapy, making it a critical option for achieving long-term metabolic stability in type 2 diabetes management.

Weight-Loss Outcomes, Timeframes, and Realistic Expectations

Semaglutide, a glucagon-like peptide-1 (GLP-1) receptor agonist, has emerged as a significant pharmaceutical advancement in the management of obesity, particularly at the 2.4 mg dose, which is characterized by clinically substantial and sustained weight loss outcomes. Clinical studies demonstrate that individuals treated with semaglutide can achieve an average weight reduction of approximately 15% of their initial body weight, and some patients may lose more than 20% [84, 105, 275]. This level of weight loss can approach the results typically associated with surgical bariatric interventions, distinguishing semaglutide as a pivotal agent in non-surgical obesity management options [84, 104, 105].

The underlying mechanisms driving the weight-loss effects of semaglutide include enhanced appetite regulation, reduced caloric intake, and delayed gastric emptying. This combination modifies how individuals perceive hunger and satiety, leading to a lower propensity for overeating [276, 277]. The efficacy of semaglutide markedly contrasts with older weight-loss medications and lifestyle interventions alone, which typically yield modest results over longer periods [103, 275]. As outlined in the STEP trials, patients receiving semaglutide 2.4 mg experienced weight loss that commenced rapidly within the initial weeks and continued progressively, peaking around months three to six of treatment [104, 105].

It is important to consider the expected timeline for weight loss with semaglutide. Initial weight loss is typically modest during the titration phase (first 4–8 weeks) before more significant therapeutic effects manifest upon reaching maintenance doses [103, 104]. Clinical observations indicate that while most weight loss can plateau after one year, adherence to treatment might enable patients to maintain or continue weight loss beyond this period [105, 278]. This sustained efficacy underscores the long-term nature of obesity management that semaglutide supports, suggesting that for optimal outcomes, treatment should be viewed as a long-term commitment rather than a short-term fix [84, 105].

Individual variability in weight loss outcomes with semaglutide remains a fundamental consideration. Factors such as baseline weight, metabolic health, age, genetic predispositions, and adherence to lifestyle modifications significantly influence results [104, 277]. Nevertheless, even a modest weight loss of at least 5–10% of initial body weight is associated with meaningful health improvements, such as enhanced glycaemic control, reduced hypertension, and decreased cardiovascular risks [278, 279]. Importantly, semaglutide also facilitates adherence to lifestyle changes by addressing psychological barriers related to food cravings and overeating, thereby promoting behavioural shifts conducive to long-term weight management success [103].

Maintaining weight loss is notably challenging; however, semaglutide's breadth of action helps counteract the physiological mechanisms that predispose individuals to regain weight after initial loss. By stabilizing appetite-regulating pathways, semaglutide not only aids in weight reduction but also contributes to weight maintenance, which is critical in treating obesity as a chronic condition [275, 276]. Consequently, the adjunctive benefits of semaglutide extend beyond weight loss to significantly improve quality of life, mobility, mood, and psychological well-being [278, 279].

Below are realistic, clinically plausible case-study timelines that illustrate how individuals may progress on semaglutide therapy over time. Each scenario reflects known therapeutic patterns, titration phases, behavioural changes, and expected weight-loss ranges seen in clinical trials such as the STEP program.

Case Study Scenario 1: "Sarah – Slow but Steady Responder"

Profile:
- 42-year-old woman
- BMI 36 kg/m^2
- Hypertension, prediabetes
- Emotional eating, irregular meal patterns

Weeks 1–4 (Titration Phase)

- Starts semaglutide at **0.25 mg weekly**.
- Mild nausea in week 2 → resolves by week 4.
- Weight change: **–1.5%**.
- Reports feeling "slightly less hungry at night."

Weeks 5–8 (0.5 mg dose)

- Appetite suppression becomes more noticeable.
- Begins naturally reducing snacking without effort.
- Weight change by week 8: **–3% total**.
- Fasting glucose improves; HbA1c decreases from 6.1% to 5.8%.

Months 3–6 (1.0 → 1.7 mg → 2.4 mg)

- Moves through titration without significant side effects.
- Experiences the strongest appetite reduction at **1.7 mg**.
- Weight loss accelerates.
- By month 6: **–10% of initial body weight**.
- Blood pressure improves enough to reduce antihypertensive medication dose.

Months 7–12 (2.4 mg maintenance)

- Weight continues to decline but more slowly.
- Cravings for sweets diminish dramatically.
- Engages more consistently in physical activity.
- By 12 months: **–15% weight loss** (~15 kg).
- Prediabetes resolves (HbA1c drops to 5.5%).

Case Study Scenario 2: "Michael – Rapid Early Responder"

Profile:

- 55-year-old man
- BMI 41 kg/m^2
- Type 2 diabetes (on metformin)
- Sedentary lifestyle

Weeks 1–4 (Titration)

- Mild nausea → managed with slower eating.
- Weight change: **–2%**.
- Reports "losing interest in large meals."

Weeks 5–8 (0.5 mg)

- Experiences rapid appetite suppression.
- Daily caloric intake drops by 25–30%.
- Weight change by week 8: **–6%**.
- Fasting glucose normalises by week 8.

Months 3–6 (1.0 → 1.7 mg → 2.4 mg)

- Strong therapeutic effect.
- HbA1c drops from 7.8% to 6.3%.
- Weight loss is continuous and linear.
- By month 6: **–13% weight loss**.

Months 7–12 (Maintenance at 2.4 mg)

• Loses an additional ~1% per month until plateau.
• By 12 months: **–18% total weight loss**.
• Diabetes improves enough to discontinue sulfonylurea.

Case Study Scenario 3: "Aisha – Gradual But Transformational Change"

Profile:
• 29-year-old woman
• BMI 33 kg/m^2
• PCOS, insulin resistance
• Long history of binge-eating tendencies

Weeks 1–4

• Experiences nausea → titration paused at week 3 for two extra weeks.
• Minimal weight loss: **–0.5%**.
• However: "my constant cravings are finally starting to calm."

Weeks 5–12 (0.5 → 1.0 mg)

• Appetite becomes stable.
• Begins recognising natural hunger cues.
• Weight loss increases steadily.
• By 12 weeks: **–5% weight loss**.
• Menstrual regularity begins to improve.

Months 3–6 (1.7 → 2.4 mg)

• Significant appetite control.
• Increased energy, improved sleep.
• By month 6: **–11% weight loss**.
• PCOS symptoms ease: reduced androgen-related symptoms.

Months 7–15 (2.4 mg maintenance)

• Weight loss continues gradually.
• Achieves **–16% total weight loss** by month 15.
• Reports major improvements in confidence, mobility, and mood.

Case Study Scenario 4: "Daniel – Modest Responder With Major Health Gains"

Profile:
• 63-year-old man
• BMI 37 kg/m^2

• Cardiovascular disease, sleep apnoea
• Limited mobility

Weeks 1–8

• Moves slowly through titration due to nausea.
• Weight loss: **–2%** by week 8.
• Sleep apnoea symptoms slightly improve.

Months 3–6 (Maintenance reached slowly)

• Weight loss accelerates modestly.
• By 6 months: **–6% weight loss**.
• Cardiologist notes improved blood pressure and reduced inflammation markers.

Months 6–12

• Weight loss is slow but steady.
• Requires continued encouragement to maintain lifestyle changes.
• By 12 months: **–9% total weight loss**.
• Despite modest weight outcomes, his:
– blood pressure improves,
– LDL decreases,
– mobility increases,
– cardiovascular risk declines.

Clinically, this level of weight loss still provides major benefits.

Case Study Scenario 5: "Elena – High Responder Approaching Bariatric-Level Loss"

Profile:
• 47-year-old woman
• BMI 44 kg/m^2
• Severe insulin resistance, fatty liver disease (MASLD)

Weeks 1–4

• Early weight loss: **–3%**.
• Strong appetite reduction.

Weeks 5–12

• Rapid reduction in caloric intake.
• By week 12: **–8% weight loss**.
• Liver enzyme levels begin improving.

Months 3–6

- Consistent, large monthly drops in weight.
- By 6 months: **–14% weight loss**.
- MRI confirms reduced liver fat content.

Months 6–12

- Maintains high responsiveness.
- By 12 months: **–21% total weight loss**.
- MASLD improves significantly.

Taken together, these case studies illustrate several important patterns in how individuals typically respond to semaglutide therapy. Weight loss tends to be modest during the first four to eight weeks, reflecting the use of low titration doses designed for acclimation rather than full therapeutic effect. More substantial changes usually emerge once patients reach higher therapeutic doses, generally between 1.0 mg and 2.4 mg, with the most pronounced effects occurring between months three and six of treatment.

By the 12-month mark, outcomes vary widely yet follow predictable ranges. Modest responders often lose around 5–10% of their initial body weight, while typical responders achieve reductions of 10–16%. High responders may exceed 17–22% weight loss, approaching magnitudes seen with certain bariatric procedures. Importantly, semaglutide's benefits extend beyond weight reduction alone. Improvements are commonly observed in glycaemic control, cardiovascular risk markers, liver fat levels, daily energy, physical functioning, eating behaviours, and overall quality of life.

Variation between individuals is expected and clinically normal. Responses are influenced by multiple factors, including adherence, metabolic health, baseline weight, genetic predispositions, and the presence of comorbid conditions. Behavioural factors—such as eating habits, psychological patterns, and engagement with lifestyle changes—also play a significant role in shaping long-term outcomes.

Cardiovascular Outcome Studies (E.G., SELECT Trial)

Cardiovascular outcome trials (CVOTs) have become critical in the regulatory landscape of diabetes and obesity treatments. This shift was catalysed by the recognition of potential cardiovascular risks associated with glucose-lowering medications in patients with type 2 diabetes and obesity. Historically, the approval of these medications relied primarily on their ability to lower blood glucose levels. However, following experiences with older drugs that posed safety concerns, regulatory authorities mandated that new agents be evaluated not only for their glycaemic control but also for their cardiovascular safety, particularly for high-risk populations [79]. Among these agents, glucagon-like peptide-1 (GLP-1) receptor agonists, especially semaglutide, have consistently demonstrated cardiovascular benefits through various CVOTs, thereby addressing both safety and efficacy concerns.

The dual nature of type 2 diabetes and obesity — where practitioners must navigate the risks of cardiovascular events alongside managing glycaemic control — highlights the importance of CVOTs. Semaglutide has exhibited significant cardiovascular protection, as shown in trials like SUSTAIN 6, which reported a 26% reduction in composite cardiovascular events compared to placebo, confirming its role not only as a glucose-lowering agent but as a medication providing broader cardiovascular benefits [40, 79, 280]. These trials underscore the critical reassessment of drug efficacy beyond glycaemic control, focusing on the real-world implications of these medications on major cardiovascular outcomes.

The SELECT Trial

Among the most pivotal studies in this arena is the SELECT trial, which marked a significant shift in exploring cardiovascular outcomes specifically for a weight-loss medication rather than diabetes management alone. The SELECT trial enrolled 17,604 adults over 45 years old, with established cardiovascular disease and a body mass index (BMI) of 27 kg/m^2 or higher, but without diabetes [281, 282]. The study aimed to determine the impact of semaglutide on major adverse cardiovascular events (MACE) over a mean follow-up of 39.8 months. The trial demonstrated that semaglutide reduced MACE by 20% compared to placebo, affirming its role in managing cardiovascular risks in overweight and obese populations [281, 283].

The SELECT trial is a landmark, global, randomised, double-blind, placebo-controlled cardiovascular outcomes study.

Key features include:

- **Population:** 17,604 adults
- **Age:** ≥45 years
- **Condition:** Overweight or obesity (BMI ≥27 kg/m^2)
- **No diabetes (HbA1c <6.5%)**
- **Established cardiovascular disease** (prior MI, stroke, or symptomatic PAD)
- **Intervention:** Semaglutide 2.4 mg weekly vs placebo
- **Duration:** Over 5 years
- **Primary endpoint:** Major adverse cardiovascular events (MACE), defined as:
  - Cardiovascular death
  - Non-fatal myocardial infarction
  - Non-fatal stroke

Furthermore, the SELECT trial is noted for being the first large-scale CVOT that evaluated the cardiovascular safety of a weight-loss medication in individuals without diabetes, thus expanding the implications of GLP-1 receptor agonists to a broader patient cohort that is often left vulnerable to cardiovascular complications [163, 205]. Previous studies focusing on glucose-lowering therapies did not encompass this population, aligning the SELECT trial's findings with contemporary clinical practice demands that recognize obesity as a critical risk factor for cardiovascular disease [144, 284].

The amalgamation of findings from previous cardiovascular outcome trials demonstrates that newer treatment paradigms in cardiovascular risk management must incorporate findings from studies like SELECT, suggesting that semaglutide's effects extend beyond glycaemic control to encompass a holistic evaluation of patient health, ultimately reducing the cardiovascular risks associated with obesity and metabolic disorders.

The SELECT trial examined the effects of semaglutide 2.4 mg on cardiovascular events and provided significant findings that are reshaping the landscape of obesity treatment as a cardiovascular intervention. One of the most notable revelations from the study is the reported 20% relative reduction in Major Adverse Cardiovascular Events (MACE) compared to placebo [282, 285]. This reduction encompassed key outcomes such as death from cardiovascular causes, non-fatal myocardial infarction, and non-fatal stroke, demonstrating a considerable effect size similar to that commonly observed with statin treatments [205]. Such results are particularly noteworthy given that they pertain to high-risk individuals—namely patients with obesity or overweight and existing cardiovascular disease but without diabetes [282, 285].

Regarding demographics, the SELECT trial illustrated that the cardiovascular benefits associated with semaglutide were consistent across various subgroups, including age, sex, baseline BMI, presence of other risk factors, and types of prior cardiovascular diseases [77]. This uniformity provides compelling evidence that semaglutide's protective cardiovascular effects are not confined to a single demographic profile, extending its applicability to diverse patient populations [76].

Furthermore, the trial underscored semaglutide's role in promoting weight loss and cardiometabolic improvements, with participants losing approximately 15.2% of body weight on average [205]. While this figure is higher than some previous studies that focused solely on obesity [84], it remains clinically significant, correlating with reduced cardiovascular risks [282]. Improvements in key cardiometabolic parameters were also documented, including reductions in blood pressure, C-reactive protein (CRP), non-HDL cholesterol, waist circumference, and various glycaemic markers, despite many participants not exhibiting diabetes at baseline [103].

Moreover, the SELECT trial yielded promising insights regarding diabetes prevention; semaglutide significantly reduced the risk of progression from high-risk glycemia to type 2 diabetes by 73% [223]. This reduction demonstrates its potential as a preventive measure, highlighting the utility of GLP-1 receptor agonists like semaglutide in managing not only obesity but also associated metabolic conditions [282].

The SELECT trial has significantly advanced our understanding of the interplay between obesity and cardiovascular risk, highlighting obesity as a considerable modifier of cardiovascular disease (CVD). Recent literature emphasizes that obesity is not simply a matter of weight but represents a distinct cardiometabolic condition with extensive systemic implications. Notably, the accumulation of visceral fat has been shown to correlate more strongly with cardiovascular risk than general measures of body weight, such as Body Mass Index (BMI) [286, 287]. Therefore, addressing visceral fat through targeted interventions can lead to substantial cardiovascular benefits, illustrating the need to incorporate obesity management into clinical cardiovascular risk assessment [288].

Additionally, there is a critical evolution in the therapeutic landscape with the regulatory approval of semaglutide (Wegovy) as a cardiovascular therapeutic agent, rather than merely a weight-loss medication. This development follows compelling evidence from the SELECT trials, which demonstrated semaglutide's efficacy in reducing cardiovascular events among individuals with obesity and established cardiovascular conditions [91, 289]. These findings signify a paradigm shift in clinical guidelines where pharmacotherapy targets not only weight reduction but also the direct mitigation of cardiovascular risks, positioning semaglutide alongside traditional CVD treatments.

Importantly, the results of the SELECT trial extend the applicability of these interventions beyond diabetic populations, demonstrating cardiovascular protective effects even in non-diabetic patients with obesity and established CVD. This broadened perspective enables healthcare providers to consider pharmacological interventions for a wider demographic, including overweight or obese adults regardless of their glycaemic control status [289, 290]. This shift aligns with recent insights advocating for a comprehensive view of obesity management within cardiovascular risk reduction strategies, emphasizing the need for effective treatment protocols that accommodate various patient profiles [287].

Recognizing obesity as a significant cardiovascular disease modifier underscores the clinical imperative to reassess treatment frameworks, integrating targeted therapies such as semaglutide into standard practice to enhance outcomes for diverse patient groups. The SELECT trials reinforce the necessity of managing visceral fat through pharmacotherapy and advocate for a holistic approach to treatment that includes patients without diabetes, ultimately aiming for improved cardiovascular health metrics across broader populations.

Other Semaglutide Cardiovascular Trials

The cardiovascular safety and efficacy of semaglutide, both injectable and oral formulations, have been established in pivotal trials such as SUSTAIN-6 and PIONEER-6, which specifically targeted patients with type 2 diabetes (T2D) at high cardiovascular risk.

In the SUSTAIN-6 trial, semaglutide was associated with a significant 26% reduction in major adverse cardiovascular events (MACE), which includes cardiovascular death, nonfatal myocardial infarction, and nonfatal stroke, compared to placebo. This trial highlighted a noteworthy decrease in the occurrence of nonfatal stroke among participants receiving semaglutide, thus establishing not only the cardiovascular safety of this treatment but also early indications of cardiovascular benefit [79, 291]. Husain et al. [164] underscore the extensive contributions of these findings to the overall understanding of the cardiovascular implications associated with GLP-1 receptor agonists, reinforcing the relevance of SUSTAIN-6 in understanding semaglutide's cardiovascular profile.

Conversely, the PIONEER-6 trial investigating oral semaglutide reported non-inferiority regarding cardiovascular safety when compared to placebo. While this trial did not yield statistically significant reductions in cardiovascular mortality, it did show trends toward benefits in this area, echoing findings from SUSTAIN-6. Aroda et al. [162] noted that the shorter duration of PIONEER-6 may have limited its ability to demonstrate superiority in outcomes compared to SUSTAIN-6. Nevertheless, both trials laid the groundwork for SELECT, the ongoing study examining the broader implications of semaglutide's cardiovascular effects [79, 291].

Further comparative analyses reveal that semaglutide's impact on cardiovascular outcomes is consistent across different patient populations. For instance, a systematic review indicated that semaglutide reduces cardiovascular risks uniformly among diverse cohorts with varying baseline cardiovascular risk profiles [164]. This consistency reinforces the general applicability and potential utility of semaglutide as a treatment option that not only manages blood glucose effectively but may also confer additional cardiovascular protection.

The evidence from SUSTAIN-6 and PIONEER-6 suggests that semaglutide is a cardiac-safe option that provides potential cardiovascular benefits, thereby supporting its role not only in glycaemic control but also in mitigating cardiovascular risk in patients with T2D.

Clinical Interpretation

Semaglutide has emerged as a significant player in cardiovascular medicine, transitioning from a metabolic therapy to a recognized disease-modifying cardiovascular drug. This transformation is supported by numerous studies outlining its benefits, which notably include weight loss, improvement in insulin sensitivity, reduction of inflammation, lowering blood pressure, improvements in lipid profiles, reduction of liver fat, and enhancement of endothelial function.

Weight loss is a prominent effect of semaglutide therapy. Clinical trials, such as the SELECT trial, demonstrated a substantial average weight loss of approximately 10% in patients, which has direct implications for reducing cardiovascular risk factors such as hypertension and dyslipidaemia [103]. This substantial weight loss has been associated with improved waist circumference and lipid profiles, contributing to an overall decrease in cardiometabolic risks related to obesity [77]. Furthermore, sustained weight loss, as observed with semaglutide, plays a critical role in improving insulin sensitivity, which is often impaired in obese patients and linked to increased cardiovascular risk [88].

Dyslipidaemia

Dyslipidaemia is a medical condition in which a person has abnormal levels of lipids (fats) in the blood. These lipids include cholesterol and triglycerides, which are essential for many bodily functions but become harmful when present in excess or in the wrong balance. Dyslipidaemia is a major risk factor for cardiovascular disease because unhealthy lipid levels contribute to the buildup of fatty plaques in arteries (atherosclerosis), increasing the risk of heart attack, stroke, and peripheral vascular disease.

Dyslipidaemia typically refers to one or more of the following:

1. High LDL cholesterol (low-density lipoprotein)

- Often called "bad cholesterol."
- High LDL contributes to plaque buildup in artery walls.

2. Low HDL cholesterol (high-density lipoprotein)

- Known as "good cholesterol."
- HDL helps remove cholesterol from the bloodstream.
- Low HDL can increase cardiovascular risk.

3. High triglycerides

- A form of fat used for energy.
- High levels are associated with insulin resistance, obesity, fatty liver, and pancreatitis.

4. High total cholesterol

- Sum of LDL, HDL, and other lipid components.

Some individuals may have a combination of these abnormalities, which increases health risks even further.

Dyslipidaemia may arise from:

1. Lifestyle Factors

- Unhealthy diet, especially high in saturated fats, trans fats, and refined carbohydrates
- Physical inactivity
- Excess body weight, especially abdominal obesity

- Tobacco use
- Excess alcohol consumption

2. Medical Conditions

- Type 2 diabetes
- Obesity
- Hypothyroidism
- Chronic kidney disease
- Polycystic ovary syndrome (PCOS)
- Non-alcoholic fatty liver disease (NAFLD/MASLD)

3. Genetic Factors

Some people inherit lipid disorders, such as familial hypercholesterolaemia, which causes very high LDL from a young age.

Abnormal lipid levels accelerate atherosclerosis — the accumulation of fatty deposits inside arteries. Over time, this:

- Narrows blood vessels
- Reduces blood flow to vital organs
- Contributes to clot formation
- Leads to serious complications such as:
    - Heart attack
    - Stroke
    - Peripheral artery disease
    - Chronic kidney disease

Dyslipidaemia often coexists with other metabolic conditions—including hypertension, insulin resistance, and obesity—further increasing risk.

A simple blood test called a lipid panel measures:

- LDL cholesterol
- HDL cholesterol
- Triglycerides
- Total cholesterol

Diagnosis also considers individual risk factors such as age, smoking, family history, and medical conditions.

Treatment focuses on lowering cardiovascular risk through:

1. Lifestyle changes

- Improved diet (e.g., Mediterranean diet)
- Regular exercise
- Weight loss
- Smoking cessation
- Reduced alcohol

2. Medications

- Statins (first-line therapy)
- Ezetimibe
- PCSK9 inhibitors
- Fibrates (for triglycerides)
- Omega-3 fatty acids

3. Management of underlying conditions

- Diabetes control
- Blood pressure control
- Treatment of NAFLD/MASLD

Dyslipidaemia is an imbalance of blood lipids—typically high LDL, high triglycerides, or low HDL—that significantly increases the risk of cardiovascular disease. It often develops alongside obesity, insulin resistance, and other metabolic disorders. Early detection and treatment through lifestyle changes and appropriate medication can greatly reduce long-term health risks and improve overall cardiovascular health.

In addition to weight loss, semaglutide has been linked to reduced inflammation and lower blood pressure. Studies indicate that significant body weight reduction correlates with a decrease in systemic inflammation markers and improved blood pressure, further lowering cardiovascular risk profiles [292]. Specifically, semaglutide appears to provide direct benefits through both metabolic changes attributable to weight loss and independent mechanisms that affect vascular tone and endothelial function, contributing to overall cardiovascular health.

Lipid improvements represent another critical aspect of semaglutide therapy. Evidence suggests that the drug assists in lowering triglycerides while increasing HDL cholesterol levels [293]. These lipid profile changes are crucial because they help mitigate the risk of developing cardiovascular diseases, especially in individuals with type 2 diabetes and obesity [22].

The impact of semaglutide on liver fat is considerable, with studies indicating a significant reduction in non-alcoholic fatty liver disease (NAFLD) among treated patients. This effect may not only enhance liver function but also contribute to improvements in insulin sensitivity and systemic inflammation, thus facilitating better cardiovascular outcomes [79]. The role of semaglutide in reducing intrahepatic fat is especially important given the association between NAFLD and increased cardiovascular risk [294].

Non-Alcoholic Fatty Liver Disease (NAFLD)

Non-alcoholic fatty liver disease (NAFLD) is increasingly recognized as a prevalent metabolic liver condition, characterized by the accumulation of excessive fat in the liver of individuals who consume little to no alcohol. This condition is notably associated with a range of metabolic disturbances including obesity, insulin resistance, type 2 diabetes, dyslipidaemia, and hypertension, forming part of the broader spectrum of metabolic syndrome [295, 296]. Epidemiologically, it affects an estimated 25–38% of adults globally, underscoring its significance as the most common chronic liver disease worldwide [295, 297]. Notably, the prevalence in individuals with obesity can reach as high as 90%, while over half of those with type 2 diabetes exhibit features of fatty liver disease [295, 296].

At the mechanistic level, the development of NAFLD is primarily driven by insulin resistance, which initiates a cascade of metabolic processes including increased fatty acid release from adipose tissue and augmented fat deposition in the liver [295, 297]. Factors such as obesity, particularly visceral fat accumulation, are critical as they exacerbate inflammation and accelerate hepatic steatosis [295, 297]. Genetic predispositions, particularly variants associated with genes like PNPLA3 and TM6SF2, further influence susceptibility and progression to more severe liver injuries, including non-alcoholic steatohepatitis (NASH) and fibrosis [298-300]. Variations in these genes have been linked to the risk of NAFLD and its histological severity, indicating a significant interaction between genetic factors and metabolic conditions [299, 301].

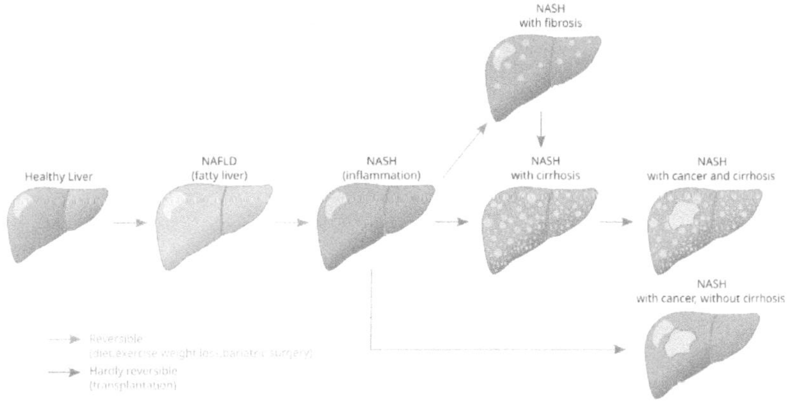

Figure 19: Liver progression for non-alcoholic fatty liver disease. Signimu, CC BY-SA 3.0, via Wikimedia Commons.

A diverse range of metabolic and lifestyle factors has been identified as risk enhancers for NAFLD, including central obesity, type 2 diabetes, dyslipidaemia, and sedentary behaviour [295, 298]. Importantly, many patients present with few to no symptoms, with detection usually occurring via liver enzyme tests or imaging studies [295, 299]. This asymptomatic nature underlines the necessity for proactive screening among high-risk populations.

Diagnosis of NAFLD typically involves a combination of blood tests, imaging techniques like ultrasound, and potentially liver biopsy for definitive assessment, especially in distinguishing simple steatosis from NASH [296, 302]. Elevated liver enzymes such as ALT and AST can indicate liver dysfunction; however, normal values do not preclude the diagnosis of NAFLD [302]. Non-invasive imaging modalities like FibroScan provide useful metrics for assessing fibrosis, while liver biopsy retains its status as the gold standard for diagnosis and staging of liver disease [295, 302].

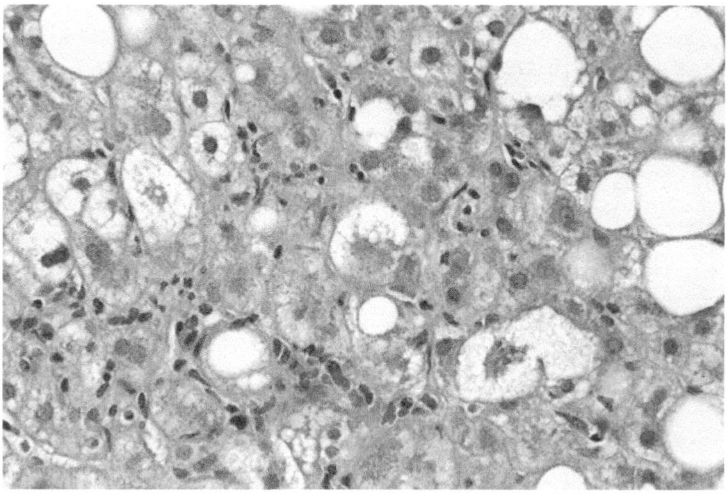

Figure 20: A microscopic image of liver tissue affected by non-alcoholic fatty liver disease (NAFLD). The large and small white spots are excess fat droplets filling liver cells (hepatocytes). NIH Image Gallery, PDM 1.0, via Flickr.

Disease progression in NAFLD tends to follow a defined pathway from simple steatosis to more severe forms like NASH, which may lead to fibrosis, cirrhosis, and potentially hepatocellular carcinoma [295, 296]. The stage of fibrosis is particularly critical as it serves as a robust predictor of long-term patient outcomes, emphasizing the connection between NAFLD and increased cardiovascular mortality [295, 296]. Cardiovascular disease remains the leading cause of death in this patient population, attributed to shared pathophysiological mechanisms linked to obesity and metabolic dysregulation [296, 299].

Management strategies centre on lifestyle modifications, particularly weight loss, which plays a pivotal role in ameliorating steatosis and inflammation [295, 302]. Currently, no specific pharmacological therapies are approved for NAFLD; however, several agents, including GLP-1 receptor agonists like semaglutide, show promise in managing hepatic fat content and promoting resolution of NASH [302, 303]. Ongoing research continues to explore the potential benefits of various medications in addressing this complex disease [295, 302].

As our understanding of NAFLD evolves, recent conceptual shifts towards categorizing these conditions as metabolic dysfunction–associated liver diseases (MASLD and MASH) reflect a growing recognition of the metabolic underpinnings of liver pathology, aiming to destigmatize NAFLD in clinical settings [295, 302].

NAFLD represents a significant global health concern linked with an array of metabolic disorders. Early detection, targeted lifestyle interventions, and ongoing research into pharmacological options present promising avenues for improving patient outcomes and curtailing the progression of this widespread disease.

Moreover, semaglutide enhances endothelial function, which is vital for maintaining vascular health. Improved endothelial function is directly correlated with lower rates of cardiovascular events and improved vascular elasticity [292]. By integrating these various benefits—weight management, improved insulin sensitivity, alterations in lipid profiles, and enhanced endothelial function—semaglutide showcases its potential as a groundbreaking cardiovascular therapy beyond its original diabetes management applications.

The SELECT trial and several other studies clearly indicate that modifications in metabolic pathways through semaglutide lead to a direct reduction in cardiovascular risk, demonstrating its effectiveness not just in diabetic populations but also in non-diabetic individuals at risk for cardiovascular diseases [77, 293]. Thus, semaglutide stands as a transformative therapy in the realm of cardiovascular and metabolic disease management.

The SELECT trial represents one of the most important cardiovascular studies of the past decade. It shows that semaglutide:

- Reduces major cardiovascular events by 20%
- Helps prevent the onset of diabetes

- Benefits a wide demographic of overweight/obese adults
- Offers a powerful, non-surgical option for cardiometabolic risk reduction
- Redefines obesity treatment as part of cardiovascular disease management

In combination with earlier SUSTAIN and PIONEER trials, SELECT establishes semaglutide as a highly effective therapy for improving metabolic health and long-term cardiovascular outcomes.

Impacts on Blood Pressure, Cholesterol, Inflammation

Semaglutide and other GLP-1 receptor agonists have gained recognition for their significant impact on glucose regulation, weight management, and broader cardiometabolic health outcomes. These medications play a crucial role in improving key cardiovascular risk factors, including blood pressure, lipid profiles, and markers of systemic inflammation, which are considered critical drivers of cardiovascular disease (CVD) [90, 304]. Such effects are closely tied to reductions in body weight, enhanced insulin sensitivity, and direct physiological interactions with the cardiovascular and immune systems.

Rigorous clinical studies indicate that semaglutide reliably lowers blood pressure, achieving reductions of approximately 4–7 mmHg for systolic and 2–5 mmHg for diastolic pressure, even among patients without hypertension [105, 166]. The efficacy of semaglutide in this area is particularly pronounced in individuals with obesity or elevated baseline blood pressure. The weight loss associated with the drug reduces vascular resistance and improves vascular health by enhancing endothelial function [91]. Mechanisms for blood pressure reduction include improved insulin sensitivity, reduced sympathetic nervous system activity, GLP-1-mediated natriuresis leading to decreased fluid volume, and overall reductions in inflammation that contribute to better vascular dynamics [305]. These modest blood pressure reductions significantly lower the risks of adverse cardiovascular outcomes such as stroke and heart failure, rendering them clinically relevant, especially for high-risk populations [166, 304].

Semaglutide lowers blood pressure through several mechanisms:

1. Weight loss

- Less body mass means less vascular resistance.
- Reduces pressure on arteries and heart workload.

2. Improved insulin sensitivity

- Reduces sympathetic nervous system activation.
- Lowers sodium retention.

3. Natriuretic effects

- GLP-1 can promote renal sodium excretion, lowering fluid volume.

4. Reduced inflammation

- Less endothelial stress and improved vascular function.

In terms of lipid metabolism, semaglutide has demonstrated favourable effects on lipid profiles, with typical reductions in triglycerides of 15–30% and reductions in LDL cholesterol by approximately 5–12% [166]. These lipid improvements occur through mechanisms such as decreased liver fat, positively influencing insulin resistance, coupled with caloric restriction and enhanced lipid metabolism due to the drug [28, 105]. The implications of these changes are notable, as they contribute to decreased risks for coronary artery disease and stroke, offering considerable metabolic advantages for those suffering from obesity-related dyslipidaemia [306].

Why cholesterol improves

1. Reduced hepatic fat

- Semaglutide decreases liver fat, lowering VLDL production.

2. Improved insulin resistance

- Less hepatic overproduction of triglycerides.

3. Reduced caloric intake

- Lowers circulating free fatty acids.

4. Weight loss

- Improves lipid metabolism at the cellular level.

A critical aspect of semaglutide's action is its impact on chronic low-grade inflammation, a condition frequently found in individuals with obesity and metabolic syndrome. This inflammation fuels cardiovascular and metabolic disorders [255]. Semaglutide has been shown to decrease inflammatory biomarkers such as C-reactive protein (CRP) and interleukin-6 (IL-6) significantly [164], while also affecting markers related to liver inflammation in patients with non-alcoholic fatty liver disease (NAFLD) [166]. The drug facilitates reductions in visceral fat, a significant source of inflammatory cytokines, and enhances metabolic function by decreasing oxidative stress and interacting directly with GLP-1 receptors on immune cells [307]. The resultant declines in inflammation are pivotal for improving vascular health and mitigating thrombotic risks [105, 255].

Why inflammation decreases

1. Reduced visceral fat

- Visceral adipose tissue produces IL-6 and inflammatory cytokines.

2. Improved metabolic function

- Normalised insulin signalling reduces inflammatory pathways.

3. Better glycaemic control

- High glucose promotes inflammation; lowering it reduces oxidative stress.

4. Direct anti-inflammatory effects

- GLP-1 receptors are present on immune cells.

The cumulative cardiometabolic benefits of semaglutide encompass reductions in blood pressure, improvements in lipid profiles, and decreases in systemic inflammation, all crucial for modifying major cardiovascular risks. These findings correlate with significant reductions in major adverse cardiovascular events as demonstrated in extensive trials such as the SELECT trial [90, 305], revealing that the advantages of semaglutide extend far beyond mere glucose control, leading to notable long-term health benefits.

Metabolic and Behavioural Changes

Metabolic and behavioural changes are central to the way semaglutide produces its clinical benefits. While its effects on glucose levels, weight, and cardiovascular risk markers are well documented, these outcomes arise from deeper shifts in how the body regulates appetite, energy use, and metabolic function. Semaglutide acts through multiple pathways—physiological, neurological, and behavioural—to reshape the metabolic environment and support long-term lifestyle change.

Metabolic Changes

Semaglutide has been shown to significantly impact appetite regulation and energy balance, primarily through mechanisms that affect central nervous system signalling and gastrointestinal function. Research indicates that activation of GLP-1 receptors in the hypothalamus plays a crucial role in mediating thirst and hunger signals, ultimately leading to reduced hunger and increased satiety [32, 103]. In detailed clinical trials, participants receiving semaglutide reported decreased self-reported hunger and food cravings, which contributed to lowered energy intake without the necessity of deliberate dietary restrictions [32, 103]. This aligns with findings suggesting that semaglutide effectively promotes weight loss partly via appetite regulation initiated in the brain [32, 157].

Additionally, semaglutide's effects on gastric emptying significantly contribute to its metabolic benefits. By slowing gastric emptying, semaglutide prolongs the time food remains in the stomach, reducing the speed of glucose absorption into the bloodstream. This action mitigates rapid postprandial blood sugar spikes and fosters more stable glucose levels throughout the day, ultimately decreasing the overall insulin demand and improving insulin sensitivity [250, 308]. The delay in gastric emptying is consistent with the physiological actions of other GLP-1 receptor agonists, providing a healthier glycaemic response post-consumption [64, 308].

Furthermore, the relationship between weight loss through semaglutide and improved insulin sensitivity is noteworthy. As body weight, particularly visceral adiposity, declines, insulin sensitivity tends to improve, which further enhances glucose management and reduces the insulin-resistance phenotype associated with obesity. Clinical observations have indicated that these metabolic changes contribute to lower fasting glucose levels, thereby alleviating the strain on pancreatic function and decreasing risks associated with chronic hyperglycaemia [278, 309]. Importantly, this connection between weight loss and insulin efficiency correlates with reduced long-term risks such as Type 2 diabetes and cardiovascular diseases [28, 278].

Visceral Adiposity

Visceral adiposity refers to the accumulation of excess fat deep within the abdominal cavity, where it surrounds vital organs such as the liver, pancreas, kidneys, and intestines. This is different from subcutaneous fat, which lies under the skin and is generally less harmful. Visceral fat is metabolically active, influencing hormones, inflammation, and organ function, and is strongly associated with a wide range of cardiometabolic diseases.

This type of fat is stored internally and is not outwardly visible in the same way as surface-level fat. Its biological activity is significant: visceral fat releases inflammatory cytokines such as IL-6 and TNF-α, as well as free fatty acids and hormones that disrupt normal metabolic processes. These substances contribute to systemic inflammation, impaired insulin sensitivity, and abnormal lipid metabolism—effects not typically seen with subcutaneous fat.

Visceral adiposity is a powerful predictor of metabolic disease. It is closely linked to insulin resistance, type 2 diabetes, dyslipidaemia (including high triglycerides and low HDL cholesterol), hypertension, non-alcoholic fatty liver disease (NAFLD/MASLD), and cardiovascular disease. Because of its internal location, visceral fat cannot be assessed accurately by body weight or BMI alone. Instead, it is commonly estimated using waist circumference, waist-to-hip ratio, or medical imaging techniques such as CT, MRI, or DEXA. Clinical features of metabolic syndrome can also serve as useful indicators.

The harm caused by visceral fat stems from its role as an active endocrine organ. It contributes to chronic low-grade inflammation, increases glucose production in the liver, alters lipid handling, disrupts hormone balance, and generates oxidative stress. Together, these mechanisms drive the development of insulin resistance and significantly increase the risk of cardiometabolic disease.

Another aspect of semaglutide's metabolic effects is its potential for lowering inflammation and improving lipid profiles, essential for cardiovascular health. Studies have noted that treatment with semaglutide results in decreased levels of inflammatory cytokines, ameliorated lipid metabolism, and reduced hepatic fat accumulation, which together signify a substantial shift towards a healthier metabolic state [309, 310]. In patients with non-alcoholic fatty liver disease (NAFLD) and insulin resistance, semaglutide's ability to improve liver enzyme levels exemplifies its therapeutic potential in supporting overall metabolic health—steadfastly reflecting reductions in hepatic fat levels and enhancing cardiovascular risk profiles [28, 310].

Semaglutide manifests substantial metabolic effects through its appetite-regulating properties and improvements in gastric emptying, insulin sensitivity, and inflammatory markers, fostering a healthier metabolic profile conducive to reducing risks associated with obesity, type 2 diabetes, and cardiovascular diseases.

Behavioural Changes

Research indicates that specific compounds and hormones can manifest substantial metabolic effects, particularly through their appetite-regulating properties, improvements in gastric emptying, insulin sensitivity, and modulation of inflammatory markers. The interplay among these factors is crucial in fostering a healthier metabolic profile that is conducive to reducing risks associated with obesity, type 2 diabetes, and cardiovascular diseases.

One of the key players in appetite regulation is glucagon-like peptide-1 (GLP-1), an incretin hormone that not only stimulates insulin secretion but also inhibits gastric emptying and contributes to increased satiety. This dual action effectively minimizes postprandial blood glucose levels and enhances insulin sensitivity, which is crucial for individuals at risk of metabolic disorders [116, 259, 311, 312]. Moreover, GLP-1 receptor agonists have been shown to exhibit cardiovascular protection, an important consideration given that patients with type 2 diabetes are at elevated risk for cardiac events [116, 312].

Furthermore, the impact of gastric emptying on insulin dynamics underscores the interconnectedness of metabolic processes. Studies show that GLP-1 significantly slows gastric emptying, which aligns with a reduction in glycaemic excursions after meals [313, 314]. These findings are supported by evidence that alterations in gastric motility can substantially affect glucose homeostasis. For instance, increased GLP-1 levels were associated with better glycaemic control and a reduction in insulin resistance, which is crucial for diabetes management and prevention [313, 314].

Additionally, appetite-regulating hormones such as ghrelin, which has an opposing action to GLP-1 by promoting hunger, and peptide YY (PYY), which contributes to satiety, also play critical roles in maintaining metabolic balance. Ghrelin's modulation of gastric emptying further emphasizes this interaction; studies have highlighted its potential to influence food intake and insulin sensitivity [315, 316].

Chronic inflammation, often tied to obesity and metabolic disorder development, can impair insulin sensitivity and exacerbate cardiometabolic risks [317]. Research has established that interventions targeting inflammatory markers can lead to improvements in insulin resistance and appetite regulation, thereby positively affecting metabolic health [318, 319]. For example, evidence suggests that hormonal alterations following bariatric surgery not only improve weight but also lead to significant enhancements in the inflammatory profile and insulin sensitivity, showcasing the profound metabolic effects of such interventions [319].

A multifaceted approach that regulates appetite through hormonal pathways, optimizes gastric emptying, and addresses insulin sensitivity can yield a healthier metabolic state. The cumulative effects of these interventions are crucial for reducing the prevalence of obesity, type 2 diabetes, and cardiovascular diseases, emphasizing the importance of ongoing research in metabolic health.

Combined Metabolic–Behavioural Impact

This medication's effectiveness lies not only in its ability to induce weight loss but also in its role in altering appetite and metabolism, thus influencing long-term health outcomes. The dual action of semaglutide is primarily attributed to its modulation of both biological and behavioural factors that drive overeating and insulin resistance. As established in clinical research, semaglutide promotes satiety and alters food preferences and reduces meal sizes. Studies have indicated that the drug significantly slows gastric emptying, which consequently diminishes appetite and leads to altered eating behaviours in individuals susceptible to obesity and metabolic disorders [84]. This biochemical modulation is foundational in reducing the biological drivers of overeating, allowing for a more manageable approach to lifestyle change compared to interventions that rely solely on willpower.

Additionally, the medication has been shown to have profound effects on metabolic processes. Semaglutide improves insulin sensitivity and influences hormonal pathways related to weight management and glucose control [320]. Impairments in the body's handling of insulin and glucose are critical contributors to both obesity and type 2 diabetes, making semaglutide's impact on these areas particularly notable. Clinical trials consistently reveal sustained reductions in body weight and improvements in glycaemic control among users of semaglutide, supporting its role as both a treatment for obesity and a means to mitigate diabetes-related complications [84, 320].

The interplay between the pharmacological effects of semaglutide and behavioural adaptation highlights the importance of addressing psychological components in obesity treatment. By alleviating the neurobiological components of cravings and hunger, semaglutide facilitates behavioural changes that are essential for achieving and maintaining healthier lifestyle practices. Notably, research has shown that patients treated with semaglutide experience not only weight loss but also improvements in psychological well-being, including reductions in symptoms of anxiety and depression [321]. These findings suggest that semaglutide does not solely act on physical parameters but also significantly influences mental health, which is crucial for patient adherence to lifestyle changes and long-term health benefits.

Furthermore, semaglutide's impact on resultant health outcomes is underscored by the complex effects it has on cardiovascular health. The medication has been linked to favourable modifications in cardiovascular risk factors such as blood pressure, lipid profiles, and overall cardiovascular health metrics, all of which contribute to improved quality of life in affected individuals [320].

The effectiveness of semaglutide results from its multifaceted approach that combines metabolic and behavioural modifications. By targeting both the biological mechanisms underlying obesity and the psychological factors that contribute to unhealthy eating behaviours, semaglutide not only helps patients achieve significant weight loss but also supports sustainable lifestyle changes and enhances overall health.

Patient Profiles: Who Responds Best?

Semaglutide produces meaningful benefits across a broad range of individuals with obesity, type 2 diabetes, or metabolic dysfunction. However, some patient profiles consistently show greater responsiveness in terms of weight loss, glycaemic improvement, metabolic normalisation, and overall cardiometabolic risk reduction. Understanding these profiles helps clinicians predict outcomes, tailor treatment plans, and set realistic expectations.

1. Individuals With Higher Baseline Body Weight or BMI

Patients with obesity—particularly those with a BMI ≥30 kg/m^2 or ≥27 kg/m^2 with comorbidities—generally experience the most substantial weight-loss responses. Higher baseline adiposity provides more "room" for metabolic improvement, and semaglutide's appetite-regulating effects tend to be particularly impactful in individuals with established overeating patterns or hyperphagia. These patients often achieve 10–20%+ weight loss during long-term therapy.

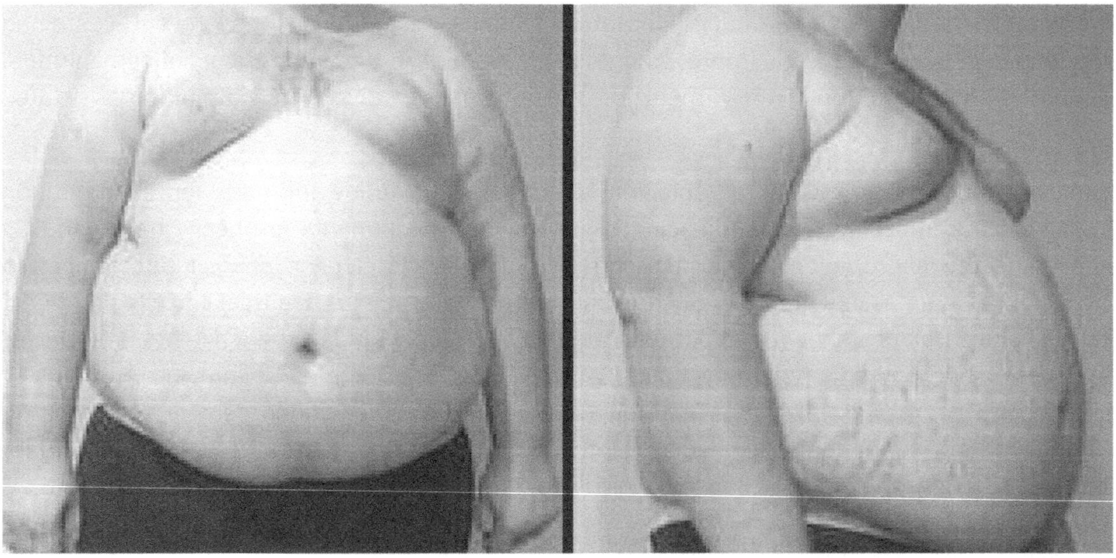

Figure 21: Obese Adult Male - Mid 20s (182kg/400lb), BMI 52.8. FatM1ke (Wikimedia Commons), Public Domain, via Picryl.

2. Patients With Significant Visceral Fat or Metabolic Syndrome

Those with visceral adiposity, central obesity, insulin resistance, high triglycerides, low HDL, or elevated blood pressure typically respond especially well. Semaglutide improves visceral fat distribution, normalises insulin signalling, and reduces inflammatory markers—all central drivers of metabolic syndrome. These patients often show improvements not only in weight, but also in waist circumference, triglycerides, blood pressure, and liver fat (NAFLD/MASLD).

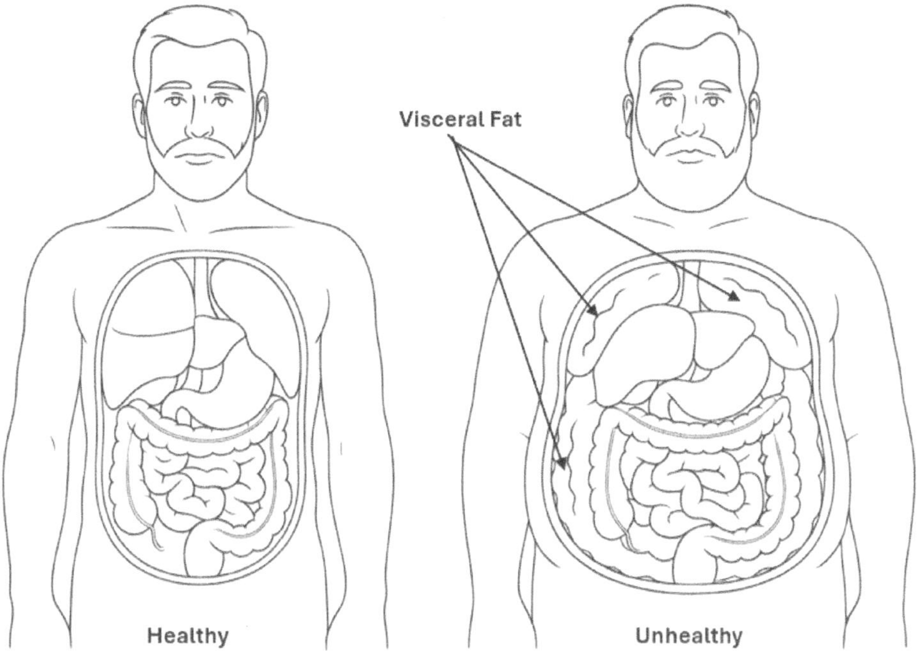

Figure 22: Visceral Fat - Fat Accumulation Around Organs.

3. Individuals With Type 2 Diabetes or Prediabetes

Patients with impaired glucose regulation—prediabetes or established type 2 diabetes—tend to see robust improvements in HbA1c, fasting glucose, post-prandial glucose, and glycaemic stability. Those with higher baseline HbA1c often experience the largest absolute reductions. Many patients with prediabetes revert to normoglycaemia, and those with type 2 diabetes may reduce or discontinue other medications, especially insulin or sulfonylureas.

4. Patients Early in Their Metabolic Disease Course

Clinical trials show that people with less advanced diabetes, earlier stages of NAFLD, or fewer long-term complications respond more strongly. Early intervention allows semaglutide to reverse metabolic dysfunction before irreversible organ damage (e.g., advanced fibrosis, long-standing β-cell decline) has occurred. Younger adults and those with shorter disease duration often achieve greater relative weight loss and metabolic change.

5. Individuals With Strong Engagement in Lifestyle Modifications

Semaglutide enhances the ability to adhere to dietary changes by reducing appetite, cravings, and emotional eating. Patients who combine medication with:

- increased physical activity
- structured nutrition plans
- behavioural therapy
- sleep optimisation

tend to experience the greatest and most durable outcomes. Weight loss of 15–20% or more is far more likely when semaglutide is paired with lifestyle adaptation rather than used alone.

6. Patients With Binge-Eating Tendencies or Dysregulated Appetite

Because semaglutide acts directly on hypothalamic appetite pathways, individuals with:

- compulsive overeating
- intense food cravings
- loss of control eating episodes

often see marked improvements. Reduced hunger, increased satiety, and slower gastric emptying support better eating patterns and long-term behavioural change.

7. Individuals Without Significant Gastrointestinal Sensitivity

Although many patients tolerate semaglutide well, those with minimal GI sensitivity—particularly people without irritable bowel syndrome, gastroparesis, or chronic reflux—tend to progress through dose escalation more smoothly and reach therapeutic doses more reliably. This leads to stronger metabolic and weight-loss results.

8. People Motivated by Health Improvement Rather Than Aesthetic Goals

Patients who engage with treatment for:

- diabetes remission

- NAFLD improvement
- cardiovascular risk reduction
- mobility and energy gains
- better long-term health

often adhere more consistently. Sustained adherence is strongly associated with greater outcomes at 6–12 months and beyond.

Chapter 6

Side Effects, Risks, and Safety Profile

As semaglutide has increasingly become a central therapy in the management of obesity and type 2 diabetes, its rapid rise in popularity has been driven by strong clinical efficacy, meaningful metabolic improvements, and impressive weight-loss outcomes. Yet, like all medications that significantly alter physiology—particularly those that affect appetite, digestion, and hormonal pathways—semaglutide comes with a characteristic safety profile that patients and clinicians must understand to ensure safe, effective, and sustainable use.

In the previous chapters, we explored semaglutide's mechanisms of action, its metabolic and behavioural effects, and the substantial clinical benefits it offers across glycaemic control, weight regulation, cardiovascular health, and liver function. This background provides important context for understanding why certain side effects occur and why some individuals are more vulnerable than others. Many of the medication's most common adverse effects—such as nausea, constipation, diarrhoea, and bloating—stem directly from the same biological mechanisms that make semaglutide effective. For most people, these symptoms are temporary and manageable, but anticipating them is essential for maintaining adherence and avoiding unnecessary discontinuation.

This chapter provides a comprehensive and practical guide to semaglutide's safety profile. It begins with the predictable gastrointestinal effects seen during dose escalation and explains the physiological reasons behind them. From there, it outlines evidence-based strategies to minimise discomfort and prevent symptom recurrence. The chapter then moves into the rarer but clinically important risks—including pancreatitis, gallbladder complications, severe gastrointestinal events, and hypoglycaemia when used with insulin or sulfonylureas—clarifying what is known, what remains uncertain, and how to recognise early warning signs.

Finally, the chapter addresses special populations where caution is warranted, including pregnant or breastfeeding individuals, adolescents, and older adults. Understanding these nuances allows both clinicians and patients to make informed decisions and ensures that semaglutide is used as safely and effectively as possible.

Taken together, the information in this chapter equips readers with a balanced, evidence-based understanding of semaglutide's side effects and risks—helping to set realistic expectations, support long-term adherence, and maximise the therapeutic benefits of this powerful medication.

Common Side Effects (Nausea, Diarrhoea, Constipation, Bloating)

Semaglutide—like all GLP-1 receptor agonists—has a predictable side-effect profile that is largely gastrointestinal in nature. These effects are dose-dependent, usually mild to moderate, and most often occur during the first weeks of treatment or during dose escalation. They generally improve as the body adapts to the medication. Below is a detailed explanation of the most common side effects: nausea, diarrhoea, constipation, and bloating, including why they happen, when they appear, and how they tend to resolve.

Common Side Effects of Semaglutide

Nausea

Nausea is a prominent side effect associated with semaglutide, a GLP-1 receptor agonist used primarily for the management of type 2 diabetes and obesity. It is reported to affect approximately 20-40% of users, depending on dosage and formulation [20, 40, 52, 322]. This gastrointestinal disturbance typically occurs during the initial weeks of treatment, especially when doses are increased, and is often described as mild to moderate in intensity [20, 40, 323]. The incidence of nausea tends to decline as the body adapts to the medication, suggesting a development of tolerance over time [40, 322, 324].

The underlying mechanism that leads to nausea with semaglutide use is primarily due to its ability to slow gastric emptying [325, 326]. This delay results in prolonged retention of food in the stomach, activating stretch receptors and satiety pathways, which can trigger nauseous sensations. Additionally, semaglutide impacts the central nervous system by altering signals within the vomiting centres, particularly in the area postrema, a region known for its role in nausea and vomiting. Studies suggest that the presence of GLP-1 receptors in this area may account for the nausea experienced by patients on such treatments [327, 328].

The onset of nausea is most commonly observed within the first four to eight weeks of treatment, aligning with initial dose escalations [20, 40, 324]. Patients may also experience early feelings of fullness and reduced appetite concurrently with nausea [20, 40, 323]. Nevertheless, severe episodes prompting discontinuation of therapy are rare, as the majority of cases are tolerable and transient [40, 322]. Notably, even when nausea occurs, the beneficial effects on appetite regulation and weight loss associated with semaglutide often contribute to patients' overall positive treatment experiences [52, 250].

As treatment progresses, the gastrointestinal system tends to adapt to the decreased motility induced by semaglutide. This adaptation leads to a gradual decline in nausea symptoms, reinforcing the idea that intolerance is often temporary [40, 225, 322]. The dynamic between gastrointestinal adaptation and alterations in central appetite regulation highlights the complexity of gastrointestinal side effects in the context of GLP-1 receptor agonists like semaglutide. The preferential outcome of these adaptations is a smoother experience for patients as they reach and maintain the therapeutic dose [40, 322, 329].

While nausea remains a significant side effect of semaglutide, its characterization as mild to moderate, onset related to dose escalation, and propensity to improve with continued treatment highlights the manageable nature of this adverse effect. Awareness of the underlying mechanisms of action, alongside patient education regarding the expected trajectory of symptoms, is vital in enhancing patient adherence and satisfaction with semaglutide therapy.

Diarrhoea

Diarrhea is a prevalent adverse effect experienced by approximately 10–20% of individuals treated with glucagon-like peptide-1 receptor agonists (GLP-1 RAs) such as semaglutide and tirzepatide. This side effect can be attributed to various mechanisms related to the pharmacological actions of these medications.

The rapid transit of intestinal contents induced by GLP-1 RAs affects fluid reabsorption in the colon, potentially leading to diarrhea. Semaglutide, in particular, influences gut motility and fluid regulation, which can result in decreased water absorption and increased stool liquidity in some patients [52, 82, 221]. Gastrointestinal effects, including diarrhea, are reported predominantly during the initial dose escalation phase of treatment. Research indicates that many patients experience these gastrointestinal adverse events (AEs) shortly after initiating therapy, and they generally tend to be relatively short-lived, often resolving within days or weeks [118, 330, 331].

Several factors may contribute to the onset of diarrhea in patients undergoing treatment with semaglutide. Notably, changes in dietary habits—often resulting from the medication's appetite-suppressing effects—may lead to smaller meal sizes or reduced fat intake, both of which can influence bowel habits [105, 332]. Moreover, transient fluctuations in gut hormone levels may exacerbate these gastrointestinal effects [20, 40, 333]. It is well documented that patients frequently report gastrointestinal symptoms during the early titration of semaglutide, with these episodes generally being mild and self-limiting as bowel habits stabilize over time [322, 334].

The management of semaglutide therapy often necessitates gradual dosage escalation to enhance tolerability and mitigate adverse effects, including diarrhea [323, 335]. Long-term studies affirm that patients generally report improvement in gastrointestinal symptoms over time, thus contributing positively to treatment adherence [105, 336].

Diarrhea in individuals treated with semaglutide and similar agents results from a complex interplay of pharmacological effects on gastrointestinal motility, dietary changes, and the body's hormonal response to the medication. These episodes are most prevalent during the initial treatment phases and typically resolve as treatment continues, facilitating better gastrointestinal tolerance and adherence to therapy.

Constipation

Constipation is a common gastrointestinal condition that can significantly affect individuals, particularly when appetite decreases, as seen in various patient populations. The underlying pathophysiology and contributing factors to constipation are multifaceted, often involving slowed gastrointestinal motility, reduced dietary fibre and fluid intake, and psychological aspects that may inhibit normal bowel habits.

The phenomenon of constipation in at-risk individuals can primarily be attributed to two main factors: slowed gastrointestinal motility and decreased fibre and fluid intake. Research indicates that reduced gastric emptying and intestinal motility are significant contributors, which can lead to infrequent stool passage and harder stools [337]. Studies suggest that significant appetite suppression often correlates with reduced dietary fibre intake, which in turn lowers stool bulk, exacerbating constipation challenges [338, 339]. Additionally, dehydration, whether intentional due to reduced thirst sensation or unintentional from dietary habits, can further slow intestinal transit time [340].

Clinically, cases of constipation are frequently observed within the first month or two of dietary changes or illness, particularly when fluid and fibre intake are inadequate [341, 342]. Patients with dietary restrictions or specific psychological pressures are at higher risk for prolonged constipation. For instance, adolescents and adults with lowered appetite control, potentially due to stress or mood disorders, display increased incidence rates of constipation [343, 344].

Certain populations are particularly susceptible to constipation, including patients on low-fibre diets and those with conditions such as Irritable Bowel Syndrome - Constipation (IBS-C) or prior instances of slow-transit constipation [337, 345]. The dietary patterns contributing to constipation are often linked to a lack of fruits, vegetables, and whole grains, which, when consumed in inadequate amounts, can lead to a significant behavioural pattern leading to chronic constipation [346, 347]. Dietary fibre is crucial, as noted in various studies, where increased fibre intake has been correlated with improved bowel movement frequency and consistency [338, 348]. Therapeutic interventions like increased dietary fibre, fluid consumption, and scheduled bowel habits remain first-line recommendations for treating functional constipation [346].

Overall, dietary modifications aimed at increasing fluid and fibre intake are efficacious in managing symptoms of constipation. Many studies advocate an integrated approach that includes not just dietary adjustments but also behavioural modifications to improve bowel habits [341, 349].

Bloating (Abdominal Distension or Fullness)

Bloating, also referred to as abdominal distension or fullness, constitutes a common yet less severe complaint that often arises during dose escalation of various therapeutic regimens. This condition is multifactorial in nature, exhibiting a complex interplay of gastric motility and sensitivity changes that can contribute to symptoms such as the sensation of tightness or fullness, mild abdominal pressure, and increased gas production.

The pathophysiology of bloating can largely be attributed to delayed gastric emptying, resulting in prolonged retention of food in the stomach, which can amplify feelings of fullness and discomfort [350, 351]. Additionally, conditions like gastroparesis, characterized by impaired gastric motility, often lead to symptoms of abdominal distension due to the accumulation of gas and stool in the gastrointestinal tract. This impairment can be coupled with slower peristalsis, compounding the bloating symptomatology as gas builds up in the intestine [352].

Changes in dietary habits, such as the consumption of smaller meals or altered macronutrient compositions, can further exacerbate bloating symptoms. For instance, modifications in diet lead to changes in the fermentation dynamics in the gut, which may produce more gas than usual, thereby increasing the sensation of bloating [353, 354]. Moreover, increased sensitivity to gut expansion may also play a significant role in the symptoms experienced by individuals, as visceral hypersensitivity has been noted in patients with functional gastrointestinal disorders like irritable bowel syndrome (IBS) [355, 356]. In these patients, the perception of distension or discomfort can be more pronounced, which may further fuel the bloating experience.

The symptoms of bloating encompass a sensation of tightness or fullness in the abdomen, accompanied by mild abdominal pressure and an increase in belching or flatulence [357]. During periods of dose adjustment, bloating is often observed to co-occur with other gastrointestinal complaints such as nausea or constipation. This symptom constellation typically improves as patients' bowel habits stabilize, suggesting that the physiological adaptations to the therapeutic changes eventually lead to symptomatic relief. The variability in symptoms is closely related to motility and sensory profiles unique to each individual, often necessitating tailored therapeutic strategies [358].

Bloating arises from a variety of mechanisms including delayed gastric emptying, altered gastrointestinal motility, increased sensitivity to abdominal distension, and dietary changes. The symptomatic features often include fullness and abdominal pressure, which may improve with stabilization of bowel habits post dose adjustment. Individual differences in gastrointestinal responses, such as visceral hypersensitivity, significantly impact the experience of bloating, necessitating a nuanced approach to management.

Why These Side Effects Occur: The Underlying Mechanism and Severity

The common gastrointestinal side effects of semaglutide—such as nausea, constipation, diarrhoea, and bloating—occur because the medication directly influences the digestive system and the brain's appetite-regulation pathways. These effects are not accidental; they are closely tied to the same mechanisms that make semaglutide effective for weight loss and glucose control. Understanding these mechanisms helps explain why these symptoms are predictable, temporary, and dose-dependent.

A major contributor is slowed gastric emptying, one of semaglutide's primary actions. The medication delays the movement of food from the stomach into the small intestine, which prolongs the feeling of fullness after eating. While this supports appetite control and reduces calorie intake, it also increases the likelihood of nausea, early satiety, bloating, and—in some individuals—constipation. As the stomach adapts to this slower emptying rate over time, these symptoms typically diminish.

Semaglutide also causes altered intestinal motility, which means it changes the speed at which the intestines move food and waste through the digestive tract. In some people, this slowing effect predominates, leading to constipation. In others, especially early in treatment or during dose changes, the intestines may speed up instead, resulting in diarrhoea. The variability reflects individual differences in gut sensitivity, baseline bowel habits, diet, hydration, and how quickly the dose is escalated.

The drug's appetite-suppressing effects also play a role. Semaglutide reduces hunger and helps people feel satisfied with smaller meals. While this is beneficial for weight loss, it also means less food enters the digestive tract. With reduced dietary volume, stool bulk decreases, making bowel movements less frequent or more difficult—another reason constipation can occur. Additionally, smaller meals can change the rhythm of digestion, contributing to sensations of fullness or bloating as the body recalibrates.

Finally, semaglutide exerts central nervous system effects, particularly in regions of the brain that regulate appetite and nausea. GLP-1 receptors are present in the area postrema—a key nausea centre. When semaglutide activates these receptors, especially at the beginning of treatment or when doses are increased, some people experience nausea or a "queasy" sensation. As the brain adjusts to these new signalling patterns, this effect generally becomes less intense.

Together, these interconnected mechanisms explain why gastrointestinal symptoms occur and why they tend to resolve with continued use. They reflect the body's adaptation to changes in digestion, appetite regulation, and metabolic signalling—effects that are central to the therapeutic benefits of semaglutide.

Patients experiencing gastrointestinal (GI) symptoms due to treatments can generally expect a progression of symptoms that adheres to well-documented timeframes. In the initial weeks of treatment, specifically Weeks 1 to 4, patients are likely to experience nausea, bloating, and mild diarrhea or constipation as low doses of medication begin to take effect [359]. This early phase is crucial as patients may struggle with the adaptation to the new medication regimen, which can heighten their symptoms [360].

As doses increase during Weeks 5 to 8, there may be a recurrence or exacerbation of symptoms, particularly noted when dosage increases occur with certain medications [359]. This phenomenon can be attributed to the escalation of pharmacological effects, which often surpasses the body's ability to acclimatize, leading to increased GI disturbances [359, 361]. Research suggests that the severity of digestive symptoms is significantly correlated with medication dosage levels, highlighting a bi-directional relationship where rising doses can exacerbate pre-existing conditions in sensitive individuals [359].

Post Week 8, and extending into Week 12, a marked improvement in symptoms is observed for most patients. By this point, a significant majority report that their symptoms either improve significantly or resolve altogether [359]. Moreover, as patients transition into the maintenance phase of their treatment, it is expected that most will experience minimal to no ongoing GI symptoms. This trend is supported by clinical trials, during which only a small percentage of patients discontinue treatment due to GI-related events, indicating that adverse impacts become less frequent and often manageable over time [359].

Table 11: Most GI symptoms follow a predictable pattern.

Time Period	What Typically Happens
Weeks 1–4	Nausea, bloating, mild diarrhoea or constipation as low doses begin
Weeks 5–8	Symptoms may recur as doses increase (especially 0.5 mg to 1 mg or 1.7 mg to 2.4 mg)
After Week 8–12	Symptoms usually improve significantly or resolve
Maintenance Phase	Most patients experience minimal to no ongoing symptoms

Clinical evaluations highlight that while the initial phases of treatment can be challenging, the majority of patients ultimately benefit from increased tolerance to medications, culminating in a sustainable health regimen. Continued monitoring and appropriate management strategies considerably mitigate the risk of discontinuation due to GI symptoms, facilitating adherence to long-term treatment plans [359, 360]. Thus, understanding the severity and duration of GI symptoms is essential in setting realistic expectations and promoting patient compliance during their treatment journeys.

Semaglutide is associated with several gastrointestinal (GI) side effects, particularly when initiated at higher doses or with rapid titration schedules. Individuals who experience nausea, bloating, or changes in bowel habits often find these symptoms exacerbated by the pace of dosage increase; rapid titration does not allow adequate time for gastrointestinal adaptation, leading to heightened adverse effects [20, 225, 362]. Specifically, clinical trials have highlighted that GI symptoms such as nausea peak early in treatment and are predominantly associated with initial dosage increases [20, 40].

Diet and eating habits are critical factors that can influence the severity of gastrointestinal symptoms in patients taking semaglutide. High-fat meals, for instance, can exacerbate nausea due to the medication's mechanism, which slows gastric emptying [363]. The prolonged presence of high-fat content in the stomach can increase discomfort and the probability of experiencing symptoms like bloating [351]. Additionally, dietary habits that include large meal sizes may further aggravate the body's response to semaglutide, complicating the management of nausea and gastrointestinal discomfort [364].

Pre-existing gastrointestinal conditions such as irritable bowel syndrome (IBS) and gastroesophageal reflux disease (GERD) also correlate with increased sensitivity to semaglutide [365, 366]. These individuals might already have underlying motility issues that are compounded by the effects of the medication, such as delayed gastric emptying, leading to more pronounced symptoms [351, 365]. Research indicates that patients with functional gastrointestinal disorders exhibit heightened reactions to pharmacological stimuli, which is particularly relevant when introducing a new treatment like semaglutide [365, 367].

The sensitivity to nausea can vary significantly among individuals, with some experiencing heightened queasiness related to their central nervous system responses to nausea stimuli. Those with a predisposition to motion sickness or medication-related nausea are likely to find the introduction of semaglutide challenging [351, 366]. Over time, with careful dose titration, many individuals see a reduction in these symptoms as the body adapts to the medication [20, 40]. Thus, while GI side effects are common, specific populations—including those with lifestyle factors, existing GI conditions, or unique physiological responses—may be more susceptible to significant discomfort when starting treatment with semaglutide.

> Semaglutide's gastrointestinal side effects appear to be modulated by various factors including the rate of dose escalation, dietary habits, existing GI conditions, and individual physiological predispositions to nausea. A tailored approach considering these variables can help manage side effects more effectively.

Clinical Relevance

These side effects:

- Are expected and usually temporary
- Are not associated with permanent gastrointestinal damage
- Can be mitigated with slow titration and dietary strategies
- Usually resolve with continued therapy as the gut adapts

Importantly, these symptoms correlate with semaglutide's therapeutic mechanism—especially appetite reduction and delayed gastric emptying—which contribute to effective weight loss and glycaemic improvements.

> Semaglutide's most common side effects—nausea, diarrhoea, constipation, and bloating—stem from predictable and reversible changes in gastrointestinal motility and appetite regulation. They are typically mild, transient, and dose-related, improving substantially once patients reach a stable dose. Understanding these effects helps patients

set realistic expectations and supports better adherence and long-term outcomes.

Strategies To Reduce Side Effects

Gastrointestinal (GI) side effects, including nausea, diarrhea, and constipation, are common challenges that can affect patients' adherence to treatment. Understanding the strategies to mitigate these side effects is essential for improving tolerability and ensuring therapy continuation. Soe strategies follow.

1. Introduce the Dose Slowly (Follow the Titration Schedule)

The most effective strategy to minimize gastrointestinal side effects is to follow a slow titration schedule as recommended by the prescribing guidelines. Initiating treatment with low doses—such as 0.25 mg weekly—allows the gastrointestinal system to adapt without immediate onset of adverse effects [225].

Rapid escalation of the dose can exacerbate symptoms such as nausea and bloating; studies indicate that patients who adhere to a gradual increase in dosage report significantly fewer gastrointestinal issues [260, 368]. This slow titration approach enhances tolerability and allows patients to achieve higher therapeutic doses safely [162].

2. Modify Eating Habits

The manner in which food is consumed greatly impacts the severity of semaglutide's gastrointestinal side effects. Recommendations for patients include eating smaller, more frequent meals rather than large portions. Dietary changes such as reducing fat intake and avoiding heavy or spicy foods can help align eating habits with semaglutide's action of slowing gastric emptying, thereby alleviating symptoms like nausea and cramping [221, 362].

Additionally, patients are encouraged to eat slowly and stop eating when they feel comfortably full. Engaging these practices can reduce the burden on the digestive system, easing symptoms and enhancing overall comfort during treatment [362].

3. Stay Hydrated

Hydration is vital, as semaglutide's side effects often lead to decreased appetite, which can result in inadequate fluid intake. Recommendations include sipping water throughout the day and increasing fluid intake when experiencing diarrhea to prevent dehydration and constipation [362]. Limiting caffeine and alcohol, which could exacerbate gastrointestinal symptoms, is also advised [221].

4. Choose Foods That Support Digestive Comfort

During the initial treatment phase, the consumption of bland and easily digestible foods can help manage gastrointestinal discomfort. Foods such as toast, rice, and non-carbonated beverages are suggested for their gentler effect on the digestive system [362]. Avoidance of carbonated beverages can further help reduce nausea and bloating [221].

5. Manage Nausea Proactively

Proactive management of nausea through home remedies can help maintain comfort. Techniques such as ginger consumption and the use of peppermint tea are supported in the literature as beneficial during the titration phase when nausea peaks [40, 362]. For persistent nausea, healthcare providers may consider prescribing anti-nausea medication temporarily [162, 369].

6. Support Bowel Regularity

To counteract semaglutide's effects on gut motility, increasing dietary fibre gradually is beneficial, as fibre can aid in promoting regular bowel movements. Additionally, staying hydrated and engaging in light physical activity, such as daily walks, can support gastrointestinal health and alleviate constipation [40, 221, 225].

7. Avoid Large Fatty Meals

High-fat meals can significantly increase the risk of nausea and bloating in patients taking semaglutide. Reducing the intake of fatty and greasy foods, including creamy sauces and fried items, can effectively mitigate these effects [221, 362]. Studies show that cutting back on such foods aligns well with semaglutide's pharmacological profile, resulting in fewer gastrointestinal disturbances [40, 64].

8. Pause Dose Escalation When Needed

If a patient experiences moderate to severe gastrointestinal side effects, it is advisable to pause dose escalation until these symptoms subside. This practice has been validated in clinical settings, where it was found to improve tolerability and patient comfort without compromising treatment efficacy [162, 221].

9. Consider Timing of Injection or Tablet

Timing can play a crucial role in managing symptoms. For instance, administering semaglutide in the evening may help alleviate nausea by shifting symptom peaks to nighttime. Conversely, taking oral semaglutide first thing in the morning can enhance absorption and mitigate variability in side effects [221, 225].

10. Maintain Gentle Activity

Light physical activity is encouraged to facilitate digestion and reduce symptoms like constipation and bloating. High-intensity workouts immediately post-meal may worsen gastrointestinal symptoms and should be avoided [40, 221, 370].

Gastrointestinal side effects from semaglutide, while common, are usually temporary. By adhering to slow dose titration, adjusting dietary habits, ensuring adequate hydration, and employing proactive management techniques, patients can significantly reduce these adverse symptoms. Each strategy aligns with the pharmacodynamics of semaglutide and supports a more comfortable treatment experience.

Serious Risks: Pancreatitis, Gallbladder Issues, Hypoglycaemia (With Sulfonylureas/Insulin), Rare GI Events

While semaglutide is generally safe and well tolerated, especially compared with older diabetes medications, clinicians and patients must be aware of several rare but serious risks. These events occur infrequently but require prompt recognition and appropriate management. The following sections outline the major risks associated with treatment: pancreatitis, gallbladder complications, hypoglycaemia (when used with insulin or sulfonylureas), and rare but significant gastrointestinal events.

Pancreatitis

Pancreatitis, or inflammation of the pancreas, poses a significant concern for patients being treated with glucagon-like peptide-1 (GLP-1) receptor agonists, including semaglutide. While extensive clinical trials have not established a direct causal link between GLP-1 receptor agonists and pancreatitis, isolated case reports and pharmacovigilance studies suggest that caution is warranted, particularly among patients exhibiting known risk factors for pancreatitis. These risk factors include a history of gallstones, elevated triglycerides, obesity, heavy alcohol use, and prolonged diabetes. For instance, Melo et al. [371] documented a case where a type 2 diabetic patient developed acute pancreatitis shortly after initiating treatment with semaglutide, emphasizing the need for vigilance in prescribing this medication to patients with heightened risks associated with pancreatitis, such as obesity and certain medications.

Pancreatitis is inflammation of the pancreas, a vital organ located behind the stomach that produces digestive enzymes and hormones such as insulin. When the pancreas becomes inflamed, these digestive enzymes can activate too early and begin damaging pancreatic tissue, leading to pain, swelling, and sometimes serious complications.

What the Pancreas Does

- **Digestive role:** Produces enzymes that help break down fats, proteins, and carbohydrates.
- **Hormonal role:** Produces insulin and glucagon, which regulate blood sugar.

When inflamed, both digestive and hormonal functions can be disrupted.

Types of Pancreatitis

1. Acute Pancreatitis
   - Sudden onset.
   - Ranges from mild discomfort to severe, life-threatening illness.
   - Often resolves with treatment, but complications can occur.
2. Chronic Pancreatitis
   - Long-term inflammation that gradually damages the pancreas.
   - Can lead to scarring, permanent enzyme loss, and diabetes.

Causes

Most common causes:

- Gallstones (block the pancreatic duct)
- Heavy alcohol use

Other causes:

- Very high triglycerides
- Certain medications
- Abdominal injury
- Autoimmune disease
- Genetic conditions
- Viral infections
- Smoking
- Post–ERCP (a medical procedure)

Some cases have no obvious cause (idiopathic pancreatitis).

Symptoms

Typical signs include:

- Severe upper abdominal pain, often radiating to the back
- Nausea and vomiting
- Fever
- Rapid heartbeat
- Tender abdomen
- Worsening pain after eating

In chronic pancreatitis:

- Persistent abdominal pain
- Weight loss
- Fatty, oily stools (steatorrhoea)

Why It's Serious

Pancreatitis can lead to complications such as:

- Pancreatic necrosis (tissue death)
- Infection
- Organ failure (in severe cases)
- Diabetes (due to damaged insulin-producing cells)
- Malabsorption (in chronic disease)
- Pseudocysts (fluid-filled sacs)

Severe pancreatitis can be life-threatening and requires hospital care.

Treatment

Acute pancreatitis management:

- Hospitalisation for IV fluids
- Pain management
- Resting the pancreas (e.g., temporary fasting)
- Treating the underlying cause (e.g., gallstone removal)

Chronic pancreatitis management:

- Enzyme supplements
- Dietary modifications (low-fat)
- Pain control
- Diabetes management
- Surgery in some cases

How Semaglutide Fits In

GLP-1 medications *rarely* cause pancreatitis, but:

- Patients with a history of pancreatitis should use caution.
- Symptoms need immediate medical evaluation.
- The drug should be stopped if pancreatitis is suspected.

Similarly, the relationship between GLP-1 receptor agonists and acute pancreatitis has been scrutinized, with findings indicating that patients on GLP-1 agonists may experience pancreatitis at rates that warrant attention, especially in the presence of such risk factors [372].

The role of GLP-1 receptors within the pancreas provides biological plausibility to these concerns, as activation of these receptors may influence pancreatic enzyme secretion or provoke localized inflammation. Elashoff et al. [373] highlighted that increased reports of pancreatitis were associated with GLP-1 therapies following initial FDA warnings about exenatide, suggesting a potential risk associated with all GLP-1 receptor agonists. Furthermore, Alenzi et al. [374] found that while a relatively small number of patients using semaglutide developed pancreatitis compared to placebo groups, the initial analysis raised caution when using these drugs in patients predisposed to pancreatitis.

Recognizing the symptoms of pancreatitis early is crucial for effective management. Patients should seek medical intervention if they experience severe abdominal pain (particularly radiating to the back), persistent vomiting, or other symptoms associated with elevated pancreatic enzymes. Guidance from the medical community stresses that semaglutide should be promptly discontinued in any instance where pancreatitis is suspected, pending further assessment [375]. It is noteworthy that the onset of pancreatitis may occur relatively soon after starting treatment with semaglutide, with cases reported as early as 23 days following the first dose [376].

Overall, while empirical evidence from large-scale studies remains inconclusive in definitively establishing a link between GLP-1 receptor agonists and pancreatitis, ongoing vigilance is essential. Clinicians are advised to remain informed about patient histories and symptomatology, ensuring that the potential benefits of these medications are carefully weighed against their risks, especially in vulnerable populations and those presenting with known risk factors for pancreatitis [377]. Regular monitoring and patient education about warning signs of pancreatitis can facilitate timely intervention and improve outcomes.

Gallbladder Issues (Cholelithiasis and Cholecystitis)

Gallbladder complications associated with semaglutide and other GLP-1 receptor agonists—including gallstones (cholelithiasis) and gallbladder inflammation (cholecystitis)—have been increasingly highlighted in clinical literature. Despite the relatively low absolute risk, this risk is significantly higher than in the general population, particularly during periods of rapid weight loss which are common with these medications. Such rapid weight loss can precipitate gallbladder changes due to several metabolic and physiological mechanisms.

Cholelithiasis (Gallstones)

Cholelithiasis refers to the formation of gallstones—solid deposits that develop inside the gallbladder. These stones can be made of cholesterol, bilirubin, or a mixture of substances. They vary in size from tiny grains to large stones several centimetres wide.

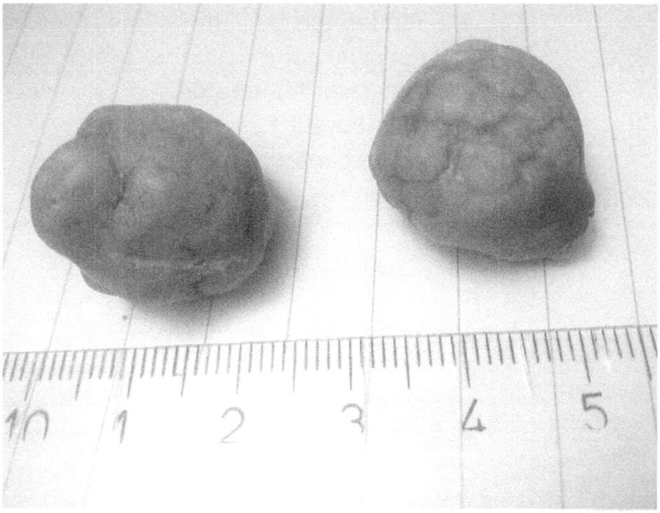

Figure 23: Gallstones can be quite large, up to an inch in diameter. On their own, they don't cause any trouble unless one blocks the bile duct that empties into the small intestine. Jakupica, CC BY-SA 4.0, via Wikimedia Commons.

Key features of cholelithiasis:

- The condition may cause no symptoms (silent gallstones).
- When symptoms occur, they usually involve:
    - Right upper abdominal pain (biliary colic)
    - Nausea or vomiting
    - Pain after eating—especially fatty meals
- Gallstones can move into the bile ducts and cause complications such as pancreatitis or cholecystitis.

What causes gallstones?

- Rapid weight loss
- Obesity
- High cholesterol
- Female sex
- Pregnancy
- Certain medications
- Family history

Cholecystitis (Gallbladder inflammation)

Cholecystitis is inflammation of the gallbladder, usually triggered by a gallstone blocking the cystic duct. This blockage traps bile inside the gallbladder, leading to swelling, irritation, and sometimes infection.

Key features of cholecystitis:

- Persistent right upper abdominal pain (more severe and prolonged than biliary colic)
- Fever or chills
- Nausea and vomiting
- Tenderness over the gallbladder when touched
- Possible complications such as infection, perforation, or gangrene if untreated

Types of cholecystitis:

- Acute cholecystitis: sudden, severe inflammation, usually caused by gallstones.
- Chronic cholecystitis: long-standing low-grade inflammation causing repeated attacks.

Relationship Between the Two

- Cholelithiasis (gallstones) is the cause in about 90–95% of cholecystitis cases.
- Not everyone with gallstones develops cholecystitis, but the presence of stones increases the risk.

Why These Conditions Matter in Semaglutide Treatment

Because semaglutide can cause rapid and significant weight loss, it increases the risk of gallstone formation, which in turn can lead to cholecystitis. Monitoring symptoms and educating patients is essential during therapy.

Rapid weight loss is known to result in increased cholesterol concentrations in bile and diminished gallbladder motility. This combination creates an environment conducive to gallstone formation, as observed in studies analysing obesity and gallstone pathogenesis. Talha et al. [378] note that severe caloric restriction during rapid weight loss surgery can lead to an increase in cholesterol saturation of gallbladder bile, promoting the precipitation of cholesterol crystals and subsequent gallstone formation. Bennion and Grundy [379] also observed that obese individuals had bile that was frequently supersaturated with cholesterol prior to weight loss, further illustrating the predisposition to gallstone development. Furthermore, Stender et al. [380]found that increased abdominal fat mass may lead to gallbladder hypomotility and bile stasis, another critical risk factor for gallstone formation.

The physiological role played by GLP-1 receptor agonists in this context is important, as these medications can impair gallbladder emptying in certain individuals, thereby enhancing the risk of stasis. Studies suggest that GLP-1 receptor agonists may slow gallbladder motility, thereby increasing the likelihood of gallstones [381]. Symptoms that patients may experience include right upper abdominal pain, nausea, and vomiting, which can escalate to severe cholecystitis requiring urgent medical attention [382]. Concerns regarding acute gallbladder events with incretin therapies have prompted recommendations for monitoring symptoms, especially in the initial months of treatment when significant weight loss occurs [381].

Clinicians must be vigilant during the first 6–12 months of therapy with GLP-1 receptor agonists, as gallbladder events need to be promptly recognized and managed to prevent more severe complications. As rapid weight loss exacerbates the risk, integrating strategies for monitoring gallbladder health can be beneficial in ensuring patient safety during GLP-1 receptor agonist treatment regimens.

While semaglutide and other GLP-1 receptor agonists present effective avenues for weight management in individuals with obesity and type 2 diabetes, there is an elevated risk of gallbladder complications, particularly during rapid weight loss phases. The interplay of weight loss, physiological changes in bile composition, and gallbladder motility, coupled with the underlying metabolic profiles of these patients, necessitates a concerted approach to risk monitoring.

Hypoglycaemia (When Used with Insulin or Sulfonylureas)

Semaglutide, a glucagon-like peptide-1 (GLP-1) receptor agonist, primarily facilitates glycaemic control through a glucose-dependent mechanism, which minimizes the risk of hypoglycaemia when administered alone. This characteristic is particularly important in managing type 2 diabetes, where the risk of hypoglycemics episodes can increase sharply when semaglutide is combined with other anti-diabetic medications, notably insulin and sulfonylureas. Insulin and sulfonylureas can provoke hypoglycaemia irrespective of blood glucose levels, thereby overshadowing the protective effects of semaglutide [20, 383].

The risk of hypoglycaemia when these medications are used together arises from overlapping pharmacodynamics. Sulfonylureas induce a continuous stimulation of pancreatic insulin secretion regardless of blood glucose levels, leading to potentially excessive insulin levels. Similarly, when semaglutide enhances overall glycaemic control, doses of basal or bolus insulin may require careful adjustment, as previously appropriate doses could become excessive [383, 384]. A systematic review highlighted that combining GLP-1 receptor agonists like semaglutide with insulin therapy necessitates careful dose adjustments to prevent hypoglycemics incidents, underlining the importance of personalized therapy based on individual patient responses [72, 385].

To mitigate these risks, healthcare providers typically initiate treatment with semaglutide alongside a careful reduction of insulin or sulfonylurea doses, followed by ongoing monitoring and further adjustments as necessary. Intensive glucose monitoring within the first 8–12 weeks of therapy is recommended, enabling timely identification and management of any hypoglycemics events [386, 387]. Educating patients to recognize early signs of hypoglycaemia—such as sweating, confusion, and weakness—allows for prompt reactions to these incidents, which is especially crucial for vulnerable populations, including older adults who may have impaired counter-regulatory responses [20, 259].

While semaglutide is noted for its low risk of inducing hypoglycaemia through its glucose-dependent mechanism, concurrent use of insulin or sulfonylureas can increase this risk. Therefore, healthcare providers must carefully manage dosing regimens and monitor glucose levels to effectively utilize the therapeutic potential of semaglutide while minimizing the likelihood of hypoglycaemic events.

Rare Gastrointestinal Events (Intestinal Obstruction, Ileus, Gastroparesis)

Semaglutide, a GLP-1 receptor agonist, has been associated with significant gastrointestinal (GI) side effects due to its pharmacological action of slowing gastric emptying and intestinal motility. Although these effects generally aid in reducing appetite and facilitating weight loss, they pose serious risks in individuals with pre-existing motility disorders such as gastroparesis, intestinal obstruction, or ileus. Such complications, though infrequent, have emerged as major concerns documented in post-marketing surveillance of semaglutide [225, 388, 389].

Intestinal Obstruction

Intestinal obstruction refers to a physical or functional blockage that prevents the normal passage of food, fluids, and gas through the intestines. The obstruction can be partial or complete, and can occur in either the small intestine or the large intestine.

Blockages may be due to:

- Mechanical causes (physical blockages), such as:
  - Adhesions from previous surgery
  - Hernias
  - Tumours
  - Strictures (narrowing)
  - Gallstone ileus
- Functional causes, where movement stops despite no physical blockage (e.g., ileus).

Symptoms:

- Severe or cramping abdominal pain
- Abdominal distension
- Nausea and vomiting
- Inability to pass stool or gas
- Dehydration

Why it is serious:

Untreated obstruction can lead to:

- Bowel ischemia (loss of blood supply)
- Perforation
- Sepsis

Immediate medical evaluation is always required.

Ileus

Ileus is a temporary loss or reduction of the normal muscular contractions (peristalsis) of the intestines, causing slowed or stopped movement of intestinal contents. Unlike mechanical obstruction, ileus is not caused by a physical blockage—the bowel simply isn't moving properly.

Common causes:

- Recent abdominal or pelvic surgery

- Severe illness or infection
- Certain medications (especially opioids)
- Electrolyte imbalances (e.g., low potassium)
- Prolonged immobility
- Abdominal inflammation (e.g., pancreatitis)

Symptoms:

- Abdominal bloating
- Nausea and vomiting
- Poor appetite
- Few or no bowel movements
- Mild to moderate abdominal discomfort

Clinical relevance:

Ileus is often reversible once the underlying cause is treated. With GLP-1 medications like semaglutide, ileus-like symptoms may occur because these drugs slow intestinal transit.

Gastroparesis

Gastroparesis is a condition in which the stomach empties much more slowly than normal due to impaired muscle contractions or nerve dysfunction. Food stays in the stomach for prolonged periods, leading to digestive symptoms.

Causes:

- Diabetes-related autonomic neuropathy (most common chronic cause)
- Viral infections
- Postsurgical nerve injury
- Medications that slow gastric emptying (including GLP-1 receptor agonists)
- Idiopathic causes (unknown origin)

Symptoms:

- Early satiety (feeling full quickly)
- Persistent nausea
- Vomiting undigested food hours after eating
- Bloating

- Upper abdominal pain
- Poor appetite and unintended weight loss

Why it occurs with semaglutide:

Semaglutide naturally slows gastric emptying as part of its mechanism of action. Most people tolerate this well, but in susceptible individuals, the effect may be exaggerated, leading to symptoms similar to gastroparesis.

Potential complications:

- Dehydration
- Malnutrition
- Fluctuating blood sugars
- Food bezoars (hardened masses) in severe cases

Reports have highlighted that patients with underlying digestive conditions, particularly those with long-standing diabetes and autonomic neuropathy, are at a higher risk for severe complications associated with semaglutide treatment. The mechanism of action whereby GLP-1 receptor agonists slow gastrointestinal transit is well-established; they do so through direct inhibition of enteric nervous pathways and modulation of gastric motility [388, 389]. Specifically, studies have demonstrated that GLP-1 receptor activation can lead to delayed gastric emptying, which in some patients results in marked symptoms such as persistent vomiting, which may escalate to dehydration, severe abdominal distension, and overall deterioration of gastrointestinal health [35, 389].

The literature suggests that the risk of these adverse events may increase with higher doses of semaglutide, especially during rapid dose escalation, as well as with consumption of large, high-fat meals or exacerbation of pre-existing dehydration [225, 388]. Importantly, healthcare providers are advised to monitor patients closely and educate them on the necessity of reporting any new or worsening GI symptoms to mitigate risks such as acute kidney injury or malnutrition stemming from delayed gastric emptying or obstruction [225, 388]. Furthermore, clinician vigilance is particularly warranted in high-risk populations that may possess genetic predispositions towards motility disturbances [225, 388].

In the case of developing symptoms such as prolonged vomiting, inability to retain fluids, or severe abdominal bloating, immediate medical attention is warranted. Guidelines indicate that in these scenarios, semaglutide administration should be paused until a thorough evaluation of the cause has been conducted and symptoms have resolved [225, 388, 389]. This approach not only underscores the necessity for proactive clinical management but also promotes a comprehensive understanding of how semaglutide's effects on gastric motility can critically impact patient safety and treatment efficacy.

Thyroid Tumour Concerns and Evidence

Concerns regarding thyroid tumours, particularly medullary thyroid carcinoma (MTC), have gained prominence in discussions surrounding glucagon-like peptide-1 receptor agonists (GLP-1 RAs), such as semaglutide. Preclinical research has indicated that exposure to high doses of these agents in rodents has led to pathological changes in thyroid C-cells, including hyperplasia and adenomas, raising red flags about potential tumorigenic effects in humans [390, 391]. The mechanism behind these findings is attributed to the higher density of GLP-1 receptors in rodent thyroid C-cells compared to humans, leading to a heightened risk of stimulation and subsequent tumour formation with GLP-1 RAs in animal models [390]. Conversely, human thyroid C-cells exhibit significantly lower GLP-1 receptor expression, suggesting that the rodent model may not be entirely applicable in predicting human outcomes [391, 392].

Medullary Thyroid Carcinoma (MTC)

Medullary thyroid carcinoma (MTC) is a rare but serious type of thyroid cancer that arises from C-cells (also known as parafollicular cells) of the thyroid gland. These cells are responsible for producing calcitonin, a hormone involved in calcium regulation. Unlike the more common forms of thyroid cancer—which arise from follicular cells—MTC behaves differently, has distinct genetic associations, and requires specific diagnostic and treatment approaches.

MTC is a neuroendocrine tumour of the thyroid. It accounts for only 3–4% of all thyroid cancers, but it is more aggressive than papillary or follicular thyroid cancers.

There are two major forms:

1. Sporadic MTC
   - Occurs randomly, with no inherited cause.
   - Represents about 75% of MTC cases.
   - Usually affects one lobe of the thyroid.
   - Typically diagnosed in adults (40–60 years old).
2. Hereditary MTC
   - Represents about 25% of cases.
   - Caused by mutations in the RET proto-oncogene.
   - Can occur as part of:
     - Multiple Endocrine Neoplasia type 2A (MEN2A)
     - Multiple Endocrine Neoplasia type 2B (MEN2B)
     - Familial MTC
   - Often diagnosed earlier in life.
   - May involve both thyroid lobes.

Because hereditary MTC is strongly genetic, family screening and early thyroid removal (prophylactic thyroidectomy) are sometimes recommended.

MTC is caused by abnormal growth of C-cells. In hereditary cases, this is driven by RET gene mutations. In sporadic cases, the cause is less well understood.
C-cells overproduce calcitonin, which becomes a useful biomarker for diagnosis and monitoring. As the tumour progresses, it can invade nearby tissues and spread (metastasise) to:

- lymph nodes
- lungs
- liver
- bones

Symptoms: Early stages may cause no symptoms. As the tumour grows, people may experience:

- A lump or swelling in the neck
- Hoarseness or voice changes
- Difficulty swallowing
- Neck pain
- Enlarged lymph nodes
- Persistent cough not linked to infection

Advanced MTC can produce hormone-related symptoms because C-cells may secrete excess calcitonin or other peptides:

- Diarrhoea
- Flushing (less common)

Diagnosis: Diagnosis typically involves:

1. Blood tests
    - Calcitonin: usually very high in MTC
    - CEA (carcinoembryonic antigen): elevated and correlates with tumour burden
2. Imaging
    - Neck ultrasound
    - CT or MRI if spread is suspected
    - Nuclear scans in some cases
3. Genetic testing
    - All patients with MTC are recommended to undergo RET mutation testing to determine hereditary vs sporadic forms.
4. Biopsy
    - Fine-needle aspiration cytology
    - Calcitonin levels in needle washout fluid can help confirm diagnosis

Treatment: The primary treatment is:
Total thyroidectomy
(removal of the entire thyroid gland)
Often combined with removal of affected lymph nodes. Unlike other thyroid cancers:

- Radioactive iodine is not effective because C-cells do not take up iodine.
- External-beam radiotherapy or targeted therapies (RET inhibitors like selpercatinib or pralsetinib) may be used for advanced disease.

Prognosis: Prognosis depends largely on:

- Stage at diagnosis
- Whether the cancer has spread
- Genetic subtype (MEN2B tends to be more aggressive)
- Calcitonin and CEA doubling times

If caught early, the 10-year survival rate is high (>90%). Advanced metastatic disease has a more guarded prognosis.

Why MTC Matters for Semaglutide

Medications like semaglutide carry a contraindication for people with:

- Personal or family history of MTC
- MEN2A or MEN2B

This warning exists because GLP-1 receptor agonists caused C-cell tumours in rodents—but this effect has not been observed in humans. Still, because hereditary MTC is highly aggressive, regulators recommend avoiding any medication that might theoretically influence C-cell behaviour.

Medullary thyroid carcinoma is a rare neuroendocrine thyroid cancer arising from C-cells that produce calcitonin. It exists in both sporadic and hereditary forms, with the hereditary type linked to RET mutations and MEN2 syndromes. MTC is diagnosed through blood biomarkers, imaging, and biopsy, and treated primarily with total thyroidectomy. Prognosis is generally good when detected early but can be serious when metastatic.

Despite the preclinical alerts, there has been no corroborative evidence from extensive human clinical trials to indicate an increased risk of thyroid cancer associated with GLP-1 RA therapy. Notable studies, including the LEADER trial for liraglutide, the SUSTAIN and PIONEER programs for semaglutide, and the REWIND trial for dulaglutide, have consistently reported no significant increase in MTC or overall thyroid neoplasms among participants [393-395]. These trials encompassing over 60,000 patient-years of observation found instances of MTC to be rare and consistent with background rates within the general population [373, 395, 396]. Importantly, the absence of C-cell hyperplasia and MTC among patients treated with liraglutide over extended periods illustrates the lack of a definitive link between GLP-1 RAs and thyroid cancer risk in humans [393, 396].

Real-world observational studies have echoed these findings, revealing a lack of increased thyroid cancer incidence correlating with GLP-1 RA usage. While certain small-scale studies hinted at a potential uptick in diagnoses of thyroid conditions, these results are often confounded by detection biases, such as increased imaging performed in populations with obesity or diabetes, suggesting that increased detection rather than an actual rise in incidence might explain these observations [392, 397]. The biological response of human thyroid cells to GLP-1 RAs, characterized by minimal receptor expression and lack of stimulation of calcitonin secretion, further supports the argument that human risks may differ significantly from those observed in animal studies [398, 399].

Regulatory bodies, however, continue to advocate for caution. The FDA mandates a boxed warning regarding the potential observed risks of thyroid tumours in animal studies, advising against the use of GLP-1 RAs in individuals with a personal or familial history of MTC or Multiple Endocrine Neoplasia type 2 (MEN2) due to the inherent increased risk of C-cell tumours in these populations [390, 391]. Patients are advised to report any thyroid-related symptoms, thus underscoring the importance of clinical vigilance, even as the overall evidence suggests a favourable safety profile for these medications in the broader population.

Rodent studies indicate an increased risk of C-cell tumours due to species-specific receptor biology associated with GLP-1 RAs, yet extensive clinical and real-world human data provide strong reassurance of safety, showing no confirmed increase in MTC. For the general population, medications like semaglutide appear safe concerning thyroid cancer risk; nonetheless, practitioners should exercise caution with high-risk individuals.

When to Stop the Medication

The decision to temporarily pause or discontinue semaglutide therapy is sometimes essential to ensure patient safety and tolerability. While semaglutide is effective for long-term management of conditions such as diabetes and obesity, there are specific situations where maintaining treatment poses a risk to the patient. These circumstances encompass severe gastrointestinal symptoms, suspected pancreatitis, gallbladder complications, severe hypoglycaemia, renal concerns, allergic reactions, pregnancy considerations, thyroid carcinoma histories, intolerability, and lack of clinical benefit.

1. **Severe or Persistent Gastrointestinal Symptoms**: Gastrointestinal side effects like nausea and vomiting are prevalent when initiating semaglutide therapy. Although these generally decrease, they can become severe or persistent, indicating a need for discontinuation. Significant gastrointestinal symptoms leading to malnutrition or dehydration may necessitate immediate evaluation to prevent further complications, including acute kidney injury due to dehydration [13, 225]. A systematic review emphasizes careful patient monitoring to mitigate risks associated with gastrointestinal side effects of semaglutide [400].

2. **Suspected or Confirmed Pancreatitis**: The discontinuation of semaglutide is critical if pancreatitis is suspected, characterized by severe abdominal pain and elevated

pancreatic enzymes. Although the connection between GLP-1 receptor agonists like semaglutide and pancreatitis remains debated, multiple case reports and clinical guidelines support caution with this medication due to its potential association with pancreatitis [13, 401, 402].

3. **Gallbladder-Related Complications**: Rapid weight fluctuations and impaired gallbladder motility linked to semaglutide treatment can elevate the risk of gallbladder issues. Presenting symptoms such as abdominal pain and persistent nausea should prompt evaluation, and treatment should be paused until assessment is complete [375, 403]. The literature stresses the importance of monitoring patients who exhibit these signs due to the potential for gallbladder complications [404].

4. **Severe Hypoglycaemia**: While semaglutide is less likely to cause hypoglycaemia when used as a standalone therapy, the risk can increase when combined with insulin or sulfonylureas. Patients experiencing recurrent or severe hypoglycaemic episodes should consider dose modification or discontinuation of semaglutide to prevent adverse outcomes [11]. Alignment of treatment regimens is crucial for maintaining safety [405].

5. **New or Worsening Kidney Problems**: Renal function may be compromised due to dehydration from gastrointestinal issues associated with semaglutide. If patients develop acute kidney injury or show rising creatinine levels, discontinuation of therapy is warranted until adequate hydration and renal assessment can be conducted [406]. Cases of acute interstitial nephritis following semaglutide usage underscore the need for thorough renal monitoring during treatment [407].

6. **Allergy or Hypersensitivity**: Instances of allergic reactions, while rare, such as rash or anaphylaxis, necessitate immediate discontinuation of semaglutide. These hypersensitivity reactions require close monitoring and a reassessment of therapeutic strategies [225, 406]. Clinicians must remain vigilant for signs of such reactions during patient management [371].

7. **Pregnancy or Breastfeeding**: Given the potential risks associated with semaglutide during pregnancy, it is imperative to discontinue the medication if pregnancy is confirmed or planned, enabling clearance of the drug from the system before conception [405]. The long half-life of semaglutide necessitates careful timing around planned pregnancies for safety [11].

8. **Diagnosed or Suspected Medullary Thyroid Carcinoma (MTC) or MEN2**: Semaglutide is contraindicated in patients with MTC or a history of MEN2 due to potential thyroid malignancies. Treatment must be halted immediately upon diagnosis to minimize risks [406].

9. **Inadequate Tolerability or Patient Preference**: Patient comfort is paramount; intolerable side effects may compel patients to discontinue semaglutide. Adjusting doses or switching to alternative therapies should be considered to balance therapeutic benefits with quality of life [11, 225].

10. **No Clinical Benefit After Adequate Trial**: If patients fail to realize significant clinical benefits after substantial treatment periods, clinicians may recommend stopping semaglutide and exploring alternative therapeutic options [405]. The necessity for ongoing evaluation of treatment efficacy is crucial for informed clinical decision-making [11].

> While semaglutide presents substantial benefits, clinicians must be prepared to make individualized adjustments or discontinuations to safeguard patient health. Such decisions are underpinned by comprehensive monitoring and assessment of pertinent side effects and risk factors.

Safety In Pregnancy, Breastfeeding, Adolescents, Older Adults

Semaglutide's safety profile varies across different life stages and populations. Because its effects extend across metabolic, hormonal, and gastrointestinal systems—and because it remains in the body for weeks after stopping—clinical guidance is highly specific for groups such as pregnant and breastfeeding individuals, adolescents, and older adults. Understanding these considerations is essential for safe prescribing and appropriate patient counselling.

Safety in Pregnancy

Semaglutide is contraindicated during pregnancy due to potential health concerns for the foetus. Evidence from animal studies indicates that GLP-1 receptor agonists, including semaglutide, can cross the placenta, which has been associated with adverse foetal outcomes such as reduced foetal weight and pregnancy loss at exposure levels comparable to or lower than therapeutic doses for humans [161, 250]. Although the direct translational value of these animal study results to human foetal development remains uncertain, the potential risks prompted regulatory agencies to recommend against the use of semaglutide during pregnancy [161, 408].

The mechanism of action of semaglutide—its ability to significantly suppress appetite and promote weight loss—could further complicate pregnancy. Adequate maternal weight gain is crucial for proper foetal development; hence, significant weight loss induced by semaglutide could adversely affect placental function and foetal growth. Regulatory reviews have highlighted that this strong appetite suppression is fundamentally incompatible with the nutritional needs associated with a healthy pregnancy [189, 408, 409].

Semaglutide's pharmacokinetics, characterized by a long half-life that allows for weekly dosing, results in the medication remaining in the body for an extended period even after the last dose—estimated to be around 5 to 7 weeks [138, 189]. Consequently, guidelines suggest that women planning a pregnancy should ideally discontinue semaglutide at least two months prior to conception. Should a pregnancy occur while on the medication, it is recommended to stop semaglutide immediately and seek medical evaluation to ensure the safety of both mother and foetus [161, 280, 408].

The available evidence underscores a strong rationale for avoiding semaglutide in pregnant women, based on its biological activity, pharmacological profile, and regulatory caution derived from animal studies, as well as the necessity for maternal nutritional adequacy during pregnancy.

Safety in Breastfeeding

The passage of medications, particularly those such as semaglutide, into human breast milk remains a critical area of inquiry for mothers managing chronic conditions such as diabetes during lactation. Semaglutide's transfer into breast milk is not well characterized in human studies. While animal research has demonstrated that semaglutide does appear in milk at low concentrations, the implications for human infants remain uncertain due to the absence of robust human data regarding its effects during breastfeeding [410].

Concerns regarding the potential impact of semaglutide on neonatal glucose regulation are significant. Adverse effects could arise from its pharmacological action, which suppresses appetite and modulates glucose metabolism, leading to potential repercussions for an infant's developing regulatory systems. Research indicates that GLP-1 receptor agonists may contribute to alterations in glucose homeostasis, which, if transferred via breastfeeding, could affect the infant's blood sugar levels adversely [410]. Furthermore, the long duration of action of semaglutide could exacerbate these risks, as the drug's metabolic effects may persist longer than its presence in milk can be monitored or controlled [410].

Another critical consideration is the impact of semaglutide on feeding patterns. Its effects on appetite regulation might lead to challenges in establishing regular feeding behaviours in infants. This could potentially interfere with both nutritional intake and overall infant growth and development. These concerns are compounded by evidence suggesting that alterations in breastfeeding experiences can influence not only immediate nutrition but also long-term health outcomes for children, including growth trajectories (Warden et al., 2025).

Due to the ambiguous safety profile of semaglutide during lactation, alternative treatments possessing established safety profiles are often recommended for postpartum glucose management. Medications such as metformin are noted for their relative safety during breastfeeding, along with lifestyle interventions aimed at weight management (Muller et al., 2023). These alternatives are preferable as they have been more extensively studied in lactating populations, providing a measure of reassurance to healthcare providers and nursing mothers alike regarding the health of both mother and infant [410].

> The limited evidence surrounding semaglutide's transfer into breast milk and its subsequent effects on breastfeeding infants underscores the necessity for cautious management and the exploration of safer alternative treatments for postpartum metabolic control.

Safety in Adolescents

Research on the use of semaglutide for managing obesity in adolescents has seen significant advancements. The STEP TEENS trial, which specifically targeted adolescents aged 12–17, demonstrated substantial weight loss and beneficial metabolic outcomes with the administration of semaglutide at a dosage of 2.4 mg weekly. These results were pivotal in leading to regulatory approvals for semaglutide, marketed as Wegovy, for adolescent obesity management in several countries, including the United States [276, 411].

However, the application of semaglutide in this age group necessitates careful clinical consideration due to several critical factors related to adolescent growth and development. Firstly, adolescents are still undergoing significant physical growth and developmental changes, which may influence their response to pharmacotherapy. Their increased nutritional demands must also be considered, as adequate nutrition is essential during this growth phase [412, 413].

Moreover, psychological considerations become paramount when prescribing weight management treatments in adolescents. Body image issues and vulnerabilities to eating disorders are pronounced during this stage, necessitating a comprehensive approach to treatment. The integration of psychological support within the treatment framework is critical for optimizing outcomes while minimizing potential adverse effects, such as exacerbation of body dissatisfaction or disordered eating patterns [413, 414].

Furthermore, the long-term effects of semaglutide on growth trajectories, puberty, and bone density in adolescents are still under investigation. Adolescents represent a unique demographic in this regard, transitioning through crucial periods of skeletal growth and hormonal changes that are essential for achieving peak bone mass [109, 415]. Clinicians are urged to monitor growth patterns closely to mitigate potential impacts on bone health, particularly since adolescence is characterized by an increased rate of bone remodelling and mineralization related to pubertal changes [416].

In practice, the administration of semaglutide is often combined with structured lifestyle interventions, including dietary adjustments and behavioural therapy, to promote holistic health and sustainable weight loss [71, 411, 417]. It is also notable that semaglutide is generally not recommended for children under the age of 12, underscoring the importance of age-appropriate treatment strategies [276, 411].

While the increasing body of research on semaglutide's efficacy in adolescents represents a significant advancement in obesity management, clinicians must adopt a multidisciplinary and cautious approach, factoring in the unique developmental and psychological challenges presented during this critical growth period.

Safety in Older Adults

Semaglutide, a glucagon-like peptide-1 receptor agonist, has demonstrated safe and effective outcomes for older adults, including those aged 65 and above, in managing obesity and diabetes. However, careful consideration is necessary in this population due to age-associated factors including reduced kidney function, altered gastric motility, and increased susceptibility to dehydration. Additionally, older adults often navigate issues related to polypharmacy and may present with frailty or reduced muscle mass, which heightens the risk for adverse effects of medications like semaglutide, as well as the appropriateness of its administration [418].

Concerns about renal function underscore the need for cautious dosing and monitoring. Research indicates that while semaglutide's safety profile is similar across various age groups, increased vigilance is necessary for older patients who inherently face higher risks of renal adverse events [418]. Moreover, there is growing evidence that older adults with type 2 diabetes may experience altered gastric emptying and motility, which can affect the drug's efficacy and pharmacokinetics. The appetite-suppressing effects of semaglutide can lead to unintended outcomes, such as excessive weight loss, sarcopenia, and nutritional deficiencies, highlighting the need for careful dose adjustment and slower titration in this vulnerable demographic [419, 420].

Excessive weight loss can result in further complications, particularly in frail older adults, where nutritional deficiencies and sarcopenia—characterized by the loss of muscle mass and strength—are prevalent. These conditions are associated with increased risks of falls and fractures, potentially compounded by dehydration often resulting from reduced caloric intake [420]. Regular monitoring of hydration, nutritional status, and body weight for those on semaglutide is therefore essential. Despite these challenges, appropriately managed semaglutide treatment has been linked to considerable improvements in glycaemic control and cardiovascular health, which can enhance overall quality of life for older adults [223, 282, 418].

Semaglutide's safety varies across special populations:

- **Pregnancy:** Not recommended; discontinue ≥2 months before conception.
- **Breastfeeding:** Avoid use due to insufficient safety data.
- **Adolescents:** Approved for obesity in ages 12–17 in some regions; requires careful monitoring.

- **Older Adults:** Generally safe but needs cautious titration and monitoring for dehydration, malnutrition, and muscle loss.

In all groups, decisions must be individualised, weighing benefits against risks and considering alternative therapies when needed.

Oral Contraceptive Pills and Semaglutide

Why Weight-Loss Drugs Are Linked to Unintended Pregnancies

Medications such as semaglutide (Wegovy/Ozempic) and tirzepatide (Mounjaro/Zepbound) have become increasingly popular as weight-loss treatments. However, growing reports of so-called *"Ozempic babies"*—unexpected pregnancies in women taking these medications—have prompted regulators like the UK's Medicines and Healthcare products Regulatory Agency (MHRA) to issue safety guidance for women of reproductive age [421]. These warnings follow at least 40 reports of unintended pregnancies among women using GLP-1–based weight-loss medications, raising concern that these drugs may interfere with the effectiveness of oral contraceptives [421].

Semaglutide and tirzepatide mimic gut hormones that regulate appetite (primarily GLP-1; tirzepatide also mimics GIP). These hormones reduce hunger by acting on brain regions involved in appetite regulation and by slowing the rate at which food leaves the stomach. This delayed gastric emptying is central to both their weight-loss effectiveness and their potential to interfere with the absorption of oral medications, including contraceptive pills [421].

Because oral contraceptives must be absorbed through the gastrointestinal tract—primarily in the small intestine—anything that delays or disrupts this process may reduce how much of the medication reaches the bloodstream. The slower a drug reaches the intestine, the later and sometimes the less effectively it is absorbed. This reduced or delayed absorption can weaken the pill's ability to suppress ovulation, thereby diminishing contraceptive reliability [421].

Research on GLP-1 medications and contraceptive interactions is still limited, but one 2024 study provides important insight. It showed that tirzepatide reduced blood levels of ethinylestradiol—a common synthetic estrogen used in combined oral contraceptives—by around 20%. It also delayed the full absorption of the hormone by two to four hours. Such reductions may compromise contraceptive efficacy [421].

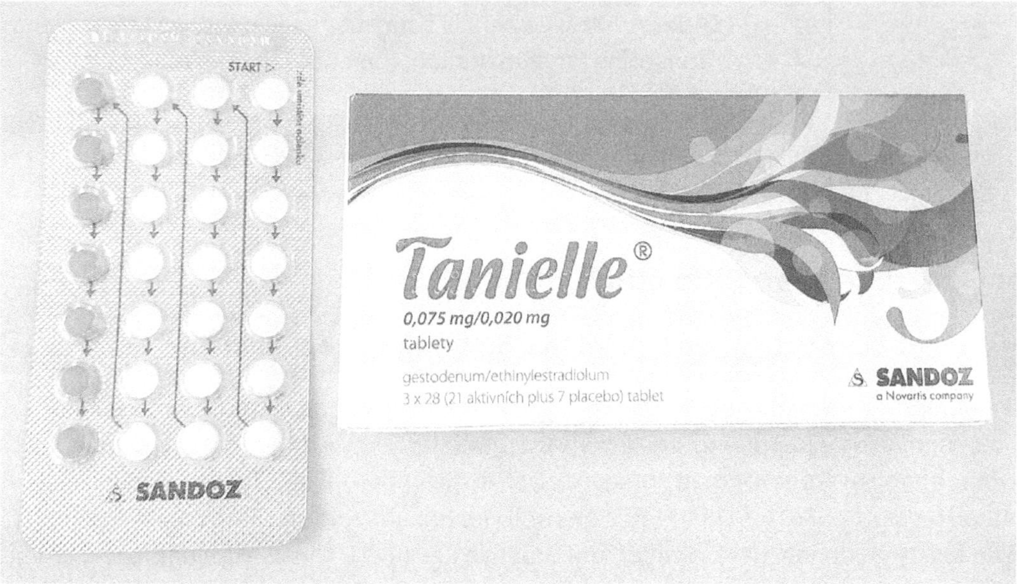

Figure 24: Tanielle is a combination birth control pill used to prevent pregnancy. Each tablet contains the hormones gestodene and ethinylestradiol, which work by preventing ovulation, thickening cervical mucus, and altering the uterine lining to stop pregnancy. The manufacturer is Sandoz, and this specific formulation may be marketed under various other brand names. Tomino de WS, CC BY-SA 4.0, via Wikimedia Commons.

Tanielle is a combination birth control pill used to prevent pregnancy. Each tablet contains the hormones gestodene and ethinylestradiol, which work by preventing ovulation, thickening cervical mucus, and altering the uterine lining to stop pregnancy. The manufacturer is Sandoz, and this specific formulation may be marketed under various other brand names. Tomino de WS, CC BY-SA 4.0, via Wikimedia Commons.

By contrast, semaglutide appeared to have a far smaller impact on ethinylestradiol absorption. The reason tirzepatide has a larger effect is not fully understood, but emerging evidence suggests that tirzepatide's influence on gastric emptying lasts longer and is more persistent than semaglutide's, leading to more pronounced changes in absorption of oral drugs [421].

Beyond delayed absorption, GLP-1 therapies—especially tirzepatide—frequently cause vomiting and diarrhoea during early treatment and dose escalations. Up to 12% of tirzepatide users experience vomiting, and 23% experience diarrhoea. These symptoms can physically expel oral medications before they are absorbed, rendering the contraceptive pill unreliable. For this reason, women taking oral contraceptives are routinely advised to use backup methods after episodes of severe vomiting or diarrhoea.

Another important factor is that weight loss—regardless of the method—can significantly improve fertility [421]. Obesity and conditions commonly associated with obesity, such as polycystic ovary syndrome (PCOS), often reduce ovulation frequency. When women lose weight using GLP-1 therapies, ovulation may resume or become more regular, increasing the likelihood of pregnancy, even when contraceptives are used correctly. This means not all unintended pregnancies in GLP-1 users are due to contraceptive failure—many result from restored fertility [421].

Current evidence suggests that only oral contraceptives are affected by GLP-1 induced changes in gastric emptying or gastrointestinal side effects [421]. Non-oral methods—such as hormonal IUDs, implants, vaginal rings, depot injections, and transdermal patches—bypass the digestive system entirely and are not impacted by GLP-1 medications. Barrier methods (such as condoms) and copper IUDs are also unaffected.

For women using the pill, additional precautions are recommended [421]:

- Use a backup non-oral method (e.g., condoms) for at least four weeks after initiating semaglutide or tirzepatide.
- Consider switching to a non-oral contraceptive if gastrointestinal side effects persist.

Because safety data on GLP-1 medications in pregnancy are extremely limited, regulators advise that women who become pregnant while using semaglutide or tirzepatide should stop the medication and consult their doctor immediately [421]. Alternative treatments will be needed, as GLP-1 therapies are not recommended during pregnancy.

Weight-loss drugs such as semaglutide and tirzepatide may increase the risk of unintended pregnancy because they:

- Delay absorption of oral contraceptives
- Reduce circulating estrogen levels (strongest effect with tirzepatide)
- Cause vomiting and diarrhoea, which disrupt medication absorption
- Improve fertility by reversing obesity-related ovulatory dysfunction

Women using oral contraceptives are therefore advised to take extra precautions during early treatment and consider non-oral contraceptive options.

Chapter 7

Semaglutide for Weight Loss: The Science and the Reality

Building on the foundations established in the previous chapters—particularly the biological, hormonal, and behavioural mechanisms that underpin obesity—this chapter expands the discussion by examining how these scientific concepts translate into real-world treatment options, decision-making, and long-term management. While earlier sections explored how semaglutide and other GLP-1 medications influence appetite regulation, metabolic health, and weight physiology, this chapter situates those effects within the broader landscape of obesity care, comparing pharmacological and surgical pathways, clarifying misconceptions, and addressing the practical realities faced by patients and clinicians alike.

Obesity is a complex, chronic disease with far-reaching health impacts, and its management requires approaches that go beyond lifestyle advice alone. Modern treatments—including semaglutide, tirzepatide, and bariatric surgery—each offer distinct mechanisms, benefits, and challenges. Yet public discourse often oversimplifies these therapies, portraying medications as "quick fixes" or surgery as a "last resort," and spreading confusion through myths, stigma, and media sensationalism. This chapter aims to correct these misconceptions by presenting an evidence-based comparison of available options and highlighting how treatment choices should align with the biology of obesity rather than outdated notions of willpower.

Readers will be guided through the scientific rationale behind GLP-1 therapy, the differences between pharmacological and surgical outcomes, and the importance of long-term maintenance in achieving durable weight loss. It also examines patient experience, safety considerations, and the role of clinicians in tailoring treatment, ensuring that obesity care is both compassionate and scientifically grounded. By understanding the realities behind these therapies, individuals and practitioners can make informed, realistic decisions that foster sustainable health improvements.

Obesity as a Chronic Disease Vs Lifestyle Problem

Obesity is increasingly recognised by major medical organisations as a chronic, relapsing, multifactorial disease, not simply the result of poor lifestyle choices. This distinction is critical because it shapes how obesity should be understood, treated, and sustained over time. Viewing obesity as a chronic disease aligns treatment with scientific evidence rather than outdated ideas about willpower or personal responsibility.

Obesity as a Chronic Disease

Obesity is increasingly recognized as a chronic disease influenced by a multifaceted interplay of biological, physiological, and environmental factors that extend beyond individual lifestyle choices. Recent literature supports the assertion that genetic predispositions, hormonal imbalances, metabolic dysfunctions, and gut microbiota contribute significantly to the development and persistence of obesity. Genetic factors account for a significant variance in obesity risk, with specific genes associated with appetite regulation, metabolism, and energy expenditure showing polymorphisms that increase susceptibility to obesity [422, 423]. Metabolic dysregulation, characterized by insulin resistance and chronic inflammation, exacerbates obesity and its related health complications, including type 2 diabetes and cardiovascular disease [424, 425].

Endocrine function plays a crucial role in obesity, particularly through hormones such as leptin, ghrelin, and insulin, which regulate appetite and energy balance. Evidence suggests that weight loss leads to hormonal changes and metabolic adaptations that defend a higher body weight set point, promoting hunger and reducing satiety signals, which contributes to weight regain [426-428]. This biological predisposition underscores the need for comprehensive and sustained treatment strategies rather than simplistic diet or lifestyle modifications, which often fail due to these physiological responses [429].

Dysregulation of appetite hormones is particularly important in understanding obesity's chronic nature. The compensatory mechanisms that arise post-weight loss often include elevated levels of ghrelin and decreased levels of leptin, leading to increased food intake and decreased energy expenditure [430, 431]. Consequently, the vast majority of individuals who lose weight experience some degree of weight regain, often within a year, due to these biological responses [426, 428]. Such patterns mimic conditions like hypertension or type 2 diabetes, illustrating the relapsing character of obesity as a chronic disease.

The ramifications of obesity extend well beyond aesthetic considerations; its association with numerous long-term health risks adds to the urgency of recognizing it as a chronic medical condition. As noted, obesity is linked to multiple serious health issues such as type 2 diabetes, non-alcoholic fatty liver disease (NAFLD), and cardiovascular conditions [424, 432]. Hence, acknowledging obesity's chronicity ensures that adequate resources and structured care are allocated within healthcare systems, shifting away from a solely behavioural perspective to one that considers the biological and environmental layers contributing to this complex condition.

Effective management of obesity thus requires lifelong interventions that encompass a blend of pharmacotherapy, dietary management, increased physical activity, and psychological support. Drugs such as semaglutide and tirzepatide exemplify advancements in pharmacological treatment, demonstrating the potential to counteract certain metabolic adaptations and support weight maintenance post-therapy [428, 429]. Additionally, behavioural modifications, alongside medical interventions, represent a holistic approach that targets the underlying biological mechanisms driving obesity and fosters sustainable outcomes [429].

Obesity should be understood as a chronic disease driven by a complex interaction of genetic, hormonal, and environmental factors. Recognizing its intricate nature and the body's resistance to weight loss is crucial in developing effective, long-term strategies for its management.

Obesity as a Lifestyle Problem (Traditional View)

The traditional view of obesity characterizes it predominantly as a lifestyle challenge, emphasizing personal choices like overeating and inactivity, and often implying that individuals simply require more willpower to attain a healthy weight. This oversimplified perspective neglects the multifactorial nature of obesity, which is influenced by an interplay of complex biological, hormonal, environmental, and psychological factors. For instance, it has been demonstrated that genetics significantly impact adiposity, challenging the notion that obesity is merely a function of personal discipline [433, 434]. Notably, environmental elements such as the "obesogenic environment"—comprising readily available, calorie-dense foods and sedentary lifestyles—further complicate the control individuals purportedly have over their weight [435, 436].

The biological factors associated with obesity are considerable. Research indicates that genetic predisposition, variations in metabolic rates, and hormonal imbalances all play pivotal roles in weight regulation [434, 437, 438]. For example, genetic variations, including those affecting the FTO gene, have been linked to dietary habits and obesity susceptibility, suggesting a biological underpinning to resistance against lifestyle changes [439]. Moreover, factors such as chronic stress and inadequate sleep can exacerbate weight gain, demonstrating that not all elements contributing to obesity are immediately modifiable through individual actions [434, 440, 441]. The distinction between the biological determinants of obesity and personal lifestyle choices thus becomes crucial for a more comprehensive understanding of the condition.

Moreover, this lifestyle-centric viewpoint perpetuates stigma and blame that can adversely affect the mental health of individuals struggling with obesity. When societal narratives attribute weight gain to personal failings, affected individuals may internalize shame, which, in turn, negatively influences their mental health and may lead to emotional eating or avoidance of seeking help [434, 442]. Reports highlight long-term weight management challenges that arise from this stigma, positing that individuals may not only feel isolated due to feelings of shame but also experience discrimination that further hampers their ability to engage in healthy behaviours [433, 434] . This aligns with findings that highlight the mental health implications of constant social judgment regarding body weight, which often lead to increased stress and negative self-image [442].

Finally, evidence suggests that a singular focus on lifestyle interventions, while important, often proves insufficient in yielding sustainable weight loss. For instance, lifestyle changes alone typically yield only minimal average weight loss—around 3-5%, with many regaining lost weight within a short time frame [442, 443]. Addressing the intrinsic biological mechanisms regulating hunger and metabolism is crucial for effective management of obesity [434, 438, 444]. As such, while personal responsibility is a component, addressing obesity demands a more nuanced strategy that considers both individual and systemic factors.

Reducing obesity to mere lifestyle choices is not only overly simplistic but also harmful, as it fails to recognize the complex interplay of biological, psychological, and social determinants of body weight. A comprehensive understanding of obesity necessitates an acknowledgment of these multifactorial influences to develop effective, compassionate public health strategies.

Why the Chronic Disease Model is Now Widely Accepted

Leading health organizations globally recognize obesity as a complex chronic disease, influenced by a multitude of biological, psychological, and social factors. The World Health Organization (WHO), along with the American Medical Association (AMA), the Australian and New Zealand Obesity Society, the Canadian Obesity Network, and the European Association for the Study of Obesity, formalized this definition based on compelling evidence underscoring the chronic nature of obesity.

A pivotal aspect of this classification stems from the understanding of body weight regulation, particularly the role of biological factors. Research suggests that obesity is not merely a result of lifestyle choices; rather, it is characterized by genetic, metabolic, and physiological processes that affect body weight regulation [445]. Studies highlight that individuals can face intrinsic biological predispositions that perpetuate weight gain and impede weight loss, aligning with findings that emphasize the chronicity of this condition, as demonstrated by high rates of recurrence post-weight loss interventions [446].

Furthermore, the significant morbidity and mortality associated with excess adiposity reinforce the urgency of addressing obesity as a chronic disease. Obesity is linked to a myriad of health complications, including cardiovascular diseases, type 2 diabetes, and certain cancers, contributing to lower quality of life and increased healthcare costs [446]. The chronicity of the disease model is supported by previously established associations between obesity and poor physical and emotional well-being, particularly among individuals with additional chronic illnesses [447].

Long-term medical interventions have shown improved outcomes for individuals managing obesity, particularly with pharmacological treatments like semaglutide, which target the biological underpinnings of the disease. Clinical trials have demonstrated that continued use of semaglutide significantly enhances weight loss maintenance, pointing to its effectiveness in the long-term management of obesity as a chronic condition [103]. This pharmacotherapy paradigm suggests that, similar to other chronic diseases, obesity may require lifelong management strategies rather than a singular focus on weight loss.

Additionally, redefining obesity as a chronic disease serves to reduce societal stigma, promoting a more compassionate approach to treatment akin to those for chronic illnesses such as hypertension or diabetes. Studies indicate that acknowledgment of obesity as a medical condition encourages both patients and healthcare providers to engage more effectively in treatment pathways, ultimately fostering a supportive environment conducive to long-term success [448, 449].

The concerted efforts of major health organizations to classify obesity as a chronic disease align with strong scientific evidence highlighting the biological regulation of body weight, the recurrence rates after weight loss, and the substantial health risks associated with obesity. These developments, combined with emerging treatment options, establish a robust framework for addressing obesity as a long-lasting health challenge requiring comprehensive medical management.

Obesity is not simply a reflection of personal choice or willpower; it is a chronic, biologically mediated disease requiring long-term, structured management. While lifestyle factors matter, they interact with powerful physiological systems that regulate hunger, satiety, metabolism, and fat storage. Recognising obesity as a chronic disease leads to:

- better care
- improved long-term outcomes
- reduced stigma
- greater access to effective treatments

This shift in understanding is fundamental to modern obesity management and underpins the use of therapies like semaglutide.

Appetite Regulation Science (Set Point Theory, Gut–Brain Axis)

Appetite regulation is governed by a highly complex biological system that involves the brain, gut, hormones, and metabolism working together to maintain body weight within a relatively stable range. Modern science shows that body weight is not simply a matter of willpower—our biology powerfully shapes hunger, satiety, cravings, and energy expenditure. Two major concepts help explain this: set point theory and the gut–brain axis.

Set Point Theory: The Body's Weight-Regulating System

Set point theory posits that individuals have a biologically determined weight range that their body actively defends, akin to homeostatic regulation of certain physiological parameters such as temperature or blood pressure. This weight range is known as the "set point" or "settling point" and reflects a form of energy homeostasis where physiological mechanisms play a crucial role in maintaining body weight. When body weight deviates from this set point, various hormonal changes occur, notably involving appetite-regulating hormones such as ghrelin, leptin, GLP-1, and PYY.

Ghrelin

Ghrelin is the body's primary *hunger hormone*. It is mainly produced in the stomach and rises before meals to stimulate appetite. When ghrelin levels increase, the brain receives a signal that the body needs food, triggering hunger and food-seeking behaviour.

Key points:

- Produced in the stomach (especially the fundus).
- Levels rise when the stomach is empty.
- Signals the hypothalamus to increase hunger.
- Falls after eating.
- Often elevated during dieting or weight loss—contributing to rebound weight gain.

Leptin

Leptin is the body's long-term *satiety (fullness) hormone*. It is produced by fat cells and tells the brain that sufficient energy is stored in the body.
Higher fat stores → higher leptin levels.
However, many people with overweight or obesity develop leptin resistance, where the brain no longer responds properly to leptin signals. This leads to increased hunger and reduced energy expenditure, despite high leptin levels.

Key points:

- Produced by adipose (fat) tissue.
- Signals long-term energy sufficiency.
- High levels should reduce appetite—but leptin resistance is common in obesity.
- Critical regulator of body weight and metabolism.

GLP-1 (Glucagon-Like Peptide-1)

GLP-1 is a gut hormone released after eating that promotes fullness, stabilises blood glucose, and slows stomach emptying. It also works directly on the brain to reduce appetite and cravings. Semaglutide and other GLP-1 receptor agonists mimic this hormone.

Key points:

- Produced in the small intestine.
- Increases satiety and reduces appetite.
- Slows gastric emptying → makes meals feel more filling.
- Enhances insulin secretion and lowers blood glucose.
- Therapeutically replicated by drugs like semaglutide and tirzepatide.

PYY (Peptide YY)

PYY is a gut hormone released from the lower small intestine and colon after eating, especially in response to protein and fibre. It signals fullness and helps regulate appetite between meals.
Key points:

- Released from the ileum and colon.
- Suppresses appetite and reduces gastric motility.
- Peaks about 1–2 hours after eating.
- Works with GLP-1 to enhance satiety.
- Often lower in individuals with obesity, contributing to overeating.

The set-point theory posits that the body maintains weight around a predetermined level, primarily regulated by mechanisms within the brain. This concept was notably articulated by William Bennett and Joel Gurin in 1982, who aimed to elucidate why many individuals struggle with long-term weight loss, as efforts to reduce body weight often lead to physiological and psychological responses that counteract these efforts [450].

In the context of weight loss, the body's response is multifaceted. The level of ghrelin, a hormone that stimulates appetite, typically increases, leading to heightened hunger and a compelling drive to regain lost weight [451]. Concurrently, the levels of satiety hormones like leptin and GLP-1 decrease, diminishing feelings of fullness from meals [452]. Research indicates that the drop in leptin levels after weight loss leads to reduced satiety, exacerbating the challenge of maintaining a lower weight [453, 454]. Metabolic adaptations also play a critical role; studies show that resting energy expenditure decreases, resulting in fewer calories being burned at rest, a phenomenon often termed "metabolic slowdown" [455]. Additionally, energy efficiency appears to increase post-weight loss, making the body more proficient at storing energy [456]. Collectively, these responses pose significant challenges for individuals attempting to sustain long-term weight loss, as they can persist for years, making lifestyle changes less effective on their own [457].

Over time, modern living conditions may promote an increase in set point levels. Factors contributing to this increase include the consumption of highly processed foods, which can lead to greater energy intake, chronic stress that can influence hormonal balances, insufficient sleep disrupting hormonal regulation, and exposure to endocrine-disrupting chemicals [458]. Genetic predispositions and the phenomenon of "weight cycling," where individuals repeatedly lose and regain weight, can also elevate the defended set point over time, complicating weight management efforts [459, 460].

In this context, medications such as semaglutide, which target the GLP-1 pathway, have been shown to aid in significantly reducing the set point by effectively lowering appetite and enhancing satiety [461]. Such pharmacological interventions may facilitate weight loss by mitigating the biological counter-responses associated with weight reduction, thereby providing a more manageable pathway toward sustainable weight loss [462].

Set point theory provides a biological and physiological framework for understanding weight regulation, highlighting both the body's protective mechanisms against weight loss and the environmental factors that may elevate these thresholds. This understanding underscores the complexity of weight management and the need for comprehensive approaches, integrating both behavioural and medical strategies, to facilitate long-term success in weight loss interventions.

The Gut–Brain Axis: How the Gut Talks to the Brain

The gut–brain axis serves as a sophisticated communication network linking the gastrointestinal tract with the brain. This intricate system involves neural, hormonal, and immune pathways that are essential for the regulation of appetite, satiety, mood, and energy balance. Hormonal signals transmitted from the gut play a pivotal role in appetite regulation, mediating sensations of hunger and fullness. Key gut hormones, including glucagon-like peptide-1 (GLP-1), peptide YY (PYY), and cholecystokinin (CCK), communicate satiety signals to the brain, while ghrelin functions as a hunger hormone, typically rising before meals and declining post-consumption [463, 464].

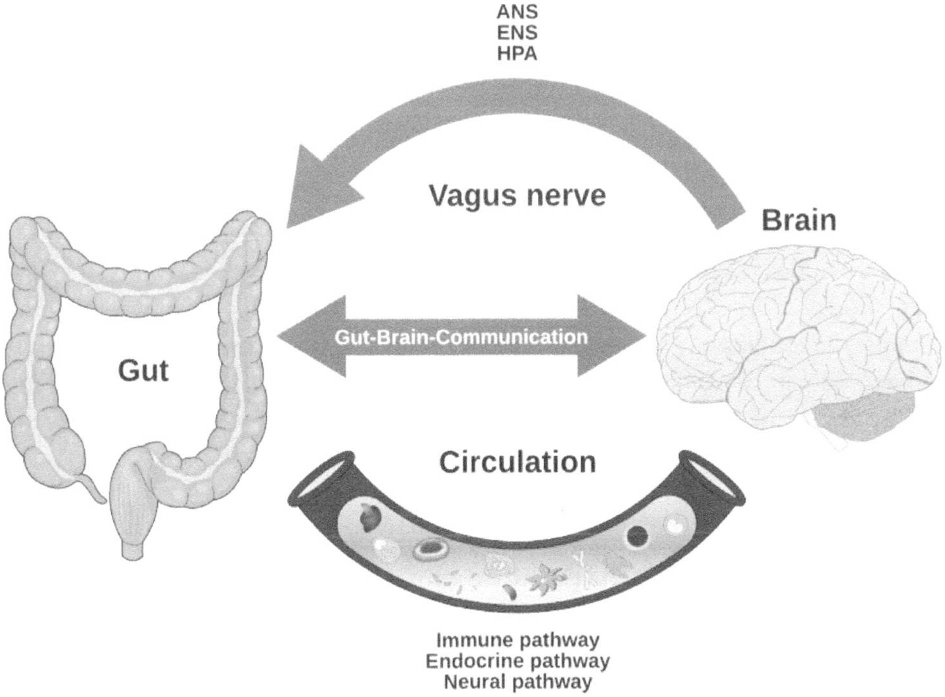

Figure 25: Schematic diagram showing the communication between the gut and brain. This is a bidirectional relationship that is strongly influenced by multiple pathways, including the autonomic nervous system (ANS), enteric nervous system (ENS), hypothalamic–pituitary–adrenal (HPA), immune pathways, endocrine pathways, and neural pathways. Suganya, Kanmani, and Byung-Soo KooThinkpinsMister PommeroyVectorization: Mrmw, CC BY-SA 4.0, via Wikimedia Commons.

Research indicates that the communication between the gut and central nervous system is dynamic, with continuous signals exchanged to modulate food intake and metabolic processes [465, 466]. This signalling is crucial in maintaining energy homeostasis, where the hypothalamus integrates sensory information regarding appetite and satiety. Activation of neurons in the hypothalamus by satiety hormones like GLP-1 has been demonstrated to suppress appetite and promote energy balance [463, 467]. Notably, obesity can disrupt the normal patterns of these hormonal signals, leading to reduced sensitivity to satiety, which intensifies feelings of hunger and increases the risk of overeating [468, 469].

The vagus nerve is another essential component of the gut-brain axis, acting as a communication highway that conveys information from the gastrointestinal tract to the brain regarding the status of food intake, nutrient content, and digestive activity. This neural pathway has been shown to facilitate the effect of gut hormones on the brain, and its appropriate functioning is critical for the regulation of energy balance [467, 470]. For instance, activation of vagal pathways can enhance the effects of GLP-1 signalling in the brain, further contributing to appetite regulation [471].

Furthermore, gut microbiota—the myriad of microorganisms residing in the intestines—plays a significant role in influencing appetite and metabolic processes through the gut-brain axis. Dysbiosis, an imbalance in the gut microbial community, can lead to alterations in gut hormone secretion, impacting appetite regulation and contributing to obesity and insulin resistance [472, 473]. This interaction emphasizes the importance of a healthy microbiota in maintaining metabolic health and a balanced appetite, as specific microbial populations are linked with increased production of satiety hormones and reduced hunger sensations [474].

Semaglutide, a GLP-1 receptor agonist, exemplifies the therapeutic potential of targeting the gut-brain axis for appetite regulation and weight management. By mimicking the effects of GLP-1, semaglutide enhances feelings of fullness, reduces hunger, and promotes increased satiety even with smaller food portions. This action is mediated through strengthened communications within the gut-brain axis, leading to improved appetite regulation, reduced cravings, and diminished reward-driven eating behaviours [33, 475]. Studies suggest that ongoing treatment with semaglutide can recalibrate the dysregulated appetite signals seen in obesity, ultimately supporting long-term weight control and metabolic health [476, 477].

Why Understanding Appetite Regulation Matters

Recognising that hunger, appetite, and weight are biologically regulated changes how obesity is treated:

- It removes the stigma associated with “lack of willpower.”
- It explains why diets alone fail for most people.
- It supports long-term, medical approaches to chronic weight management.

- It highlights the powerful role of medications like semaglutide in correcting underlying biology.

> Appetite regulation is a sophisticated biological system governed by set point mechanisms and gut–brain signalling. Obesity arises when this system becomes dysregulated, causing persistent hunger, reduced satiety, stronger cravings, and a higher defended body weight. Understanding these mechanisms shows why obesity is a chronic disease—not a lifestyle failure—and why therapies that target these pathways, such as semaglutide, are so effective in restoring healthy appetite control.

Why GLP-1 Medications Work When Diets Often Fail

GLP-1 medications, such as semaglutide, provide a novel and potentially more effective approach to weight management compared to traditional dieting methods. Traditional dieting primarily relies on willpower and behavioural changes; however, the biological framework of obesity involves complex physiological processes that significantly hinder sustained weight loss [32]. Research indicates that GLP-1 therapies act on the central nervous system and various hormonal pathways involved in appetite regulation, hunger suppression, and energy metabolism [478]. For example, a clinical study demonstrated that semaglutide significantly reduces self-reported hunger and food cravings, leading to a decrease in overall energy intake during meal times [31]. This ability to influence biological processes provides a more sustainable approach to weight management, as it helps individuals overcome their body's natural defences against weight regain [479].

The mechanisms by which GLP-1 medications facilitate weight loss are diverse and target multiple factors driving obesity. One critical adaptation observed in individuals attempting weight loss through dieting is the body's response to perceived starvation, which includes an increase in hunger hormones like ghrelin and a decrease in satiety signals, such as GLP-1 and leptin [480]. This hormonal imbalance, coupled with a slowed metabolism and intensified cravings, creates a significant barrier to achieving lasting weight loss [480]. Semaglutide counteracts these mechanisms by restoring satiety signals and reducing hunger through its action on GLP-1 receptors in the hypothalamus and other brain regions, leading to improved appetite regulation [478]. Furthermore, GLP-1 medications have been shown to reduce gastric emptying, contributing to prolonged feelings of fullness [31].

Additionally, GLP-1 treatments reduce the body's "set point," a term that describes the weight range that the body biologically defends against deviations [32]. Research indicates that treatment with semaglutide leads to reductions in visceral fat and improvements in insulin sensitivity, which collectively support the maintenance of a lower body weight [105]. The normalization of appetite regulation through GLP-1 therapies helps stabilize metabolic processes that might otherwise promote weight regain following diet-induced weight loss [481]. Clinical trials have demonstrated that semaglutide can achieve weight loss percentages of around 15%

or more in many participants, which exceeds the typical results associated with conventional dieting, often resulting only in 3-5% weight loss that is frequently regained [479, 482].

Additionally, the benefits of GLP-1 medications extend beyond weight loss, addressing chronic conditions commonly associated with obesity. For instance, they improve insulin sensitivity and lower systemic inflammation markers, addressing underlying metabolic dysfunction often seen in individuals with overweight and obesity [105, 483]. Traditional diets alone often neglect these aspects, leaving individuals without the metabolic advantages conferred by GLP-1 treatments [482]. Evidence suggests that GLP-1 therapies also reduce emotional and reward-driven eating by acting on neural pathways, which helps mitigate compulsive eating behaviours [484].

GLP-1 medications like semaglutide represent a shift in obesity treatment by addressing the biological and hormonal underpinnings of weight management. Unlike traditional dieting, which often emphasizes willpower and behavioural change, GLP-1 therapies focus on restoring hormonal balance and supporting metabolic efficiency, ultimately leading to sustainable weight loss and improved metabolic health. This comprehensive approach recognizes obesity as a chronic disease requiring interventions that manage its intrinsic biological drivers, underscoring the limitations of dietary-only strategies in achieving lasting success.

Comparing Semaglutide to Bariatric Surgery Outcomes

Semaglutide and bariatric surgery both produce far more weight loss than lifestyle change alone, but they do so in very different ways and with different magnitudes, risks, and long-term implications. Thinking of them as "either/or" options can be misleading – they sit on a spectrum of obesity treatments, from least to most intensive.

Typical Weight-Loss Outcomes

The weight-loss outcomes associated with the use of semaglutide (2.4 mg weekly, marketed as Wegovy) and bariatric surgery demonstrate contrasting approaches and results, with both modalities providing significant benefits for individuals struggling with obesity.

In the context of semaglutide, recent evidence from the STEP trials, particularly STEP 1 and STEP 5, indicates that participants can achieve an average weight loss of approximately 15% of their initial body weight after 68 weeks of treatment, with many individuals experiencing weight reductions in the range of 15–20% and some exceeding 20% [154, 205]. Specifically, during the STEP 1 trial, a notable mean reduction was reported at 15.2% for patients without diabetes, highlighting the efficacy of semaglutide in this population [205]. Furthermore, the weight loss occurs gradually over 6 to 12 months, with a plateau typically reached around one year; however, this weight loss is maintained only as long as the treatment continues, as evidenced by studies showing participants regaining approximately two-thirds of their lost weight upon discontinuation of the medication [109].

Conversely, bariatric surgery, including procedures such as sleeve gastrectomy and Roux-en-Y gastric bypass, typically results in superior weight loss outcomes. Sleeve gastrectomy generally leads to a 50–60% excess weight loss, translating to approximately 25–30% of total body weight lost [485]. Roux-en-Y gastric bypass is associated with even greater excess weight loss, achieving 60–70%, equivalent to around 25–35% of total body weight [485].

Sleeve Gastrectomy (Vertical Sleeve Gastrectomy – VSG)

Sleeve gastrectomy is a bariatric (weight-loss) surgery in which approximately 70–80% of the stomach is surgically removed, leaving a narrow, tube-shaped “sleeve.” The remaining stomach holds far less food and produces fewer hunger hormones—especially ghrelin, which is mainly made in the part of the stomach that is removed.

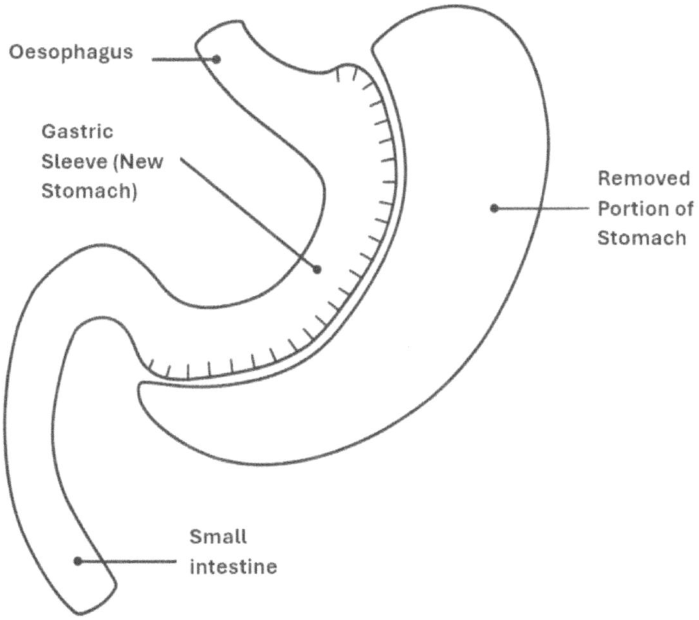

Figure 26: Gastric sleeve surgery.

How it works:

- Restrictive: the smaller stomach limits food intake.
- Hormonal: reduction in ghrelin lowers appetite and helps regulate hunger.
- Metabolic: improves insulin sensitivity and reduces liver fat.

Key features:

- Does not involve rerouting the intestines.
- Generally simpler and lower-risk than gastric bypass.
- Produces ~25–30% total body-weight loss on average.
- Permanent, non-reversible procedure.

Roux-en-Y Gastric Bypass (RYGB)

Roux-en-Y gastric bypass is a more complex bariatric surgery that changes both the stomach size and the digestive pathway. Surgeons create a small stomach pouch (about the size of an egg) and connect it directly to the small intestine, bypassing the majority of the stomach and the first segment of the small bowel (duodenum).

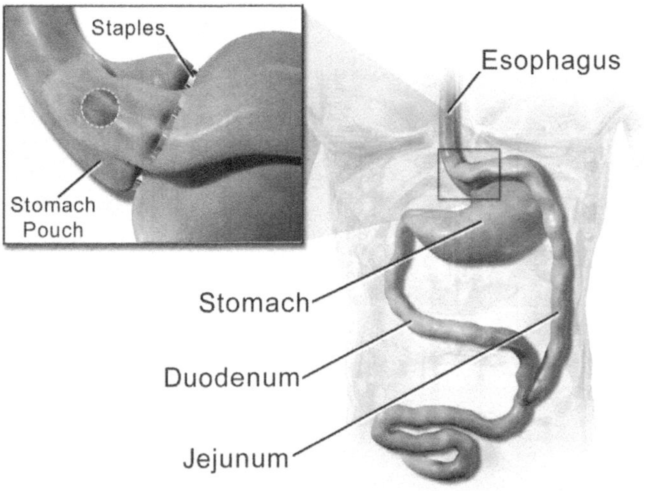

Figure 27: Roux-en-Y Gastric Bypass. Blausen.com staff (2014). "Medical gallery of Blausen Medical 2014". WikiJournal of Medicine 1 (2). DOI:10.15347/wjm/2014.010. ISSN 2002-4436., CC BY 3.0, via Wikimedia Commons.

How it works:

- Restrictive: small pouch dramatically limits meal size.
- Malabsorptive: bypassing part of the intestine reduces calorie and nutrient absorption.

- Hormonal: powerful changes in gut hormones (GLP-1, PYY, others) reduce hunger and improve glucose metabolism.

Key features:

- Produces ~25–35% total body-weight loss, often greater than sleeve gastrectomy.
- Has the strongest evidence for type 2 diabetes remission.
- Requires lifelong nutrient supplementation (B12, iron, calcium, vitamin D, etc.).
- Higher surgical complexity and risk than sleeve gastrectomy.
- Generally not reversible.

These surgical interventions yield the fastest weight loss within the first 6 to 12 months, with long-term studies indicating that many patients are able to maintain 20–30% of their total body weight loss even a decade after surgery [486].

When comparing the two treatment modalities, semaglutide can approach the lower-end surgical results for high responders, indicating that its pharmacological approach provides a viable alternative for weight management, especially among individuals who may not qualify for or prefer to avoid surgery [103]. However, on average, bariatric surgery remains the more effective long-term solution for significant weight loss, providing greater and more sustained results over time when considering the cumulative data from clinical outcomes [109, 485].

While semaglutide represents a promising pharmacological option for weight loss, particularly in terms of accessibility and ease of use, surgical interventions continue to demonstrate more substantial and durable weight loss outcomes for patients struggling with obesity.

Durability of Results

The durability of results from medical interventions for weight management is a significant consideration, notably in the context of semaglutide and bariatric surgery. Semaglutide, a GLP-1 receptor agonist, has shown considerable promise in achieving weight loss; however, the sustainability of this weight loss raises important questions about the long-term implications of its use.

Studies indicate that semaglutide's effect on weight loss is contingent upon continuous use. When semaglutide treatment is discontinued, individuals commonly experience weight regain, with studies showing that many regain a substantial portion of their lost weight within a year if no additional interventions are implemented [103, 105, 154]. This underscores the notion that semaglutide should be viewed as a long-term therapeutic option, similar to chronic medications for conditions such as hypertension or hyperlipidaemia [84, 118]. Specifically, research indicates substantial variability in long-term weight maintenance, indicating a need for further insights into the mechanisms by which semaglutide fosters weight loss and mitigates regain following discontinuation [223, 487].

Comparatively, bariatric surgery presents a fundamentally different approach, leading to permanent physiological alterations in the gastrointestinal tract that influence hormone levels and satiety. While some weight regain occurs within two to five years post-surgery, patients generally maintain a significant net loss from their baseline weight [105, 488, 489]. The advantages of surgery extend beyond weight loss; long-term metabolic benefits such as improved glycaemic control and reductions in the risk of hypertension and mortality tend to persist despite some degree of weight regain [487, 490]. This contrasts with semaglutide, where the absence of treatment often leads to gradual weight regain and potential returns to pre-treatment metabolic states [84, 154, 491].

While both semaglutide and bariatric surgery effectively facilitate weight loss, the durability of these results differs markedly. Semaglutide requires ongoing use to maintain its effects and minimize weight regain, reinforcing its classification as a chronic therapy. In contrast, bariatric surgery tends to result in lasting physiological changes that can provide enduring benefits even if some weight is regained after the initial loss. Therefore, the choice between these two modalities should take into account the patient's long-term management preferences and the potential need for continuous treatment with pharmacotherapy.

Effects on Type 2 Diabetes and Metabolic Health

Semaglutide, a glucagon-like peptide-1 (GLP-1) receptor agonist, has been shown to significantly impact the management of type 2 diabetes and metabolic health. Clinical studies indicate that semaglutide can achieve reductions in glycated haemoglobin (HbA1c) ranging from approximately 1.0% to 2.0%, with many patients successfully reaching guideline glycaemic targets [72, 492]. Furthermore, a meta-analysis suggests that patients utilizing semaglutide often experience substantial weight loss alongside these improvements in glycaemic control, which is particularly pronounced in those with a recent diagnosis of diabetes [80]. Although some patients may achieve diabetes remission, resulting in normal glycemia without the use of additional medications, the extent and sustainability of such remission can vary [72, 492].

Beyond glycaemic control, semaglutide has been associated with improvements in various cardiometabolic parameters. Studies have demonstrated reductions in blood pressure, triglycerides, low-density lipoprotein (LDL) cholesterol levels, and liver fat, addressing critical features associated with non-alcoholic fatty liver disease (NAFLD) [274, 492]. Additionally, its effects extend to reducing systemic inflammation and cardiovascular risk markers, showcasing its multifaceted role in managing type 2 diabetes [99].

Conversely, bariatric surgery remains a pivotal intervention in the context of diabetes management. Its effectiveness in inducing diabetes remission is substantial, with remission rates reported between 40% and 80%, highly variable depending on characteristics such as surgical procedure type, patient demographics, and disease duration [493, 494]. Surgical interventions not only often provide enduring remission of type 2 diabetes but are also associated with lower long-term mortality and reduced risk of cardiovascular events, renal disease, fatty liver disease progression, and certain cancers [495, 496]. While the beneficial effects of bariatric surgery can be lasting, some patients may experience relapse years later, often correlated with weight regain [494].

> Both semaglutide and bariatric surgery have demonstrated profound impacts on cardiometabolic health in individuals with type 2 diabetes. While semaglutide offers significant medical benefits without the need for surgical intervention, particularly in risk reduction of cardiovascular events and improvements in metabolic health, bariatric surgery currently holds the most robust evidence for long-term diabetes remission. This comparative efficacy highlights the importance of individualized approaches to diabetes management, integrating pharmacological and surgical options as appropriate for specific patient contexts.

Risks, Side Effects, and Recovery

Semaglutide, a glucagon-like peptide-1 receptor agonist, has gained popularity in the treatment of obesity and type 2 diabetes due to its efficacy in weight loss and glycaemic control. However, it is essential to recognize both the common side effects associated with its use and the serious risks that may arise under certain conditions.

Common Side Effects

The gastrointestinal (GI) side effects of semaglutide are well-documented and include nausea, vomiting, diarrhea, constipation, abdominal discomfort, and bloating. These adverse events are often dose-dependent and may be mitigated through gradual dose escalation and dietary modifications during treatment initiation. For instance, clinical trials have consistently reported that these GI events are the most commonly observed adverse occurrences, notably in participants receiving semaglutide compared to placebo [32, 40, 497]. Additionally, a systematic review indicated that gastrointestinal disorders were also the leading side effects in long-term studies involving semaglutide for weight management [417].

Serious Risks

While semaglutide is generally well-tolerated, some serious but less frequent risks are associated with its use. These include potential cases of pancreatitis, gallbladder disease, and renal impairment due to dehydration, exacerbated by the GI side effects that may lead to decreased fluid intake. The evidence suggests that individuals using GLP-1 receptor agonists like semaglutide may be at an increased risk for gallbladder-related diseases [498] and pancreatitis [499]. Furthermore, there is a theoretical risk of thyroid tumours in individuals with specific genetic predispositions, a concern noted in studies involving GLP-1 receptor agonists [500]. Importantly, no significant aesthetic risks or surgical complications are explicitly associated with semaglutide use, differentiating it from surgical interventions for obesity [501].

Bariatric Surgery Considerations

Contrasting with semaglutide, bariatric surgery (such as gastric bypass) carries more substantial immediate risks and recovery considerations. Short-term risks of surgery include bleeding, infection, and anastomotic leaks, with potential complications such as blood clots and anaesthesia-related issues [502]. Long-term risks involve nutrient deficiencies (e.g., iron, vitamin B12, calcium), dumping syndrome, reflux, bowel obstructions, and hernias—conditions that necessitate continuous monitoring and potentially further surgical interventions. Recovery from bariatric surgery can be lengthy and requires patients to engage in lifelong nutritional supplementation [501]. Thus, while surgery may be more effective for some individuals in achieving substantial weight loss, it comes with higher initial risks compared to the non-invasive nature of a pharmacological approach with semaglutide.

Risk Trade-offs

When comparing the two treatment options, it becomes evident that while surgical procedures entail a higher upfront risk, they eliminate the need for ongoing medication and the associated costs of injectable treatments. Conversely, semaglutide's procedural risk profile is lower; however, it requires long-term commitment to daily management and side effect monitoring, adding another layer of complexity to patient management over time [501]. Clinical decision-making should weigh these factors based on individual patient circumstances, preferences, and tolerance for risk.

Both semaglutide and bariatric surgery present unique benefits and challenges. By understanding the side effects and risks associated with these interventions, patients and healthcare providers can better manage expectations and treatment outcomes.

Reversibility and Flexibility

Semaglutide, a glucagon-like peptide-1 (GLP-1) receptor agonist, has gained significant attention in the treatment of obesity due to its unique combination of reversibility and flexibility in administration. Unlike bariatric surgery, which permanently alters stomach anatomy, semaglutide's treatment is fully reversible; patients can cease or adjust their dosages based on response and side effects. Studies show that during the Semaglutide Treatment Effect in People with Obesity (STEP) trials, gradual dose titration is feasible, allowing healthcare providers to tailor treatment effectively over time to meet individual health goals [32, 84, 233].

In clinical trials, semaglutide has demonstrated significant weight loss among participants, with an average reduction of approximately 14.9% body weight over 68 weeks [32, 103, 109]. However, upon discontinuation, patients often experience weight regain, emphasizing the importance of ongoing lifestyle interventions alongside pharmacotherapy [109]. This contrasts starkly with bariatric surgery, which is generally irreversible and comes with inherent risks associated with surgical interventions. While surgery may result in significant weight loss without reliance on medication adherence, the anatomical changes are permanent, and any revisions are complex and fraught with additional risks [88].

Moreover, the flexibility of semaglutide allows for combined therapies, wherein it can be administered alongside other antidiabetic medications or lifestyle interventions to maximize weight loss and improve overall health outcomes [84, 503]. For example, combination therapy with agents like cagrilintide alongside semaglutide has shown potential for further augmenting weight loss [33]. This adaptable dosage and regimen set semaglutide apart from bariatric interventions, which do not offer similar opportunities for adjustment based on individual patient responses.

Cagrilintide, an investigational medication developed by Novo Nordisk, is designed for weight management and belongs to the class of amylin analogues. These hormone-based drugs mimic the action of amylin, a naturally occurring peptide that is co-secreted alongside insulin from pancreatic β-cells. Both preclinical and clinical research demonstrates that cagrilintide holds significant promise in enhancing satiety, reducing cravings, slowing gastric emptying, and ultimately contributing to weight management solutions, especially in combination with GLP-1 receptor agonists such as semaglutide [33, 503].

Cagrilintide is engineered to be a long-acting agent, extending the action of amylin in the body compared to its natural, short-lived counterpart. The therapeutic mechanism of cagrilintide involves targeting amylin receptors in both the brain and gastrointestinal tract. This dual engagement significantly contributes to feelings of fullness and regulates appetite and glucose metabolic pathways, making it a potent adjunct to existing GLP-1 therapies [503, 504]. Clinical studies, particularly a phase 1B trial, demonstrated that when paired with semaglutide, cagrilintide can lead to a more substantial weight loss effect—up to an additional 7.4% in body weight for those already on semaglutide, resulting in a total loss of approximately 17.1% [33, 503, 504].

The combination of cagrilintide with semaglutide, termed CagriSema, is particularly noteworthy. Preliminary research indicates that patients receiving this combination therapy can experience weight losses exceeding 25%, with some individuals achieving reductions of 30% or more, comparable to outcomes from bariatric surgery [505, 506]. CagriSema integrates the appetite suppression and gastric motility benefits of both agents, leading to normalized eating behaviours and improved glycemic control in patients with obesity and type 2 diabetes [506]. Early phase trials have shown promising data, highlighting the potential of CagriSema as one of the leading non-surgical obesity treatments currently under investigation [503, 506].

In terms of safety, the adverse effects associated with cagrilintide are generally similar to those observed with GLP-1 analogues, primarily involving gastrointestinal symptoms like nausea and vomiting, which are often dose-dependent [33, 507]. These side effects tend to improve with careful titration of the dose, with no major safety concerns reported so far, although additional long-term studies are in progress to fully assess the medication's safety profile [33, 507].

The development of cagrilintide—and especially its combination therapy with semaglutide—has significant implications for the management of obesity, particularly in patients who do not adequately respond to existing GLP-1 treatments or those requiring more profound weight loss interventions [503, 506]. Given that cagrilintide targets a different hormonal pathway than other obesity therapeutics, it is particularly suited for patients with severe obesity or those exhibiting hedonic eating behaviours [506]. Overall, cagrilintide represents a promising advancement in the field of obesity treatment, particularly when combined with other therapeutic agents like semaglutide.

Semaglutide represents a comprehensive and adaptable approach to obesity management, providing the ability to tailor dosing and treatment duration based on patient needs and responses while also allowing for the potential to cease treatment if necessary. The inherent reversibility of the treatment stands in stark contrast to the rigid permanency associated with bariatric surgery, promoting a broader accessibility for various patient populations.

Patient Experience and Practical Considerations

Semaglutide: Overview and Patient Considerations

Administered either as a weekly injection or in a lower-dose oral tablet format, semaglutide provides patients with flexible dosing options [409, 508]. The need for hospital admissions or general anaesthetics is eliminated, making it a less invasive alternative to bariatric surgery. Furthermore, the absence of hospital stays can reduce the emotional and logistical burdens associated with surgical options [52, 409].

As with most medications, semaglutide does have a profile of potential side effects, primarily gastrointestinal (GI) in nature. These adverse effects are often pronounced during the initial titration phase once treatment begins [20, 154]. It is critical for clinicians to monitor tolerability closely, as rapid dose escalations can exacerbate these effects, potentially leading to complications like gastroparesis [225]. The side effects can deter patients, thus emphasizing the necessity for proper patient education to aid in managing expectations and compliance [20, 509].

Access to semaglutide poses a significant challenge, primarily due to cost considerations. In many countries, the medication is not universally covered by health insurance plans, which may result in substantial out-of-pocket expenses for patients [509]. The practical implications of these factors can impact the accessibility of semaglutide therapy for various populations, especially those with mild to moderate obesity or individuals who may be ineligible or unprepared for surgical interventions [52].

Bariatric Surgery: Considerations and Patient Experience

In contrast, bariatric surgery represents a major life event characterized by extensive pre-operative preparations, requiring hospital stays that can vary in length based on the surgical approach and individual patient recovery [52, 229]. Post-surgery, patients must commit to lasting changes in eating behaviours and engage in long-term follow-up care to ensure success in weight management and overall health [20].

The criteria for eligibility for surgery are generally stringent, often limiting this option to individuals with a BMI of 40 or more, or those with a BMI of 35 accompanied by significant comorbidities [88, 229]. Surgical interventions are typically considered once non-surgical approaches, such as pharmacotherapy, have failed to provide adequate results [20]. While the surgical options may provide greater immediate results in sustained weight loss and comorbidity improvement compared to medications like semaglutide, they involve risks and lifestyle changes that can be daunting [103].

Moreover, semaglutide's efficacy can complement surgical options for patients experiencing weight regain or stasis after initial success post-operation [52, 154]. This integrative approach highlights the potential for pharmacological agents to provide substantial continuous support in managing obesity alongside surgical interventions.

> Both semaglutide and bariatric surgery present viable, albeit distinct, approaches for managing obesity and type 2 diabetes. The choice between them is influenced by various factors including patient preferences, medical eligibility, financial considerations, and the experience of side effects. An informed decision based on a thorough understanding of these variables can empower patients to choose the option that best aligns with their health goals and lifestyle.

How Clinicians Tend to Position Them

Clinicians often utilize semaglutide as a pharmacologic intervention for individuals struggling with obesity and/or type 2 diabetes, typically categorizing it as a first-line treatment for patients not ready for surgical options. Semaglutide has demonstrated significant efficacy in weight management and glycaemic control, making it an attractive alternative for patients whose conditions require more than lifestyle modifications but who do not meet the criteria for or are hesitant about undergoing bariatric surgery [160, 510, 511]. This approach is substantiated by evidence showing semaglutide's effectiveness in achieving substantial weight loss, with studies reporting reductions in body weight of approximately 14% to 15% within a year of administration [160, 512].

Conversely, bariatric surgery is often positioned as the most intense and effective intervention for individuals with severe obesity, particularly when patients exhibit high body mass index (BMI) levels or advanced complications of diabetes, or when medical management fails to achieve desired outcomes [513-515]. Studies show that these surgical interventions lead to significant and sustained weight loss, with results indicating a reduction of over 30% of baseline weight in some cases [516, 517]. The comparative efficacy of bariatric procedures over conventional medical therapies suggests that surgery may be the preferred option in cases of advanced obesity, where non-surgical interventions have not succeeded [514, 517]. A review of outcomes after bariatric surgery emphasizes its capacity to improve not only weight loss but also obesity-related comorbidities significantly, with a notable decrease in cardiovascular events and diabetic complications over the long term [518].

Importantly, a growing trend in clinical practice sees semaglutide and bariatric surgery not as mutually exclusive options but rather as complementary strategies within a comprehensive obesity management program. Patients may initiate semaglutide therapy to achieve weight loss prior to surgery, which could reduce surgical risks and enhance postoperative outcomes [510, 519, 520]. For patients who experience weight regain after bariatric surgery, semaglutide has shown promise as an effective pharmacological adjunct that helps sustain weight loss and improve metabolic parameters such as glycemia and lipid profiles [510, 519]. Recent evidence indicates that utilizing semaglutide for weight management in conjunction with surgical procedures might optimize weight control and overall patient health, thereby reinforcing a multidisciplinary approach in obesity management [521].

> The current landscape of obesity management reflects a dual approach where pharmacological interventions like semaglutide and surgical options are integrated, enhancing the potential for effective weight loss and improved health outcomes among patients with obesity and type 2 diabetes.

Long-Term Maintenance and What Happens After Stopping

Understanding the implications of discontinuing semaglutide is important for both clinicians and patients. As obesity is a chronic, relapsing metabolic disease, the benefits of semaglutide only persist while the medication is administered; once treatment ceases, weight regain is common due to the re-emergence of biological drivers of obesity [71, 109].

Upon achieving the target dosing of semaglutide—typically 2.4 mg weekly—patients not only experience weight loss but also subjective improvements in appetite regulation, craving control, and metabolic health markers such as insulin sensitivity and blood pressure [84, 103]. Research has demonstrated sustained weight loss among patients on semaglutide, with studies indicating approximately a 15% reduction in body weight at one year and about 14.9% at 68 weeks in the STEP 1 trial [105]. After an active weight-loss phase in the initial months of therapy, participants often reach a weight plateau, maintaining a new lower set point. The STEP 1 trial found that, upon cessation of semaglutide, a substantial proportion of participants regained weight rapidly, with an average regain of about two-thirds of the lost weight within a year [109].

Physiological mechanisms behind this weight regain include alterations in hunger and satiety hormones, where ghrelin levels increase and satiety hormones decrease after discontinuation [109]. The abrupt withdrawal of semaglutide can lead to heightened appetite and cravings, alongside slower metabolism and decreased energy expenditure [109]. Consequently, individuals who achieved higher weight loss or who have underlying metabolic conditions may experience more pronounced weight regain upon discontinuation [193], as their bodies are biologically predisposed to resist deviations from previous weight set points.

To counteract weight regain after halting semaglutide, patients may need to implement structured lifestyle interventions, including dietary adjustments emphasizing high-protein, low-calorie eating, consistent physical activity, and behavioural support strategies [71]. Furthermore, transitioning to alternative therapeutic agents such as tirzepatide or orlistat may help maintain weight loss benefits [103]. However, the success rate without continued pharmacological support remains low, emphasizing the chronic nature of obesity management.

Tirzepatide

Tirzepatide is a dual-incretin medication developed by Eli Lilly for the treatment of type 2 diabetes and obesity. It is a once-weekly injectable drug that activates both:

- GLP-1 receptors (glucagon-like peptide-1), and
- GIP receptors (glucose-dependent insulinotropic polypeptide).

This "dual agonist" action makes tirzepatide more potent than traditional GLP-1–only medications such as semaglutide.

Tirzepatide helps with weight loss and metabolic control by:

- significantly reducing appetite and food cravings
- slowing gastric emptying
- enhancing insulin sensitivity
- lowering blood glucose levels
- reducing body fat, especially visceral fat

Clinical trials show tirzepatide can produce 15–25% body-weight reduction, making it one of the most effective non-surgical treatments available.

Orlistat

Orlistat is an older weight-loss medication that works very differently from GLP-1 drugs. It is a lipase inhibitor, taken orally as a capsule. Orlistat blocks the action of gastrointestinal lipase enzymes, preventing the absorption of about 30% of dietary fat. The unabsorbed fat is excreted through the bowel.

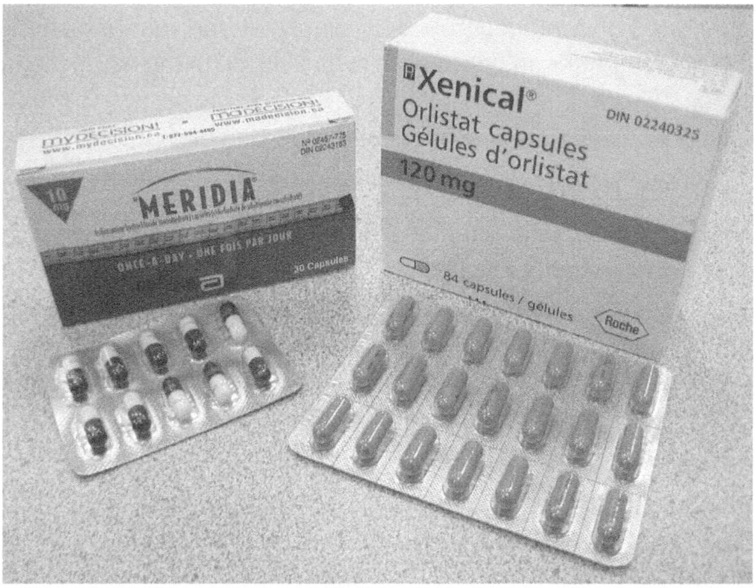

Figure 28: Medication used for obesity - Orlistat and sibutramine. James Heilman, MD, CC BY-SA 3.0, via Wikimedia Commons.

Main effects:

- modest weight loss (typically 5–7%)
- improvement in cholesterol and blood pressure related to lower fat intake

Side effects:

Orlistat commonly causes gastrointestinal symptoms due to unabsorbed fat, including:

- oily stools
- urgent bowel movements
- flatulence with leakage
- abdominal discomfort

These effects are more pronounced when meals contain higher amounts of fat.

While semaglutide facilitates significant weight loss and metabolic enhancements during its administration, the cessation of treatment prompts a return to pre-treatment biological states that favour weight regain. This underscores the necessity for ongoing management that may include either the resumption of semaglutide or alternative therapies, thereby reinforcing the concept of obesity as a chronic disease requiring continuous intervention [84, 193].

Myths, Misconceptions, And Media Hype

The rise of semaglutide as a treatment for weight management has indeed generated significant global attention, which has simultaneously surfaced various myths, misconceptions, and exaggerated narratives surrounding its use. Although semaglutide is backed by substantial clinical evidence indicating its efficacy and safety for weight loss, public discourse often distorts its role, framing it as a "miracle drug" that does not require accompanying behavioural adjustments. Media portrayals frequently spotlight dramatic transformations and endorsements by celebrities, potentially misleading individuals into thinking that significant weight loss can occur effortlessly. However, substantial evidence indicates that semaglutide's efficacy is maximized when it is integrated with behavioural modifications, such as improved dietary habits and regular exercise [32, 497].

Moreover, some media narratives erroneously characterize semaglutide as a short-term, cosmetic solution rather than recognizing obesity as a chronic, relapsing condition. Clinical trials, including those summarized in the STEP program, demonstrate that semaglutide is intended for long-term management of obesity, akin to pharmacotherapy for other chronic conditions like hypertension or diabetes [105, 522]. These narratives often trivialize the complexity of obesity treatment and contribute to stigma, further obscuring the condition's medical seriousness [522, 523].

Concerns regarding safety are also prevalent, with media sometimes amplifying fears regarding severe side effects such as thyroid cancer or gastroparesis without adequately contextualizing these risks. While semaglutide does have known adverse effects, particularly gastrointestinal disturbances, research illustrates that it maintains a favourable safety profile when used as directed. Large-scale clinical trials have shown that, while adverse effects can occur, they are generally mild and reversible [223, 522]. Reports conflating rare adverse occurrences with confirmed risks can exacerbate public anxiety and hinder informed decision-making about the medication.

Another commonly held belief is that discontinuing semaglutide leads to immediate weight regain or lasting metabolic detriment. In truth, research has established that the biological mechanisms regulating appetite can rebound once the medication is halted, reflecting the chronic nature of obesity rather than a flaw intrinsic to the treatment itself [109, 524]. Understanding this rebound effect is critical for setting realistic expectations around treatment and ensuring adherence to a recommended comprehensive obesity management strategy.

Additionally, misconceptions persist regarding the universal applicability of semaglutide, leading to unrealistic expectations among those who may not be ideal candidates for treatment. Important clinical contraindications, such as a history of multiple endocrine neoplasia type 2 (MEN2) and potential pregnancy risks, are frequently overlooked in public discussions [109, 524].

This can create a false narrative that semaglutide is suitable for anyone looking to lose weight, disregarding the need for careful assessment by healthcare professionals.

Lastly, the framing of semaglutide as simply a trend—a "Hollywood secret" or an anti-aging treatment—can trivialize its medical role and foster negative stigma for patients relying on it for legitimate health reasons. This kind of media portrayal detracts from the understanding that obesity is a chronic disease requiring a nuanced and comprehensive approach to treatment [523, 525]. Addressing these misconceptions is essential for cultivating a more informed and compassionate dialogue around obesity management and treatments like semaglutide.

Chapter 8

Diet, Nutrition, and Lifestyle While Taking Semaglutide

Successful use of semaglutide involves more than taking a weekly injection—it requires understanding how diet, hydration, movement, and daily habits interact with the medication's physiological effects. Because semaglutide slows gastric emptying, reduces appetite, and alters gut–brain signalling, many individuals experience significant changes in how they feel, eat, and respond to food. This chapter provides practical, evidence-based guidance to help patients navigate these changes safely and comfortably.

While semaglutide is a powerful tool for weight loss and metabolic improvement, its benefits are maximised when paired with thoughtful nutrition strategies, supportive lifestyle routines, and structured physical activity. Dietary choices can reduce or worsen common gastrointestinal side effects such as nausea, bloating, constipation, and early fullness. Similarly, hydration, fibre intake, and meal timing play key roles in digestive comfort and long-term adherence. Exercise enhances metabolic efficiency, preserves muscle mass, and accelerates fat loss—creating a synergy that supports healthier body composition and more sustainable outcomes.

This chapter also explores behavioural tools such as mindful eating, hunger-cue awareness, and portion regulation, which help individuals build lasting habits beyond the period of medication use. Finally, we examine how alcohol, caffeine, and commonly used substances like THC and CBD may influence side effects, metabolism, and safety during treatment.

Together, these nutrition and lifestyle strategies empower individuals to work with semaglutide rather than against it—maximising benefits, minimising discomfort, and laying the foundation for long-term health and weight-management success.

Nutrition Strategies for Nausea Prevention

Nausea is indeed a prevalent side effect associated with semaglutide therapy, especially during the initial phases of treatment or subsequent dose adjustments. The mechanism behind this occurs largely because semaglutide slows gastric emptying and modifies gut-brain signalling pathways, making gastric motility slower and potentially increasing the sensitivity of the stomach to food intake [308, 526]. As a result, changes in meal size, composition, and even the rate of eating can significantly influence the perception of nausea among patients [527].

Implementing targeted nutrition strategies emerges as a viable approach to mitigating these side effects. For instance, adhering to smaller and more frequent meals instead of larger portions can reduce gastric load and help prevent feelings of excessive fullness, which can exacerbate nausea due to semaglutide's effect on gastric emptying [527, 528]. Recommendations indicate that patients could benefit from reducing their overall meal volume by 20–30%, maintaining nutritional adequacy while enhancing comfort during and after meals [529]. Furthermore, consuming meals slowly and stopping immediately when fullness is sensed allows for more manageable digestion, accommodating the slower gastric clearance associated with GLP-1 receptor agonists [528].

When it comes to food choices, selecting gentler, easily digestible items is crucial. Studies suggest that bland, low-fat foods—such as toast, crackers, and rice—are less likely to trigger nausea than high-fat or spicy meals, which can further delay gastric emptying and complicate symptoms [308, 527]. Patients often report that soft foods and simple carbohydrates are better tolerated during episodes of nausea, while reintroducing more complex foods gradually as their condition stabilizes [528]. This dietary adaptation works synergistically with semaglutide's pharmacological effects, enhancing patient comfort and adherence to treatment protocols.

Hydration habits constitute another vital aspect of managing nausea. Instead of consuming large quantities of fluids in one go, which can lead to a sensation of bloating and fullness, it is advisable for patients to sip fluids throughout the day. Selecting beverages such as water, herbal teas, and ginger-infused drinks can provide solace, as these are often well tolerated compared to carbonated or sweetened beverages, which may aggravate nausea [527, 528].

Strategically timing meals around medication doses can also minimize discomfort. Patients might find relief by eating before administering their semaglutide injection or adjusting their meal timing on days when nausea is particularly pronounced [526, 530]. For those utilizing oral semaglutide, taking the medication on an empty stomach and delaying food intake by a short period may alleviate symptoms of nausea [530].

Lastly, maintaining proper eating behaviours can greatly influence symptom management. Practices such as avoiding recumbency immediately post-meal and refraining from skipping meals or consuming large late-night meals further promote smooth digestion and reduce the likelihood of nausea [527, 528]. Simple remedies like ginger tea or consuming small protein snacks can also help ease discomfort in between meals [530].

Effectively managing nausea during semaglutide therapy revolves around a combination of adopting appropriate dietary strategies, focusing on meal timing, and fostering healthy eating behaviours—all aimed at harmonizing with semaglutide's physiological effects and improving overall treatment adherence.

Recommended Eating Patterns (E.G., Mediterranean, High-Protein)

Semaglutide has demonstrated significant efficacy in reducing appetite and regulating hunger signals. However, sustained success in weight management necessitates the adoption of dietary strategies that prioritize metabolic health, preserve muscle mass, and minimize gastrointestinal side effects associated with the medication. Effective dietary patterns, such as the Mediterranean diet and high-protein eating strategies, are aligned with semaglutide's functional mechanisms, contributing to both weight loss and overall well-being.

The Mediterranean diet emphasizes whole foods, including lean proteins (such as fish and legumes), fruits, vegetables, nuts, and healthy fats, particularly olive oil. Research shows that such a dietary pattern is rich in fibre and antioxidants, fostering cardiovascular health, reducing inflammation, and enhancing satiety—all critical for effective weight management [531, 532]. Specifically, the combination of healthy fats (primarily monounsaturated), moderate protein intake, and low-glycaemic index carbohydrates aids in stabilizing blood sugar levels and may mitigate gastrointestinal discomfort, which is particularly relevant for users of semaglutide as they may experience such side effects [531, 533]. The flexibility and non-restrictive nature of the Mediterranean diet promote adherence, making it feasible for long-term implementation among individuals undergoing treatment with semaglutide [532].

Incorporating a high-protein eating pattern enhances the weight loss benefits experienced with semaglutide. Protein has superior satiating effects compared to other macronutrients, effectively curbing hunger and assisting in the preservation of lean muscle mass—an important consideration during rapid weight loss phases [534, 535]. Evidence indicates that ensuring adequate protein at each meal, sourced from foods such as poultry, fish, tofu, beans, and dairy products, supports sustained energy levels and appetite stability, and may also reduce occurrences of gastrointestinal distress compared to high-fat meals [536]. Clinical recommendations suggest a daily intake of approximately 1.0–1.2 grams of protein per kilogram of body weight to optimize weight management while accommodating individual energy needs [532, 536].

Balanced, low-glycaemic eating patterns are critical for effective appetite regulation, particularly in conjunction with semaglutide treatment. Consuming carbohydrates that digest slowly—like legumes, whole grains, and various vegetables—supports stable blood sugar levels and fullness cues, thus preventing spikes and dips that can lead to increased cravings [531, 537]. This strategy not only complements the delayed gastric emptying associated with semaglutide but also helps reduce the risk of nausea or discomfort [533, 538]. Reducing ultra-processed foods and refined carbohydrate intake further supports appetite control, reinforcing the necessary dietary behaviours for sustainable weight loss.

Structured meal patterns, such as consuming smaller meals combined with healthy snacks, may benefit individuals during semaglutide's dose-escalation phase. This method prevents excessive gastric overload that may exacerbate gastrointestinal symptoms while ensuring nutritional adequacy [539]. As individuals adapt and their appetite stabilizes, the frequency of meals can naturally decrease, provided they continue consuming nutrient-dense foods to mitigate the risk of dietary deficiencies [537]. While semaglutide does not prescribe specific dietary guidelines, integrating these balanced, health-focused eating patterns enhances optimal outcomes in weight management and metabolic health.

Both the Mediterranean diet and high-protein dietary patterns present robust, evidence-based frameworks that align with semaglutide's appetite-regulating properties. They facilitate satiety, muscle mass preservation, blood sugar stabilization, and minimized gastrointestinal disturbances—all essential components for achieving sustainable weight loss and health outcomes.

Foods That Help or Worsen Side Effects

The management of side effects associated with semaglutide, a glucagon-like peptide-1 receptor agonist frequently used in the treatment of type 2 diabetes and obesity, involves considerable consideration of dietary choices. Semaglutide alters gastric emptying and appetite signals, making the dietary context critical for mitigating gastrointestinal side effects such as nausea, bloating, diarrhea, and constipation.

Foods That Help Reduce Side Effects

Easily digestible food options are recommended to relieve nausea and digestive discomfort during the early phases of semaglutide treatment. Foods such as crackers, dry toast, plain rice, and broth-based soups provide gentle nourishment for an irritable stomach [20]. Incorporating ginger into the diet, whether through ginger tea, chews, or biscuits, may be beneficial due to its recognized anti-emetic properties [540]. Cold or room-temperature foods, including yogurt and smoothies, often prove easier to tolerate than hot or strongly aromatic meals [31].

Gradually increasing the intake of dietary fibre through vegetables, oats, legumes, chia seeds, or psyllium husk is crucial for promoting bowel regularity and relieving constipation [31]. Additionally, hydrating foods like watermelon and cucumbers help maintain fluid balance and contribute to gastrointestinal health, especially when diarrhea is present [308]. Lean proteins, such as fish, eggs, and chicken, provide nutritional benefits while being easier to digest compared to richer, fatty options [41]. Smaller, more frequent meals can also help prevent overloading the gastrointestinal tract, which is typically associated with large meal portions [20].

Foods That May Worsen Side Effects

Conversely, certain food types can exacerbate gastrointestinal side effects during treatment with semaglutide. High-fat and greasy foods, such as fried items and fatty meats, are known to increase nausea and bloating since they remain longer in the stomach due to slowed gastric emptying [20]. Similarly, overly sweetened foods can draw water into the gut, worsening nausea and potentially causing diarrhea due to their rapid absorption and effects on blood sugar levels [540].

Highly processed foods, carbonated beverages, and large meal portions contribute to digestive discomfort as they are often more difficult to digest [41]. Alcohol is identified as a potential irritant that may impair gastric lining integrity and worsen symptoms of nausea and dehydration [541]. Additionally, spicy dishes and foods rich in sugar or acids may provoke reflux and irritation in sensitive individuals [20].

Putting It into Practice

Patients using semaglutide typically report improved tolerance to a wider variety of foods over time, as the body adapts to the medication [542]. Identifying personal dietary triggers is essential for individuals, allowing them to make necessary adjustments to enhance their comfort during treatment. Strategies such as eating at a slower pace, stopping intake when comfortably full, and ensuring proper hydration further help to minimize gastrointestinal issues associated with the medication [478].

Through informed dietary choices—focusing on foods that ease gastrointestinal discomfort while avoiding those that induce adverse effects—individuals can enhance their treatment experience with semaglutide, underscoring the importance of diet in managing side effects associated with this medication.

Hydration, Fibre, And Bowel Health

Hydration, fibre intake, and bowel health are particularly critical for patients undergoing treatment with semaglutide, a medication that can significantly affect gastric emptying and intestinal motility. This discussion synthesizes the evidence surrounding how these factors can mitigate common gastrointestinal side effects associated with semaglutide.

Importance of Hydration

Proper hydration plays a vital role in digestive health, particularly for patients on semaglutide, where slowed gastrointestinal transit can lead to complications such as constipation and bloating. Studies indicate that adequate water intake is fundamental for maintaining bowel regularity and preventing discomfort during treatment [543]. Recommendations for hydration typically suggest a daily intake of 1.5 to 2.5 litres of water, though exact needs vary based on body size, activity level, and environmental conditions [544].

It is critical to support hydration through regular fluid consumption rather than consuming large quantities at once, which can overwhelm the digestive system [545]. Increased fluid intake is advised if patients experience gastrointestinal symptoms like nausea or diarrhea, as hydration helps maintain not only bowel health but also overall physiological balance, including kidney function and appetite regulation, particularly during weight loss phases prompted by semaglutide therapy [546]. Thus, hydration is often the first and most effective strategy for alleviating constipation related to this medication [543].

Role of Fibre Intake

Fibre intake is another crucial component that contributes significantly to bowel health. A balanced fibre diet aids in regulating bowel movements and enhancing gut health, which is particularly necessary for individuals on semaglutide who may experience altered gastrointestinal motility. The general recommendation is to consume between 25 to 38 grams of fibre daily, but it is essential to introduce fibre gradually to prevent gas, cramping, and bloating that can accompany rapid increases in fibre [547].

The inclusion of both soluble and insoluble fibres in the diet can benefit individuals experiencing constipation. Soluble fibre, found in foods such as oats and legumes, absorbs water and forms a gel that can ease stool passage, while insoluble fibre, found in whole grains and vegetables, adds bulk and promotes intestinal movement [548]. Care should be taken to increase fibre intake over several weeks to minimize discomfort, ensuring that the adjustments support overall digestive health while being mindful of the slowed gastric emptying associated with semaglutide [545].

Managing Bowel Health

Management of bowel health for patients on semaglutide should focus on strategies to prevent common issues like constipation and bloating. Recommendations to counteract these effects include:

- **Increasing Water Intake**: As discussed, sufficient hydration is paramount to prevent hard stools and constipation [543].
- **Incorporating Soluble Fibre**: Foods such as chia seeds and psyllium can facilitate smoother bowel movements [549].
- **Eating Smaller, More Frequent Meals**: This can reduce gastrointestinal pressure and discomfort [550].
- **Minimizing Fatty Foods and Processed Snacks**: These can exacerbate bloating and digestive discomfort [551].
- **Routine Physical Activity**: Regular movement can enhance bowel motility and should be encouraged [548].

For cases exacerbated by constipation despite following these strategies, low-dose osmotic laxatives can be effective and are generally well-tolerated [547]. Additionally, recognizing the role of gradual dietary changes can significantly affect comfort during treatment and lead to a more sustainable long-term approach to managing bowel health [548].

> The interplay between hydration, fibre intake, and bowel health is crucial for successfully managing gastrointestinal side effects in patients on semaglutide. Adequate hydration, a balanced approach to fibre consumption, and proactive management of dietary choices can enhance overall comfort and compliance during treatment. Effective bowel management not only alleviates discomfort but also promotes adherence to therapeutic interventions aimed at achieving weight loss and improving metabolic health.

Exercise Considerations and Metabolic Synergy

The integration of exercise with semaglutide therapy offers a effective strategy to enhance metabolic health, particularly in individuals seeking weight loss and improved body composition. Semaglutide, a glucagon-like peptide-1 (GLP-1) receptor agonist, primarily functions by reducing appetite and facilitating weight loss. To enhance the benefits of this medication, incorporating exercise is essential, as it strengthens metabolic effects and helps alleviate some side effects associated with semaglutide therapy.

Exercise and Its Role in Semaglutide Therapy

Semaglutide significantly reduces caloric intake, which may lead to a decrease in metabolic rate due to lower energy availability. Exercise plays a vital role in counteracting this effect by helping to preserve lean muscle mass and maintain a higher metabolic rate during the treatment process. Regular physical activity, especially resistance training, is important. Evidence suggests that individuals engaging in resistance training during semaglutide treatment can significantly improve their lean body mass and metabolic health, thereby preventing the metabolic slowdown typically associated with weight loss [552, 553].

Combining dietary protein with exercise can further enhance muscle preservation. Experts recommend a protein intake of 1.2–1.6 g/kg body weight daily, which works synergistically with resistance training to maintain muscle integrity during periods of caloric restriction [554, 555]. This combined approach can significantly reduce the risk of muscle loss, a common consequence of rapid weight loss induced by medications like semaglutide [556, 557].

Cardiovascular and Metabolic Health Improvements

In addition to muscle maintenance, aerobic exercise significantly contributes to cardiovascular health. Studies indicate that aerobic activities, such as brisk walking, cycling, or swimming, can improve lipid profiles, lower blood pressure, and enhance insulin sensitivity, complementing the effects of semaglutide therapy [558, 559]. Guidelines recommend engaging in at least 150 minutes of moderate-intensity aerobic exercise weekly to achieve optimal health benefits and support weight maintenance following weight loss interventions [560].

Recommended weekly targets (based on international guidelines):

- **150 minutes of moderate-intensity** exercise (e.g., brisk walking, cycling, swimming), OR
- **75 minutes of vigorous-intensity** exercise (e.g., running, high-intensity intervals)

Activity can be spread throughout the week in 10–30 minute sessions.

The physiological responses to exercise also include a reduction in visceral fat, which is crucial because semaglutide has been shown to improve insulin sensitivity and control blood glucose levels. Research indicates that combining exercise with weight loss can lead to greater reductions in visceral fat and enhanced glucose tolerance compared to either intervention alone [561-563].

Exercise and Side Effect Management

Moreover, exercise can help manage common side effects of semaglutide therapy, including nausea and constipation. Light physical activity, such as walking after meals, can enhance gastric motility and alleviate discomfort, thereby promoting better adherence to the treatment regimen [559]. However, it is important to note that intense physical activity immediately after injection may exacerbate nausea, suggesting that a more tailored approach to exercise scheduling is necessary for optimal comfort [553, 560].

The Synergistic Effects of Exercise and Semaglutide

The interaction between exercise and semaglutide creates a synergistic effect that is greater than the sum of their individual benefits. This combination promotes fat loss, particularly visceral fat, while also supporting better long-term weight-loss maintenance and enhancing metabolic health [556, 560]. Individuals who actively engage in both pharmacological treatment and structured exercise programs tend to experience greater and more sustained improvements in body weight, body composition, and overall health status than those relying solely on medication [556, 557, 564].

Exercise should be viewed as a crucial component of semaglutide therapy for individuals aiming to improve their metabolic health and achieve weight-loss goals. By preserving muscle mass, supporting cardiovascular health, and managing side effects, structured exercise enhances the efficacy of semaglutide, illustrating a powerful metabolic

synergy critical for long-term weight management and improved health outcomes.

Below are exercise case study scenarios that demonstrate how individuals can integrate structured physical activity with semaglutide therapy to maximise metabolic health, preserve muscle mass, and improve long-term weight-loss outcomes. Each scenario illustrates different levels of fitness, comorbidities, goals, and real-world challenges.

Case Study Scenario 1: The Beginner with Obesity and Joint Pain

Profile

- **Age:** 52
- **Sex:** Female
- **Starting BMI:** 38
- **Conditions:** Knee osteoarthritis, hypertension, dyslipidaemia
- **Semaglutide Dose:** Titrated to 2.4 mg weekly
- **Challenges:** Low fitness, fear of exercise, nausea in early dose escalation

Exercise Strategy

- Begin with low-impact movement:
  - 10–15 minutes slow walking twice daily
  - Light chair-based exercises for lower body
- Introduce aquatic exercise by week 4:
  - 30 minutes pool walking or light swimming 3× weekly
- Progress to resistance training in week 8:
  - 2× weekly, 20–30 minutes
  - Focus on leg strength: sit-to-stand, resistance bands, step-ups

Outcomes After 12 Weeks

- Weight loss: 8% of total body weight
- Pain reduced enough to walk 5 km/week
- Improved blood pressure and cholesterol
- Nausea reduced through slower eating + walking after meals

Learning Points

Gentle, joint-friendly exercise significantly boosts metabolic benefits while preventing muscle loss and improving mobility—key factors for long-term success.

Case Study Scenario 2: The Busy Professional Losing Muscle Mass on Semaglutide

Profile

- **Age:** 41
- **Sex:** Male
- **Starting BMI:** 33
- **Semaglutide Dose:** 1.0 mg weekly
- **Conditions:** None
- **Challenges:**
  - Rapid appetite suppression → very low caloric intake
  - Fatigue → risk of lean mass loss
  - Minimal time for exercise

Exercise Strategy

- Introduce short "micro sessions" to fit schedule:
  - 10 minutes resistance circuits (push-ups, rows, squats) daily
  - 1–2 longer 30-minute sessions on weekends
- Focus on protein intake: 1.4 g/kg/day
- Add standing desk breaks + 10-minute post-meal walks

Outcomes After 16 Weeks

- Weight loss: 12%, mostly fat
- Lean muscle preserved due to consistent strength training
- Energy levels improved with structured protein intake
- Better glycaemic control and reduced visceral fat

Learning Points

Time-efficient strength training preserves muscle and prevents metabolic slowdown, even with reduced calorie intake induced by semaglutide.

Case Study Scenario 3: The Patient with Type 2 Diabetes & Visceral Obesity

Profile

- **Age:** 60
- **Sex:** Male
- **Starting BMI:** 36
- **Conditions:** Type 2 diabetes, fatty liver (MASLD), sleep apnoea
- **Semaglutide Dose:** 2.4 mg weekly

Exercise Strategy

- Begin with aerobic training to reduce visceral fat:
    - 30 minutes brisk walking 5× weekly
- Add resistance training by week 4:
    - 2× weekly (machines preferred for safety)
- Incorporate core-strength and posture work to improve breathing during sleep
- Maintain moderate intensity (RPE 4–6)

Outcomes After 24 Weeks

- Weight loss: 15%
- Marked reduction in visceral fat (waist circumference ↓ 10 cm)
- Liver markers (ALT, AST) improved
- HbA1c reduced by 1.2%
- Sleep apnoea symptoms improved

Learning Points

Aerobic training + semaglutide rapidly reduces visceral fat, improving metabolic disease and liver health.

Case Study Scenario 4: The Highly Motivated Individual Wanting Maximal Fat Loss

Profile

- **Age:** 29
- **Sex:** Female
- **Starting BMI:** 32
- **Semaglutide Dose:** 2.4 mg weekly
- **Goal:** Significant fat loss + visible muscle definition
- **Challenges:** Nausea early in therapy, tendency to under-eat

Exercise Strategy

- Hybrid training program:
    - Strength training 3× weekly (progressive overload)
    - High-intensity interval training (HIIT) 1–2× weekly
    - Daily walking target: 8,000–10,000 steps
- Ensure adequate nutrient intake:
    - 1.6 g/kg protein
    - High hydration
    - Electrolyte support on heavy workout days

Outcomes After 20 Weeks

- Weight loss: 14%
- Significant fat loss with muscle definition maintained
- Improved strength and cardiovascular fitness
- Side effects managed by post-meal walking and avoiding large meals

Learning Points

Structured resistance + HIIT + high protein ensures high-quality weight loss (fat loss > muscle loss).

Case Study Scenario 5: Older Adult Prioritising Mobility and Bone Health

Profile

- **Age:** 68
- **Sex:** Female
- **Starting BMI:** 35
- **Conditions:** Osteopenia, mild hypertension
- **Semaglutide Dose:** 0.5 mg weekly

Exercise Strategy

- Focus on weight-bearing exercise:
  - Walking 20–30 minutes daily
  - Light hiking on weekends
- Add strength training to improve bone density:
  - 2× weekly small weights, resistance bands
- Add balance and mobility training: Tai chi, yoga
- Avoid high-intensity work due to dizziness early in titration

Outcomes After 12 Months

- Weight loss: **10%**, slower but steady
- Improved bone density markers
- Reduced fall risk
- More independence and reduced need for blood pressure medication

Learning Points

In older adults, maintaining muscle and bone strength is as important as weight loss; semaglutide + tailored exercise improves function and reduces long-term health risks.

Case Study Scenario 6: Patient Struggling with Nausea During Dose Escalation

Profile

- **Age:** 45
- **Sex:** Female
- **BMI:** 40
- **Challenges:**
    - Moderate-to-severe nausea after dose increases
    - Bloating and constipation
    - Fear of exercising due to discomfort

Exercise Strategy

- Begin with gentle walking after meals (10 minutes) to improve gastric motility
- Avoid intense workouts on injection days
- Start light mobility + stretching on "high-nausea days"
- Introduce resistance bands gradually as symptoms improve
- Encourage hydration + electrolyte balance

Outcomes After 10 Weeks

- Weight loss: **7%**
- Significant reduction in nausea through light movement
- Increased exercise tolerance
- Improved mental health and energy

Learning Points

Gentle, consistent activity can *reduce* semaglutide side effects and encourage gradual progression to more structured training.

Case Study Scenario 7: Former Athlete Returning to Training

Profile

- **Age:** 38
- **Sex:** Male
- **BMI:** 34
- **History:** High-level athlete until early 30s
- **Challenges:**

  - High expectations
  - Low fitness after years of inactivity

Exercise Strategy

- Restart with moderate-intensity cardio: cycling + elliptical
- Build to strength training 4× weekly
- Introduce interval training after week 8
- Focus on protein intake to support muscle regrowth

Outcomes After 12 Weeks

- Weight loss: 11%
- Rapid gains in strength and aerobic capacity
- Better mood, motivation, and adherence

Learning Points

Semaglutide helps regulate hunger, allowing former athletes to train consistently without overeating or compensatory hunger spikes.

Behavioural Strategies (Mindful Eating, Hunger Cues, Portion Sizing)

Behavioural strategies are vital for maximizing the benefits of semaglutide and supporting long-term weight management success. While semaglutide significantly reduces appetite and "food noise," it is critical to recognize that behavioural habits ultimately shape outcomes, particularly when the body starts to adapt to the treatment or if the medication is discontinued [32, 565]. Therefore, establishing sustainable eating patterns through mindful eating, awareness of hunger cues, and appropriate portion sizing can effectively reinforce the physiological effects of semaglutide.

Mindful Eating

Mindful eating entails heightened awareness of the eating process, including sensory aspects of food and internal signals of hunger and fullness. This practice helps dismantle patterns rooted in emotional or automatic eating that individuals may exhibit before commencing GLP-1 therapy [105, 565]. Key principles of mindful eating include eating slowly and without distractions, which can significantly reduce instances of nausea associated with rapid eating, often experienced during semaglutide treatment [32, 105]. This practice encourages individuals to notice various aspects of food, such as flavours and textures, and to pause mid-meal to assess satiety levels, promoting an intuitive response to hunger and fullness cues that semaglutide amplifies. As therapy progresses, and the focus shifts from weight loss to maintenance, mindful eating remains an effective tool for balancing intake and enhancing awareness of physiological signals [103, 565].

Recognizing Hunger and Fullness Cues

While semaglutide effectively suppresses appetite, it can lead to a misunderstanding of hunger signals, necessitating the development of skills to identify different types of hunger cues. Distinguishing physical hunger—characterized by sensations such as mild stomach rumbling—from emotional or habitual triggers is essential for maintaining a balanced intake [32, 565]. Recognizing the fullness cues, which are influenced by semaglutide, helps individuals learn to stop eating at a point of comfortable fullness rather than relying on external cues, such as an empty plate or social eating contexts. Consequently, awareness of these cues can minimize overeating behaviours that may provoke nausea and bloating, thus aiding in weight stabilization and reducing potential side effects of the medication [103, 566].

Portion Sizing

Semaglutide has been shown to decrease appetite and slow gastric emptying, enabling most individuals to comfortably manage smaller portion sizes [32, 105, 565]. By actively engaging in portion control, individuals can further enhance their comfort and reinforce sustainable eating patterns essential for weight maintenance. Practical strategies such as using smaller plates and serving half portions before assessing hunger levels can fundamentally shift visual and psychological perceptions of portion sizes [103, 105]. Prioritizing protein and vegetables while adjusting starchy food intake further supports nutritional balance while allowing for caloric reduction without sacrificing nutritional value [105, 565, 567].

Why Behavioural Strategies Matter Even with Reduced Appetite

Despite semaglutide's effectiveness in modifying biological predictors of eating, behavioural strategies continue to play a crucial role in weight management. Behavioural patterns may linger, and appetite can partially resurge, particularly after discontinuing treatment [105]. Frequent overeating, especially of calorically dense foods, can still evoke symptoms like nausea [32, 105]. Therefore, fostering consistent behavioural changes alongside pharmacological intervention is essential for achieving long-term weight loss and preventing pitfalls such as under-eating or subsequent weight regain. Learning to effectively respond to hunger cues helps prevent metabolic decline and muscle loss often associated with unintentional caloric restriction [103, 566]. In conclusion, integrating mindful eating practices, awareness of hunger and fullness cues, and intentional portion control fortifies semaglutide's metabolic effects, paving the way for sustainable and healthy eating habits that extend beyond the duration of medication use.

Alcohol, Caffeine, and Substance Interactions

Understanding the interactions between semaglutide, alcohol, caffeine, and recreational substances such as cannabis is critical for patients using semaglutide for the management of type 2 diabetes and obesity. While semaglutide itself does not have significant direct drug-drug interactions with these substances, important clinical implications arise from their combined use regarding safety, glycaemic control, and the management of side effects.

Interaction between Alcohol and Semaglutide

Alcohol can exacerbate symptoms associated with semaglutide, particularly gastrointestinal discomfort and glucose control. For example, both alcohol consumption and semaglutide can irritate the stomach lining and delay gastric emptying, potentially leading to heightened nausea and vomiting, especially during the initial dose escalation of semaglutide therapy [568]. Moreover, the risk of hypoglycaemia increases when alcohol is introduced to the regimen, particularly for individuals who may also be using insulin or sulfonylureas alongside semaglutide [569]. Since alcohol can impair the liver's capacity to release glucose into the bloodstream, individuals may experience masked symptoms of low blood sugar, complicating diabetes management [569].

Additionally, the appetite-suppressive effects of semaglutide may be influenced by alcohol, which could lead to inadequate nutrient intake [570]. This risk is particularly relevant for individuals with pre-existing conditions such as non-alcoholic fatty liver disease, where alcohol may worsen liver inflammation [571]. Experts recommend limiting alcohol intake during semaglutide treatment to minimize these risks, particularly during dose titration, and advise against drinking on an empty stomach [572].

Interaction between Caffeine and Semaglutide

Caffeine, a common stimulant, does not interfere with the pharmacodynamics of semaglutide but can amplify certain side effects. For instance, caffeine may heighten gastrointestinal irritation, exacerbating nausea or reflux, especially when consumed in large quantities or on an empty stomach [573]. This complication can be particularly troubling for patients adjusting to semaglutide, as early stages of treatment often include gastrointestinal side effects.

Moreover, caffeine has mixed effects on appetite regulation; while it might temporarily suppress appetite, this can lead to rebound hunger when its effects diminish, potentially complicating the weight management aspect of semaglutide therapy [574]. The diuretic nature of caffeine can also contribute to dehydration and worsen constipation—common side effects associated with semaglutide [575]. Therefore, moderation in caffeine consumption is advised—generally recommending no more than 1-2 cups of moderately caffeinated beverages per day [573].

Interaction between Cannabis and Semaglutide

The interaction between cannabis (THC and CBD) and semaglutide is complex. THC is known to stimulate appetite, which could counteract semaglutide's appetite-suppressing effects, potentially leading to unwanted weight gain [576, 577]. Additionally, cannabis edibles can further slow gastric emptying, increasing the likelihood of nausea, a side effect some users may already experience from semaglutide [569].

THC (tetrahydrocannabinol) and CBD (cannabidiol) are the two most well-known active compounds found in the *Cannabis sativa* plant. Although they come from the same plant, they have very different effects on the brain and body, which is why they are used for different medical and recreational purposes.

THC (Tetrahydrocannabinol)

THC is the main psychoactive compound in cannabis—meaning it is responsible for the "high" or altered mental state associated with marijuana use.

Key Characteristics:

- Produces euphoria, relaxation, altered perception
- Stimulates appetite ("the munchies")
- Can impair memory, concentration, reaction time
- May increase anxiety or paranoia in some individuals
- Has analgesic (pain-relieving) properties
- Can reduce nausea and vomiting

How It Works:

THC binds strongly to CB1 receptors in the brain, which regulate:

- pleasure
- memory
- coordination
- appetite
- time perception

This explains the noticeable cognitive and psychological effects.

Common Uses:

- Recreational use
- Pain management
- Appetite stimulation
- Nausea control (e.g., chemotherapy)

CBD (Cannabidiol)

CBD is non-psychoactive, meaning it does not create a "high." It has calming and therapeutic properties without altering cognition.

Key Characteristics:

- Does *not* impair thinking or cause intoxication
- Reduces anxiety and stress
- Has anti-inflammatory and analgesic effects
- May improve sleep

- Can reduce seizures (FDA-approved in epilepsy treatment)
- May counteract some negative effects of THC (anxiety, paranoia)

How It Works:

CBD interacts more gently with the body's endocannabinoid system, particularly:

- CB2 receptors (immune and inflammatory pathways)
- serotonin receptors
- pain modulation pathways

It does *not* strongly bind to CB1 receptors, which is why it doesn't cause a high.

Common Uses:

- Anxiety and stress reduction
- Sleep support
- Pain and inflammation
- Epilepsy (especially childhood epilepsies such as Dravet and Lennox-Gastaut syndrome)
- Muscle relaxation

THC vs CBD: Quick Comparison

Feature	THC	CBD
Psychoactive?	Yes (causes a high)	No
Appetite	Increases appetite	Neutral or mild decrease
Anxiety	May increase anxiety in some	Often reduces anxiety
Pain relief	Strong	Moderate
Legal status	Strictly regulated	Widely legal in many regions
Medical uses	Pain, nausea, appetite stimulation	Anxiety, epilepsy, inflammation

Conversely, there is anecdotal evidence suggesting that CBD might alleviate nausea, offering potential therapeutic benefits for some patients [578]. However, the overall safety and efficacy of combining these substances during semaglutide treatment require further empirical investigation.

Other Recreational Substances

It is important to recognize that recreational drugs like cocaine, methamphetamine, and MDMA pose significant risks for patients on semaglutide, predominantly due to their impact on cardiovascular health and appetite suppression [569, 578]. These substances can induce severe elevations in heart rate and blood pressure, complicating semaglutide's therapeutic effects, especially since semaglutide may result in decreased blood pressure [570].

Given these numerous potential interactions and side effects, a strong recommendation exists for patients on semaglutide to avoid the use of recreational stimulant drugs to safeguard against adverse outcomes associated with hypoglycaemia and unhealthy appetite management [574].

> Careful monitoring and management of alcohol, caffeine, and recreational substance use are essential when prescribing semaglutide. The nuanced interactions among these compounds highlight the importance of patient education regarding lifestyle habits that could either challenge or enhance the therapeutic efficacy of semaglutide.

Summary

Alcohol

✓ Safe in moderation
✗ May worsen nausea
✗ Risk of hypoglycaemia with diabetes medications
✗ Not ideal during titration

Caffeine

✓ Safe in moderate doses
✗ Can worsen nausea and dehydration
✗ Avoid high-caffeine beverages

Cannabis

✓ Generally safe
✗ May counteract appetite suppression
✗ Edibles worsen GI symptoms

Nicotine

✓ No direct interaction
✗ Raises cardiovascular risk

Recreational stimulants

✗ Strongly discouraged
✗ High cardiovascular and dehydration risk

Chapter 9

Semaglutide in Diabetes Management

Managing type 2 diabetes has evolved significantly over the past decade, shifting from a glucose-centric model to a broader, multifactorial approach that targets weight, cardiovascular health, kidney protection, and metabolic regulation. Semaglutide—a GLP-1 receptor agonist—has become one of the most important additions to this modern therapeutic toolkit. Unlike older medications that primarily lower blood glucose, semaglutide acts across multiple pathways, improving appetite regulation, insulin sensitivity, inflammation, cardiovascular risk markers, and body weight. These wide-ranging benefits position semaglutide not only as a glucose-lowering medication but as a true disease-modifying therapy.

This chapter explores how semaglutide fits within the broader diabetes-management pathway, particularly in relation to cornerstone treatments such as metformin, SGLT2 inhibitors, and insulin. It explains when semaglutide should be added, how other medications should be adjusted, and why GLP-1–based therapies are increasingly being used earlier in the treatment journey. Through real-world case studies, the chapter demonstrates how semaglutide can intensify therapy when glucose control is inadequate, reduce reliance on insulin, and provide powerful cardiometabolic protection.

By examining evidence-based mechanisms, clinical guidelines, and practical prescribing strategies, this chapter provides a comprehensive understanding of semaglutide's role in preventing complications and improving long-term outcomes for people living with type 2 diabetes.

Role Relative to Metformin, SGLT2 Inhibitors, Insulin

Semaglutide plays an increasingly important role in type 2 diabetes management due to its dual ability to improve glycaemic control and promote substantial weight loss. Its place in therapy is best understood in the context of the broader diabetes treatment pathway, particularly how it compares and complements cornerstone therapies such as metformin, SGLT2 inhibitors, and insulin.

Semaglutide and Metformin: When and Why to Add GLP-1 Therapy

Getting to Know Semaglutide and Other GLP-1–Based Medications

Metformin is widely recognized as the first-line therapy for type 2 diabetes mellitus (T2DM) globally, which stems from its demonstrated effectiveness in lowering blood glucose levels, its favourable safety profile, low cost, weight neutrality, and associated cardiovascular benefits. This is corroborated by multiple guidelines and research studies, indicating that metformin significantly aids in achieving glycaemic control and improving overall health outcomes for individuals with T2DM [579-581]. Its efficacy was initially established through landmark studies, such as the UK Prospective Diabetes Study (UKPDS), which highlighted both its glucose-lowering capabilities and its role in reducing cardiovascular mortality among overweight populations [579, 580].

Metformin

Metformin is an oral medication classified as a biguanide. It is used to:

- lower high blood glucose
- improve insulin sensitivity
- reduce the risk of diabetes complications
- support long-term metabolic health

It is especially effective in people with insulin resistance, obesity, and early type 2 diabetes.

Metformin does not stimulate insulin production; instead, it improves how the body uses and processes glucose.

Metformin improves blood glucose control through several interconnected metabolic pathways, with its primary effects occurring in the liver, muscles, and gastrointestinal system. Its most significant action is the reduction of glucose production in the liver. In people with type 2 diabetes, the liver often produces excessive glucose—especially overnight—which leads to elevated fasting blood sugar. Metformin suppresses this overproduction by reducing gluconeogenesis, improving the liver's response to insulin, and decreasing unnecessary glucose release. This mechanism accounts for the majority of metformin's glucose-lowering effect.

In addition to regulating liver function, metformin enhances insulin sensitivity in muscle and other tissues. Insulin resistance is a hallmark of type 2 diabetes, meaning cells do not respond effectively to insulin, leaving glucose circulating in the bloodstream. Metformin helps increase glucose uptake into muscle cells, enables insulin to work more efficiently, and gradually lowers circulating insulin levels. These improvements support better metabolic control and reduce overall physiological stress on the body.

Metformin also acts on the gastrointestinal tract. It slows the absorption of glucose in the intestine and alters the gut microbiome in ways that positively influence metabolism. Some evidence suggests it may modestly increase natural GLP-1 secretion, which can enhance satiety and glucose regulation. These gut-related actions explain why gastrointestinal symptoms—such as nausea, bloating, or diarrhoea—are relatively common when patients first start metformin.

Beyond its primary metabolic effects, metformin offers several additional clinical benefits. It is weight neutral and may even promote mild weight loss, unlike many older diabetes medications. It carries a very low risk of hypoglycaemia because it does not stimulate insulin secretion. Long-term data show cardiovascular protection, with reduced rates of heart attack and stroke. Metformin is also considered safe for extended use, backed by decades of evidence, and emerging research suggests it may lower the risk of certain cancers.

Metformin is used widely across metabolic conditions. It remains the first-line treatment for type 2 diabetes and is also prescribed for prediabetes to delay or prevent progression to diabetes. In polycystic ovary syndrome (PCOS), metformin improves insulin resistance and supports ovulation. It is also used in individuals with obesity-related insulin resistance to help improve metabolic function.

Despite these advantages, metformin alone may not suffice for many patients over time, prompting the need for additional therapies. For those whose HbA1c levels remain above target despite adequate metformin dosing, or when weight loss or cardiovascular risk is a clinical priority, the addition of glucagon-like peptide-1 (GLP-1) receptor agonists, such as semaglutide, becomes a salient option. Semaglutide has been especially noted for achieving substantial HbA1c reduction while promoting weight loss and reducing cardiovascular risks [40, 77, 582]. The evidence from meta-analyses and randomized controlled trials suggests that GLP-1 receptor agonists not only enhance glycaemic control but also confer cardiovascular benefits [52, 77, 583].

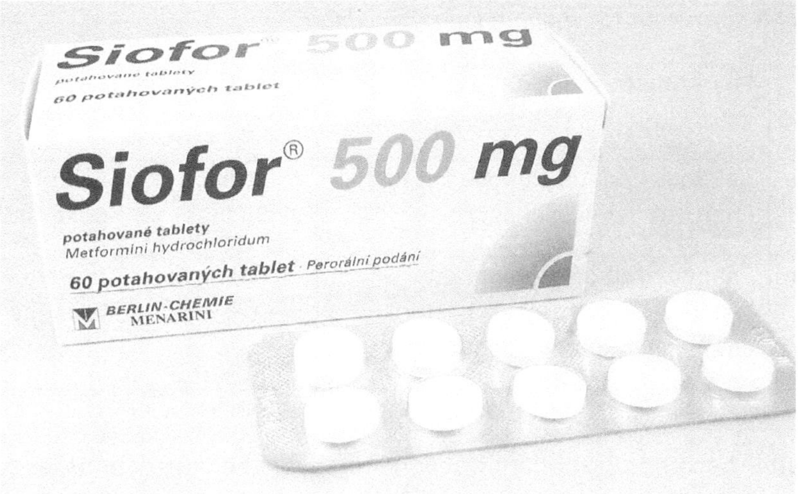

Figure 29: Siofor, proprietary medicinal product, 1 tablet contains 500 mg of metformin. Manufacturer Berlin-Chemie. Tomino de WS, CC BY-SA 4.0, via Wikimedia Commons.

In situations where patients either cannot tolerate metformin or where it is contraindicated, the initiation of GLP-1 receptor agonists like semaglutide is recommended. For instance, explorative analyses from clinical trials have indicated that semaglutide leads to significant reductions in both HbA1c and body weight, alongside improvements in cardiovascular risk profiles [46, 52, 582]. This dual benefit makes semaglutide a valuable option for patients facing these specific circumstances.

Semaglutide is commonly introduced when:

- HbA1c remains above target despite adequate metformin dosing
- Weight loss is a clinical priority
- Cardiovascular risk is elevated
- Metformin is not tolerated or contraindicated

Given the multifaceted approach to managing T2DM, healthcare professionals frequently consider the introduction of therapies such as semaglutide under the aforementioned scenarios—targeting adequate glycaemic control, prioritizing weight management, addressing cardiovascular concerns, or accommodating for metformin intolerance.

Table 12: How Metformin and Semaglutide actions differ.

Medication	Mechanism	Effect on Weight	Key Benefits
Metformin	Reduces hepatic glucose output; improves insulin sensitivity	Neutral or slight loss	Long-term safety, low cost
Semaglutide	Enhances glucose-dependent insulin secretion; slows gastric emptying; reduces appetite	Significant weight loss	Powerful glycaemic lowering and CV protection

Semaglutide often becomes the preferred second-line agent because it provides stronger HbA1c reduction and clinically meaningful weight loss, addressing two core drivers of diabetes progression.

Semaglutide and SGLT2 Inhibitors: Complementary Effects

SGLT2 inhibitors, including empagliflozin and dapagliflozin, are essential medications in diabetes management, offering benefits beyond glycaemic control, such as improvements in cardiovascular health, chronic kidney disease (CKD), and heart failure outcomes. Evidence supports the cardiovascular benefits of these agents, with studies indicating significant reductions in major adverse cardiovascular events (MACE) and hospitalizations for heart failure associated with these medications [584-587]. Both empagliflozin and dapagliflozin have been shown to reduce hospitalization for heart failure and provide renal protective effects across diverse populations [587-589]. Specifically, the EMPEROR trials demonstrated significant reductions in the combined risk of cardiovascular death or hospitalization for heart failure in patients administered empagliflozin, irrespective of diabetes status or left ventricular ejection fraction [585, 586].

Empagliflozin and Dapagliflozin

Empagliflozin and dapagliflozin are medications used to treat type 2 diabetes and improve cardiovascular and kidney health. They belong to a drug class called SGLT2 inhibitors (sodium–glucose co-transporter 2 inhibitors), which work by helping the kidneys remove excess glucose from the bloodstream through urine.

Empagliflozin

- Brand names: Jardiance, Glyxambi (combination), Synjardy (with metformin)
- Manufacturer: Boehringer Ingelheim / Eli Lilly

- Approved for:
    - Type 2 diabetes
    - Heart failure (with reduced or preserved ejection fraction)
    - Chronic kidney disease (CKD)
    - Reducing risk of cardiovascular death in adults with type 2 diabetes and heart disease

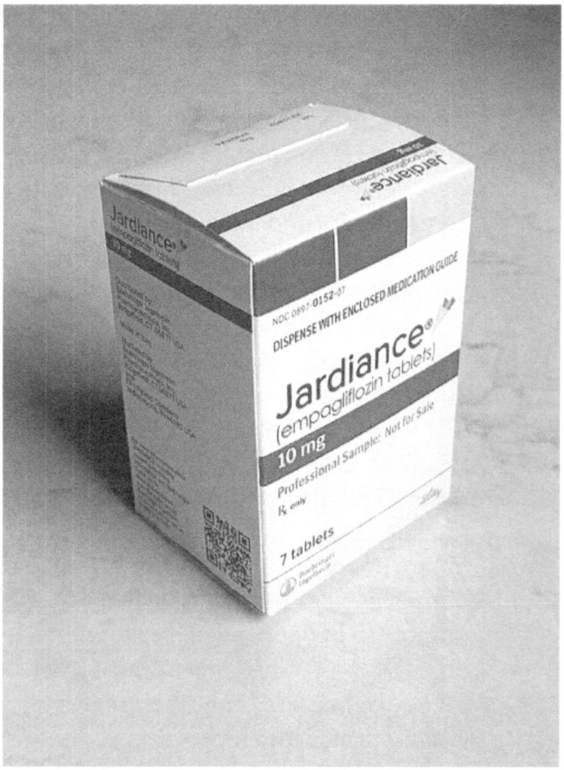

Figure 30: A box of Jardiance (empagliflozin) 10mg tablets. Grendelkhan, CC BY-SA 4.0, via Wikimedia Commons.

Dapagliflozin

- Brand names: Farxiga (US) / Forxiga (global)
- Manufacturer: AstraZeneca
- Approved for:
    - Type 2 diabetes
    - Heart failure (HFrEF and HFpEF)
    - Chronic kidney disease (CKD)

- Reducing risk of hospitalisation for heart failure

Both medications were originally designed for glucose control but are now widely used for their cardiovascular and renal protective effects, even in people without diabetes.

Empagliflozin and dapagliflozin work by blocking SGLT2 transporters in the kidneys. Under normal circumstances, these transporters reabsorb glucose from the urine back into the bloodstream. When SGLT2 is inhibited, more glucose is excreted through urine, which leads to lower blood glucose levels, reduced circulating insulin, and a daily loss of approximately 200–300 calories. These medications also cause a small reduction in blood pressure and lower filtration pressure within the kidneys, providing additional renal protection. Because their mechanism does not rely on insulin, they carry a low risk of hypoglycaemia and pair well with other glucose-lowering treatments, including metformin, semaglutide, and insulin.

The health benefits of these medications extend well beyond glucose control. Both empagliflozin and dapagliflozin reduce HbA1c by around 0.5–1.0%, particularly in individuals with insulin resistance. They also support modest weight loss—typically 2–3 kilograms—due to caloric loss via glucose excretion. Blood pressure reduction is another recognised benefit, with systolic pressure dropping by an average of 3–5 mmHg and diastolic pressure by 1–2 mmHg. Importantly, these drugs provide strong cardiovascular protection, lowering the risk of heart failure hospitalisation and, in the case of empagliflozin, reducing cardiovascular death. They also improve symptoms and long-term outcomes in people with heart failure, even in the absence of diabetes.

Kidney protection is another major therapeutic advantage. SGLT2 inhibitors slow the progression of chronic kidney disease, reduce proteinuria (albumin leakage), and lower the risk of requiring dialysis. For this reason, both empagliflozin and dapagliflozin are now considered foundational therapy in CKD management.

Despite their benefits, these medications can cause side effects, largely related to glucose excretion in urine. Common issues include genital yeast infections—more frequent in women—urinary tract infections, increased urination, and dehydration or dizziness due to mild diuretic effects. Rare but serious risks include euglycaemic diabetic ketoacidosis (DKA), Fournier's gangrene (a severe perineal infection), and significant volume depletion in frail or elderly individuals.

There are also situations where SGLT2 inhibitors should not be used. They are typically avoided in people with type 1 diabetes because of the high risk of DKA, in those with severe kidney impairment (eGFR below 20–25 mL/min, depending on the specific drug), individuals with recurrent genital infections, and those susceptible to dehydration or low blood pressure.

Summary

Feature	Empagliflozin	Dapagliflozin
Class	SGLT2 inhibitor	SGLT2 inhibitor
Main Use	Type 2 diabetes; heart/renal protection	Type 2 diabetes; heart/renal protection
Weight Loss	Modest (2–3 kg)	Modest (2–3 kg)
Heart Benefits	Strongest evidence for ↓ cardiovascular death	Strongest evidence for ↓ hospitalisation for heart failure
Kidney Benefits	Proven in CKD	Proven in CKD

These agents primarily exert their glucose-lowering effects by inhibiting the SGLT2 protein in the renal proximal tubule, which decreases glucose reabsorption and increases glucose excretion in the urine. This mechanism aids glycaemic control while also inducing favourable diuretic and natriuretic effects, contributing to cardiovascular and renal benefits [590, 591]. Notably, combining SGLT2 inhibitors with glucagon-like peptide-1 (GLP-1) receptor agonists, such as semaglutide, demonstrates a synergistic approach. While SGLT2 inhibitors promote glucose elimination and weight loss through osmotic diuresis, semaglutide enhances insulin secretion, suppresses glucagon secretion, slows gastric emptying, and reduces appetite, leading to greater improvements in glycaemic control, weight management, and a lower risk of hypoglycaemia compared to either treatment alone [585, 592, 593].

This combined therapeutic strategy yields multiple benefits, characterized by additive reductions in HbA1c levels, enhanced weight loss, improved cardiovascular risk profiles, and low incidences of hypoglycaemia when these agents are not used in conjunction with insulin or sulfonylureas [594, 595]. Given these complementary actions, the combination of SGLT2 inhibitors and GLP-1 receptor agonists is increasingly regarded as a comprehensive metabolic optimization strategy, particularly in patients with obesity, cardiovascular disease, or CKD, where managing glycaemia and reducing cardiovascular risk are paramount [584, 596].

The distinct mechanisms of action of SGLT2 inhibitors and GLP-1 receptor agonists support a comprehensive strategy for managing type 2 diabetes and its associated complications, ultimately contributing to improved patient outcomes and quality of life for individuals with diabetes and coexisting conditions.

Semaglutide and Insulin: When GLP-1 Therapy May Replace or Reduce Insulin

Insulin therapy remains a cornerstone in the management of advanced or decompensated diabetes; however, it is often associated with several adverse effects, including weight gain, hypoglycaemia, and increasing insulin requirements over time. Large doses of exogenous insulin can lead to hyperinsulinaemia and an average weight gain in individuals with Type 2 diabetes (T2D) of approximately 3-9% over baseline weight [597]. Additionally, traditional insulin regimens have been shown to increase the risk of hypoglycaemia, particularly when high doses are used without adequate monitoring [386]. Consequently, there is often a progressive increase in total daily insulin requirements, underscoring the complexity and potential ineffectiveness of prolonged insulin therapy alone [598].

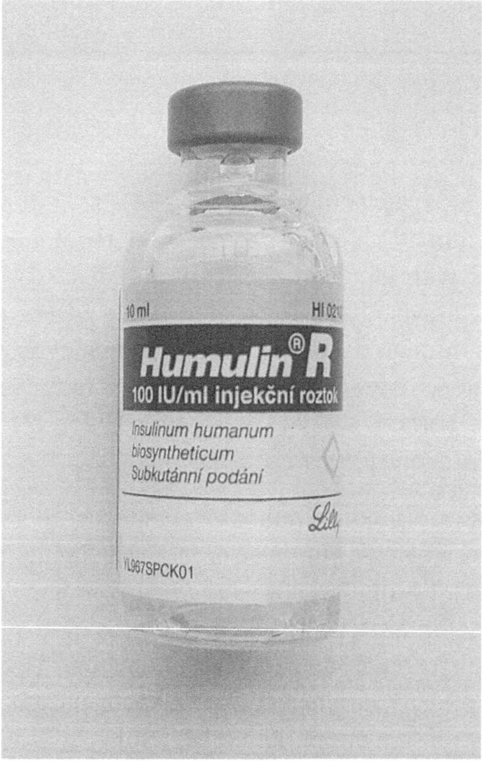

Figure 31: Human insulin 100IU/ml vial. Wesalius, CC BY 4.0, via Wikimedia Commons.

Semaglutide presents a compelling alternative or adjunct to traditional insulin therapy. It has been shown that adding semaglutide, a GLP-1 receptor agonist, can significantly reduce the need for insulin doses, with reductions reported between 20% and 40% in daily requirements [383, 599]. Moreover, semaglutide facilitates weight loss, contrasting with the weight gain typically associated with insulin therapy [599]. Its mechanism allows for improved post-prandial control and a decreased risk of hypoglycaemia due to its glucose-dependent insulinotropic effects [600]. In clinical trials, semaglutide has been shown to improve HbA1c levels more effectively than simply increasing insulin doses, while also promoting a reduction in body weight, which can help mitigate long-term cardiovascular risks associated with diabetes [599].

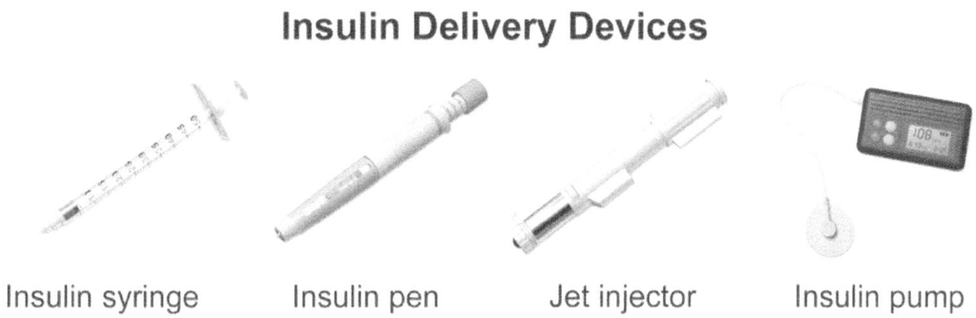

Figure 32: Insulin Delivery Devices. BruceBlaus, CC BY-SA 4.0, via Wikimedia Commons.

The recommendation to consider semaglutide before initiating insulin therapy is supported by clinical guidelines, particularly when HbA1c levels are not excessively high and when catabolic symptoms are not present [383, 599]. This paradigm shift highlights the recognition that GLP-1 therapies may address underlying metabolic dysfunction with fewer risks than intensifying insulin therapy, as they offer a simplified approach to managing diabetes more effectively [601]. In cases where traditional insulin regimens prove inadequate for glycaemic control, switching to or combining semaglutide with basal insulin may enhance overall treatment outcomes with fewer adverse effects [386, 599].

While insulin therapy remains crucial for patients with advanced diabetes, the drawbacks of weight gain, hypoglycaemia, and progressively increasing insulin doses pose considerable challenges. Semaglutide, as a complementary treatment, provides a valuable option to optimize diabetes management by alleviating these issues, promoting weight loss, and enhancing glycaemic control without heightening the risk of hypoglycaemia.

Table 13: Summary - Where Semaglutide Fits in Diabetes Treatment.

Therapy	Typical Position in Treatment Pathway	Weight Impact	Hypoglycaemia Risk	Cardiometabolic Benefits
Metformin	First line	Neutral	Very low	Moderate
SGLT2 inhibitors	Add-on after metformin	Mild loss	Very low	Strong CV & renal benefits
Semaglutide (GLP-1 RA)	Preferred second/third line; sometimes first-line if weight/CV risk high	Significant loss	Very low	Strong metabolic & CV benefits
Insulin	Reserved for advanced disease or severe hyperglycaemia	Gain	Moderate–high	Essential when needed

In modern diabetes management, semaglutide is often used before insulin and alongside metformin or SGLT2 inhibitors, reflecting its potent glycaemic, cardiovascular, and weight-loss benefits.

How to Adjust Other Medications

The initiation of semaglutide in diabetes and weight management necessitates careful adjustment of other medications, particularly insulin and sulfonylureas, due to semaglutide's capacity to improve insulin sensitivity, lower blood glucose, and reduce appetite. This multifaceted effect can significantly alter glycaemic control and treatment requirements, emphasizing the importance of these adjustments being made under professional supervision [602, 603].

Insulin Adjustments: Semaglutide often reduces blood glucose levels sufficiently to warrant a decrease in insulin dosages, particularly prandial insulins. When semaglutide is introduced, the risk of hypoglycaemia can increase, as evidenced by findings that highlight the need for a decrease of 10-20% in basal insulin and a more substantial reduction (20-40%) in prandial insulin doses [383, 603, 604]. This recommendation is derived from a variety of clinical trials that show considerable benefits and a lower risk of hypoglycaemia when such reductions are implemented at the initiation of semaglutide therapy [601, 605].

Sulfonylureas: Similar adjustments are warranted for sulfonylureas, which stimulate insulin secretion independently of blood glucose levels, thus leading to an increased risk of hypoglycaemia when combined with semaglutide. The typical practice is to reduce the sulfonylurea dose substantially (by 25-50%) or discontinue it altogether when starting semaglutide, as the latter improves endogenous insulin effectiveness [385, 601]. Clinical evidence indicates that this adjustment can mitigate the hypoglycaemic risk while maintaining effective glycaemic control [601, 605].

Sulfonylureas are among the oldest and most widely used oral medications for managing type 2 diabetes. They work by stimulating the pancreas to release more insulin, which lowers blood glucose levels. Although they are effective and affordable, sulfonylureas come with notable limitations—particularly the risks of hypoglycaemia and weight gain. For this reason, their use has declined in favour of newer, safer medications such as GLP-1 receptor agonists (e.g., semaglutide) and SGLT2 inhibitors. Understanding how sulfonylureas work and where they fit in modern diabetes care is essential for safe clinical practice.

Sulfonylureas belong to a class of drugs known as insulin secretagogues, meaning they trigger insulin release from pancreatic β-cells regardless of the person's current blood glucose level. Common medications in this class include gliclazide, glipizide, glimepiride, and glyburide (glibenclamide). They are typically taken once or twice daily and have remained popular due to their rapid glucose-lowering effects and low cost.

These medications work directly on the pancreas. By binding to sulfonylurea receptors (SUR1) on β-cells, they close potassium channels, causing depolarisation of the cell membrane. This, in turn, opens calcium channels, leading to insulin secretion—even when blood glucose is normal or low. Because this mechanism is glucose-independent, sulfonylureas can quickly reduce high blood sugar but also increase the risk of dangerous hypoglycaemia.

Sulfonylureas retain several important benefits. They are highly effective at lowering HbA1c, typically achieving reductions of around 1–1.5%, which is comparable to metformin. They are also inexpensive and widely accessible, making them a practical option in settings where newer drugs may not be available. Their effect is fast, with many patients experiencing improved glucose levels within days.

However, sulfonylureas carry several limitations and risks. Hypoglycaemia is the most significant concern, as these medications stimulate insulin release irrespective of glucose levels. Symptoms such as shaking, sweating, dizziness, confusion, and, in severe cases, loss of consciousness can occur. The risk is heightened in older adults, individuals with kidney impairment, people who skip meals, and those taking semaglutide or insulin alongside a sulfonylurea. Because of this, dose adjustments are often required when semaglutide is introduced.

Weight gain is another common drawback. Chronic insulin stimulation encourages fat storage, leading to weight increases of 1–3 kg on average. This can be counterproductive in people with obesity or insulin resistance. Additionally, sulfonylureas tend to lose effectiveness over time as pancreatic β-cells fatigue, often necessitating additional medications or a switch to newer therapeutic options. While older sulfonylureas were associated with increased cardiovascular risk, modern agents are considered safer—though they still do not provide the heart and kidney protection seen with newer drug classes.

Sulfonylureas are generally unsuitable for individuals with unpredictable eating patterns, a high risk of hypoglycaemia, significant kidney impairment, frailty, or those who are aiming for weight loss. They are also problematic when used concurrently with semaglutide unless carefully dose-adjusted. Despite this, sulfonylureas remain useful in certain situations, such as when patients cannot afford newer agents, when rapid blood glucose reduction is required, or as short-term therapy in individuals with preserved pancreatic function.

In summary, sulfonylureas are effective and inexpensive diabetes medications that increase insulin secretion and improve glycaemic control. However, their risks—especially hypoglycaemia and weight gain—and their gradual loss of effectiveness limit their long-term utility. When used alongside modern therapies such as semaglutide, careful dose reduction or discontinuation is often needed to maintain safety and optimise outcomes.

Metformin and SGLT2 Inhibitors: Notably, metformin typically does not require dosage adjustments when starting semaglutide due to its complementary mechanism of action, which aids in weight management and supports insulin sensitivity with a low risk of hypoglycaemia [604, 606]. In contrast, SGLT2 inhibitors (e.g., empagliflozin) often pair well with semaglutide, showing no necessary adjustments while offering additive cardiovascular benefits [383, 606].

Other Medications: The initiation of semaglutide may necessitate indirect adjustments to antihypertensives and lipid-lowering medications due to weight loss and improvements in insulin sensitivity that can lower blood pressure and lipid levels [604, 607]. Psychological medications known for contributing to weight gain may also need re-evaluation during semaglutide therapy [605].

Monitoring Protocols: It's critical to include robust monitoring practices during the initial weeks of semaglutide treatment. Frequent checks on glucose levels (utilizing finger-stick or continuous glucose monitoring) are imperative to guide further medication adjustments and ensure safety [20, 605].

> The integration of semaglutide into diabetes management strategies necessitates substantial adjustments to other pharmacological agents to mitigate risks such as hypoglycaemia and to optimize therapeutic outcomes. These adjustments should reflect established clinical guidelines and be carried out under close medical supervision.

Case Studies Showing Treatment Intensification

Below are several case studies illustrating treatment intensification in type 2 diabetes using semaglutide. Each scenario shows how semaglutide fits into modern diabetes management pathways—particularly when metformin or other oral agents are no longer sufficient.

Case Study 1: Metformin Failure → Add Semaglutide

Patient Profile

- **Age:** 52
- **BMI:** 33
- **HbA1c:** 8.3%
- **Current treatment:** Metformin 1000 mg twice daily
- **Comorbidities:** Hypertension, NAFLD

Clinical Challenge

Despite maximal metformin dosing and lifestyle changes, HbA1c remains above target. Patient reports strong appetite, late-night snacking, and difficulty losing weight.

Treatment Intensification

Step 1: Add semaglutide 0.25 mg weekly → titrate to 1.0 mg over 8 weeks.
Step 2: Continue metformin.
Step 3: Provide education on nausea management and smaller meals.

Outcomes (12–16 weeks)

- HbA1c ↓ from 8.3% → 6.7%
- Weight ↓ 7% of initial body weight
- Liver enzymes improved (ALT ↓)

- Blood pressure modestly reduced

Key Teaching Point

Semaglutide is a highly effective second-line agent when metformin alone is inadequate, offering glycaemic and weight-loss benefits without increasing hypoglycaemia risk.

Case Study 2: Metformin + Sulfonylurea → Hypoglycaemia Risk After Semaglutide Start

Patient Profile

- **Age:** 68
- **BMI:** 29
- **HbA1c:** 9.1%
- **Current treatment:** Metformin + gliclazide
- **Comorbidities:** Early CKD (eGFR 55), osteoarthritis

Clinical Challenge

High HbA1c requires intensification. Sulfonylurea poses hypoglycaemia risk, especially in older adults.

Treatment Intensification

Step 1: Start semaglutide 0.25 mg → up-titrate.
Step 2: Reduce gliclazide dose by 50% immediately.
Step 3: Stop gliclazide completely once semaglutide reaches 0.5 mg.

Outcomes (3–4 months)

- HbA1c ↓ from 9.1% → 7.0%
- Hypoglycaemia episodes dropped to zero
- Weight ↓ 4 kg
- Kidney function stable

Key Teaching Point

When adding semaglutide to a sulfonylurea, dose reduction or discontinuation is essential to prevent hypoglycaemia.

Case Study 3: Metformin + SGLT2 Inhibitor → Inadequate Control → Add Semaglutide

Patient Profile

- **Age:** 44
- **BMI:** 38
- **HbA1c:** 8.7%
- **Current treatment:** Metformin + empagliflozin
- **Comorbidities:** PCOS, dyslipidaemia

Clinical Challenge

Despite dual therapy, HbA1c remains high. Weight loss is a priority.

Treatment Intensification

Step 1: Add semaglutide while continuing both metformin and SGLT2 inhibitor.
Step 2: Monitor hydration (SGLT2 inhibitors cause mild diuresis).
Step 3: Reinforce protein intake and resistance training.

Outcomes (6 months)

- HbA1c ↓ to 6.3%
- Weight ↓ 12%
- Triglycerides ↓ 30%
- Menstrual cycle becomes regular due to improved insulin resistance

Key Teaching Point

The combination of Metformin + SGLT2 inhibitor + GLP-1 RA is one of the most effective non-insulin regimens for glucose control, weight loss, and cardiometabolic health.

Case Study 4: Longstanding Diabetes on Basal Insulin → Switch to Semaglutide-Based Regimen

Patient Profile

- **Age:** 61
- **BMI:** 32
- **HbA1c:** 9.4%
- **Current treatment:**
    - Metformin

  - Basal insulin 40 units nightly

- **Comorbidities:** Hypertension, diabetic neuropathy

Clinical Challenge

Insulin doses are increasing, weight is rising, and HbA1c remains high. Patient desires to lower insulin use.

Treatment Intensification

Step 1: Add semaglutide 0.25 mg weekly.
Step 2: Reduce basal insulin by 20% to avoid hypoglycaemia.
Step 3: Titrate semaglutide to 1.0 mg.

Outcomes (4–6 months)

- HbA1c ↓ to 7.1%
- Insulin dose ↓ from 40 units → 10 units
- Weight ↓ 8%
- Fewer nocturnal hypoglycaemia episodes

Key Teaching Point

Semaglutide can allow insulin de-escalation, improving glycaemia and weight outcomes while reducing risks.

Case Study 5: Severe Obesity + Diabetes → High-Dose Semaglutide for Dual Benefit

Patient Profile

- **Age:** 37
- **BMI:** 45
- **HbA1c:** 7.9%
- **Current treatment:** Metformin only
- **Comorbidities:** Sleep apnoea, NAFLD

Clinical Challenge

Obesity is the primary metabolic driver. Patient prefers non-surgical weight loss.

Treatment Intensification

Step 1: Use semaglutide titrated to 2.4 mg (Wegovy) for weight management and glucose control.
Step 2: Introduce resistance exercise plan to preserve muscle.

Outcomes (1 year)

- HbA1c ↓ to 5.9% (near remission range)
- Weight ↓ 20%
- Liver fat markedly reduced
- Sleep apnoea symptoms improved

Key Teaching Point

High-dose semaglutide (Wegovy) offers powerful glycaemic improvement even in individuals with severe obesity and early diabetes.

Case Study 6: Intensification in a Patient Declining Insulin Therapy

Patient Profile

- **Age:** 58
- **BMI:** 31
- **HbA1c:** 10.2%
- **Current treatment:** Metformin + sitagliptin (DPP-4 inhibitor)
- **Comorbidities:** Hyperlipidaemia

Clinical Challenge

Patient strongly prefers to avoid insulin. DPP-4 inhibitor offers limited benefit.

Treatment Intensification

Step 1: Stop sitagliptin (DPP-4 inhibitors should not be combined with GLP-1 RAs).
Step 2: Start semaglutide.
Step 3: Reinforce lifestyle and glucose monitoring.

Outcomes (3–6 months)

- HbA1c ↓ from 10.2% → 7.4%
- Weight ↓ 6%
- Marked reduction in post-meal glucose spikes

Key Teaching Point

Semaglutide is often the best next step before insulin, particularly in patients who want a non-insulin option.

Case Study 7: Diabetes With Cardiovascular Disease → Add Semaglutide for Cardio-Protection

Patient Profile

- **Age:** 72
- **BMI:** 28
- **HbA1c:** 7.5%
- **Current treatment:** Metformin + SGLT2 inhibitor
- **Comorbidities:** Previous heart attack, peripheral artery disease

Clinical Challenge

Glucose control is acceptable—but cardiovascular risk is very high.

Treatment Intensification

Step 1: Add semaglutide 0.25 mg → 1.0 mg.
Step 2: Continue SGLT2 inhibitor for heart/kidney protection.

Outcomes (6–12 months)

- Modest weight loss (4–5 kg)
- HbA1c ↓ to 6.5%
- Improved walking distance due to reduced claudication
- Cardiovascular risk reduction supported by evidence (SUSTAIN-6, SELECT trials)

Key Teaching Point

Semaglutide is used not just for glucose control but also for cardiovascular risk reduction, even in patients with good baseline glycaemia.

Across multiple patient scenarios, several consistent patterns emerge regarding the use of semaglutide in diabetes management and treatment intensification.

1. Semaglutide reliably improves glycaemic control—even in difficult cases.

Patients with HbA1c levels ranging from moderate elevation (7.5–8.5%) to very high (>10%) experienced substantial reductions, often reaching or approaching target levels within 3–6 months. This demonstrates semaglutide's strong glucose-lowering effect across different disease severities and backgrounds.

2. Significant weight loss is a consistent secondary benefit.

Weight reductions ranged from 4–20%, with the largest losses seen at higher semaglutide doses or when combined with structured lifestyle strategies. This weight loss contributed to improvements in blood pressure, lipid profiles, NAFLD, and sleep apnoea.

3. Semaglutide supports treatment simplification by reducing insulin requirements.

In patients previously on basal insulin, adding semaglutide led to marked insulin dose reductions and fewer hypoglycaemia episodes, demonstrating its ability to de-escalate insulin therapy while still improving glycaemia.

4. Sulfonylurea use requires caution and dose reduction to prevent hypoglycaemia.

Case studies confirm that hypoglycaemia risk rises significantly when sulfonylureas and semaglutide are combined. Safe practice involves reducing or discontinuing sulfonylureas once semaglutide is introduced.

5. Combining semaglutide with SGLT2 inhibitors provides powerful metabolic synergy.

This combination produced some of the most impressive improvements in HbA1c, weight, triglycerides, insulin resistance, menstrual regularity (in PCOS), and cardiometabolic outcomes—highlighting a modern, highly effective non-insulin regimen.

6. Semaglutide can be an alternative to starting insulin.

In patients reluctant to initiate insulin—or whose β-cell function remains adequate—semaglutide provides a strong, non-insulin path to improve control, often reducing HbA1c dramatically.

7. Benefits extend beyond glycaemia to cardiovascular and hepatic health.

Patients with cardiovascular disease, NAFLD, dyslipidaemia, or metabolic syndrome showed measurable improvements in:

- liver enzymes
- triglycerides
- blood pressure
- walking tolerance
- cardiovascular risk markers

This aligns with major trials showing GLP-1 receptor agonists reduce cardiovascular events.

8. Semaglutide is suitable across a wide range of patient profiles.

The cases demonstrate its efficacy in:

- older adults
- individuals with CKD
- severe obesity
- PCOS
- long-standing diabetes
- early diabetes
- high cardiovascular risk groups

This versatility underscores semaglutide's value as a comprehensive metabolic therapy.

The case studies collectively show that semaglutide:

- is a powerful tool for glycaemic control,
- consistently delivers meaningful weight loss,
- reduces cardiovascular and metabolic risks,
- allows tapering of higher-risk medications (especially sulfonylureas and insulin), and
- works synergistically with other modern therapies.

Hypoglycaemia Risk

Semaglutide is widely recognized for its efficacy in managing type 2 diabetes mellitus (T2DM) with a notably low risk of hypoglycaemia when used as monotherapy. This safety profile arises from several mechanisms governing its action. Firstly, semaglutide stimulates insulin secretion in a glucose-dependent manner, meaning it activates insulin release only when blood glucose levels are elevated, thus effectively avoiding hypoglycaemic episodes [52, 217, 608]. Secondly, it reduces glucagon secretion similarly in a glucose-dependent manner, allowing normal glucagon responses when blood sugar levels are low [217, 608]. Lastly, semaglutide's ability to enhance postprandial glucose regulation without inducing excessive insulin secretion is particularly advantageous [608].

The low hypoglycaemia risk is especially beneficial for vulnerable populations, such as older adults who may struggle with hypoglycaemia awareness and patients with prolonged diabetes histories who are more at risk for severe hypoglycaemia [609, 610]. Clinical studies affirm that semaglutide maintains a significantly lower incidence of hypoglycaemia compared to traditional therapies, particularly when used in combination with non-insulin medications like metformin and SGLT2 inhibitors, which tend to have complementary mechanisms that do not excessively lower blood sugar [51, 608].

While semaglutide is generally safe as a standalone treatment, the risk of hypoglycaemia can increase significantly when combined with other glucose-lowering agents that act independently of blood glucose levels. For example, sulfonylureas (e.g., gliclazide, glimepiride) can induce hypoglycaemia due to their ability to stimulate insulin secretion irrespective of blood glucose status, which may lead to dangerously low glucose levels, particularly when semaglutide is improving overall glucose control [20, 609]. The management of patients on these combinations may often require dose reductions of sulfonylureas by 50–100% [20, 150]. Similarly, the concurrent use of insulin can present challenges, as improved glycaemic control through semaglutide may render previously appropriate insulin doses excessive, typically requiring reductions of 10–30% for basal insulin when initiating therapy [20, 150].

Another crucial factor that could exacerbate hypoglycaemia risk when using semaglutide is reduced calorie intake, a common result of appetite suppression induced by GLP-1 receptor agonists [217, 608]. Patients might skip meals or consume very few calories, which can enhance the potential for hypoglycaemic events, especially in conjunction with insulin or sulfonylureas [608].

Vulnerable patient populations, including older adults with impaired awareness of hypoglycaemia, patients with renal insufficiency where insulin effects last longer, or those with irregular meal patterns or engaging in intense physical activity, require vigilant monitoring to mitigate the risk of hypoglycaemia [52, 610].

To prevent hypoglycaemia in patients on semaglutide therapy, several strategies can be employed: adjusting insulin or sulfonylurea dosages at the initiation of semaglutide treatment; ensuring regular and structured meal intake; increasing the frequency of glucose monitoring, especially in the early treatment stages; and educating patients on managing potential hypoglycaemic episodes and recognizing early symptoms [20, 150, 609]. Thoughtful management of these factors enables patients to maximize the benefits of semaglutide, enhancing glycaemic control while minimizing hypoglycaemia risk.

Semaglutide stands out as a safe option for diabetes management with a minimal risk of inducing hypoglycaemia when used as monotherapy or in conjunction with non-insulin agents. Nonetheless, awareness, careful monitoring, and proactive adjustments are essential when semaglutide is combined with other insulinotropic agents or in situations that may precipitate reduced calorie intake to ensure safety and optimize therapeutic outcomes.

Semaglutide Vs Tirzepatide in Diabetes Outcomes

The comparison between semaglutide and tirzepatide, two important medications for managing type 2 diabetes, highlights key differences in their mechanisms of action, efficacy in reducing HbA1c levels, and effects on weight loss and insulin sensitivity.

Mechanisms of Action: Tirzepatide is unique due to its dual mechanism, mimicking both glucagon-like peptide-1 (GLP-1) and glucose-dependent insulinotropic peptide (GIP) receptors. This dual action enhances its pharmacological effects compared to semaglutide, which selectively targets the GLP-1 receptor. The GIP component in tirzepatide has been shown to enhance insulin secretion and improve insulin sensitivity better than GLP-1 receptor agonists alone, thus providing a synergistic incretin effect that is not replicated by GLP-1 agonists [611-613].

Tirzepatide is marketed under two main brand names, depending on the therapeutic indication:

1. Mounjaro®
Indication: Type 2 diabetes
Manufacturer: Eli Lilly
Purpose:

- Improves glycaemic control
- Often used off-label for weight loss in some regions

2. Zepbound®
Indication: Chronic weight management (obesity or overweight with comorbidities)
Manufacturer: Eli Lilly
Purpose:

- FDA-approved specifically for weight loss
- Higher titration doses used compared with diabetes indication

HbA1c Reduction: Clinical trials, especially within the SURPASS program, indicate that tirzepatide consistently results in greater reductions in HbA1c levels compared to semaglutide. For example, tirzepatide treatment provides HbA1c reductions between 2.0% and 2.5%, with up to 92% of participants attaining HbA1c levels below 7.0% [3, 614]. Conversely, semaglutide leads to reductions of about 1.0% to 1.8%, with approximately 70–80% of patients reaching the same target [3, 615].

Weight Loss Effects: Both medications promote weight loss, yet tirzepatide appears to be more effective, facilitating an average weight reduction of 10-15%, and some patients may lose more than 20% at higher doses [614, 616]. In contrast, semaglutide yields around 5-7% weight loss at the 1.0 mg dose, with its higher dose formulation (2.4 mg for obesity management) achieving approximately 10-16% [617, 618]. The superior weight loss with tirzepatide is attributed to its dual action, which enhances appetite suppression and boosts fat metabolism [613, 619].

Improvement in Insulin Sensitivity and Beta-Cell Function: Research suggests that tirzepatide improves insulin sensitivity and beta-cell function more significantly than semaglutide, shown by lower fasting insulin levels and substantial reductions in fasting glucose [611, 620]. While semaglutide also improves insulin resistance, tirzepatide's effects are more pronounced, making it more suitable for patients with severe insulin resistance [619, 621].

Impact on Liver Fat and Non-Alcoholic Fatty Liver Disease (NAFLD): Studies indicate that tirzepatide reduces liver fat and improves conditions related to NAFLD more effectively than semaglutide, with reductions of 30-60% for tirzepatide versus 15-30% for semaglutide [614, 617]. This is particularly important given the high prevalence of liver disease in type 2 diabetes populations.

Cardiovascular Outcomes: Current findings show that semaglutide has established benefits for cardiovascular health, significantly lowering rates of major adverse cardiovascular events (MACE) [622]. However, comprehensive data regarding tirzepatide's cardiovascular effects is still forthcoming and may indicate comparable or superior outcomes once available [614, 623]. Preliminary evidence suggests improvements in weight, blood pressure, and lipid profiles with tirzepatide, hinting at potential cardiovascular benefits as well [611, 617].

Tolerability and Side Effects: Both semaglutide and tirzepatide are associated with gastrointestinal side effects such as nausea, vomiting, and diarrhea. However, tirzepatide may cause higher rates of nausea during initial dosing compared to semaglutide [611, 621]. The risk of hypoglycaemia remains low for both medications when not used alongside insulin or sulfonylureas [621, 624].

> While both semaglutide and tirzepatide are effective in managing type 2 diabetes, tirzepatide generally demonstrates superior efficacy, particularly in reducing HbA1c levels, promoting weight loss, and enhancing insulin sensitivity. This makes tirzepatide a compelling option for patients requiring intensive diabetes management, especially those with elevated HbA1c levels and significant insulin resistance.

Table 14: Summary: Semaglutide vs Tirzepatide for Diabetes.

Feature	Semaglutide	Tirzepatide
Mechanism	GLP-1 RA	Dual GIP + GLP-1 RA
HbA1c reduction	–1.0% to –1.8%	–2.0% to –2.5%
Weight loss	5–7% (diabetes dose)	10–15%
Insulin sensitivity	Improves	Improves more strongly
Fat reduction	Significant	Greater, especially visceral fat
Cardiovascular evidence	Strong, proven	Pending
Side effects	Well-established	Slightly more GI symptoms
Overall efficacy	Very strong	Stronger

Role in Preventing Diabetic Complications

Semaglutide has emerged as a pivotal therapeutic option in the management of type 2 diabetes, primarily because of its multifaceted effects that extend beyond simple blood glucose regulation. This glucagon-like peptide-1 (GLP-1) receptor agonist not only aids in glycaemic control but also plays a significant role in mitigating the progression of various diabetes-related complications, which include vascular, renal, ocular, and neurological impairments [18, 79]. The damage caused by diabetes impacts the blood vessels, nerves, kidneys, eyes, and heart over time, underscoring the importance of holistic management strategies that encompass not only glucose levels but also weight, blood pressure, and systemic inflammation [625].

A substantial body of clinical evidence, particularly the SUSTAIN-6 trial, underlines semaglutide's efficacy in providing cardiovascular protection, demonstrating a significant reduction in risks associated with heart attack, stroke, and cardiovascular mortality among patients with type 2 diabetes and pre-existing cardiovascular conditions. Notably, these cardiovascular benefits are realized without the hypoglycaemic risks commonly associated with other diabetes treatments [79, 626]. Moreover, semaglutide contributes to cardiovascular health by effectively improving lipid profiles and reducing visceral fat, which are critical factors in managing cardiovascular disease [627].

Furthermore, semaglutide has shown protective effects on kidney function, indicating its potential to prevent the onset and progression of chronic kidney disease (CKD). Long-term administration has been linked to improvements in markers of kidney health, thereby positioning semaglutide as a cornerstone in nephroprotective strategies for diabetic patients [628]. A recent expert perspective emphasizes the incorporation of GLP-1 receptor agonists, including semaglutide, into clinical guidelines aimed at managing diabetic kidney disease [628].

In terms of ocular health, semaglutide effectively lowers the risk of diabetic retinopathy through better glycaemic control [130]. However, caution is warranted for patients with advanced forms of the condition, as rapid improvements in glucose control can lead to transient worsening of retinopathy [626].

The medication also addresses the challenge of diabetic neuropathy, a common complication resulting from prolonged hyperglycaemia, which leads to nerve damage and associated symptoms like pain and numbness. By improving glucose stability and reducing inflammation, semaglutide has shown promise in decreasing the incidence of neuropathic symptoms [625].

Moreover, semaglutide's benefits extend to liver health, particularly in conditions like non-alcoholic fatty liver disease (NAFLD) and non-alcoholic steatohepatitis (NASH), which are prevalent in diabetic populations. Clinical studies highlight its role in reducing liver fat and improving liver function markers, thereby addressing a significant metabolic challenge in diabetes management [629, 630].

Lastly, semaglutide enhances vascular health, crucial for preventing diabetic foot complications, which are a significant source of morbidity in diabetes. Its effects on improving wound healing, reducing inflammation, and enhancing circulation are instrumental in minimizing the risks of ulcers and subsequent amputations [631].

Semaglutide transcends its primary role of glucose-lowering to emerge as a comprehensive disease-modifying agent in diabetes management. Its multifactorial benefits, spanning cardiovascular, renal, ocular, neurological, and hepatic health, underscore its significance in preserving metabolic health and preventing long-term complications associated with diabetes.

Chapter 10

Pharmacology and Drug Interactions

Understanding how a medication behaves inside the body—how it is absorbed, distributed, metabolised, and eliminated—is essential for safe and effective clinical use. This is especially true for long-acting therapies like semaglutide, where extended duration, delayed gastric emptying, and unique metabolic pathways influence everything from dosing schedules to drug-drug interactions. For many patients, semaglutide is added to already complex treatment regimens, making it crucial that clinicians appreciate the pharmacological features that underpin its benefits, limitations, and safety profile.

This chapter explores the key pharmacokinetic properties of semaglutide, including its high bioavailability, long half-life, slow absorption profile, and protein-based metabolism. These characteristics explain why semaglutide maintains steady plasma levels, requires only once-weekly dosing, and demonstrates minimal interactions with medications metabolised via the cytochrome P450 system. The chapter also examines how delayed gastric emptying affects the timing and absorption of certain oral medications—an especially important consideration for drugs requiring precise or rapid onset of action, such as oral contraceptives, levothyroxine, pain medicines, and selected CNS-active agents.

In addition, special attention is given to drug interactions involving insulin, sulfonylureas, and meglitinides, where the risk of hypoglycaemia increases significantly when combined with semaglutide. Practical guidance is provided on dose adjustments, monitoring, and clinical decision-making in these scenarios.

Finally, the chapter discusses how renal and hepatic function influence semaglutide pharmacology, and why the medication is generally safe in these populations despite the heightened vulnerability of patients with organ impairment. The issue of polypharmacy in older adults—one of the most common and clinically challenging contexts for semaglutide use—is also addressed, offering strategies to minimise risk and ensure safe integration into complex medication regimens.

Together, these sections provide a framework for understanding how semaglutide behaves in real-world clinical settings and how to optimise its use for safety, efficacy, and long-term therapeutic success.

Absorption, Half-Life, Metabolism, Elimination

Getting to Know Semaglutide and Other GLP-1–Based Medications

Semaglutide is a synthetic analogue of human glucagon-like peptide-1 (GLP-1), designed to enhance therapeutic efficacy while maintaining the fundamental functionalities associated with natural GLP-1. Notably, semaglutide shares approximately 94% sequence homology with native GLP-1, and several structural modifications have been made to extend its stability and action in vivo, allowing for once-weekly dosing rather than daily administration [60, 632].

One significant modification involves the truncation of the first six amino acids from the GLP-1 sequence. This truncation does not compromise its binding capability to GLP-1 receptors and is essential for optimizing the drug's clinical properties [60, 632]. Additionally, semaglutide features critical substitutions at positions 8 and 34, wherein the alanine (Ala) at position 8 is replaced with 2-aminoisobutyric acid, and the lysine (Lys) at position 34 is substituted with arginine (Arg). These modifications prevent proteolytic degradation by dipeptidyl peptidase-4 (DPP-4), significantly enhancing the compound's longevity and pharmacokinetic profile in the systemic circulation [60, 632].

Moreover, the amino acid at GLP-1 position 26 is acylated with a C-18 fatty acid chain. This modification boosts the hydrophobicity of the molecule and facilitates strong binding to serum albumin, creating a reservoir effect that prolongs the drug's half-life and, consequently, its glucose-regulating properties [60, 632]. This mechanism underlines the drug's ability to maintain significant levels of activity over an extended duration, allowing for less frequent dosing compared to previous GLP-1 analogues.

The structural alterations fundamentally transform semaglutide into a long-acting GLP-1 analogue that retains full agonistic activity at the GLP-1 receptor while overcoming the rapid metabolic degradation seen with its native counterpart or earlier formulations. These advancements contribute to improved outcomes in glycaemic control and appetite regulation, thereby offering substantial benefits for individuals managing type 2 diabetes and obesity [60, 632].

> Semaglutide's modifications—including the N-terminal truncation, strategic amino acid substitutions, and fatty acid acylation—collectively enhance its pharmacological profile, marking a significant advancement in GLP-1 receptor agonists. These innovations allow semaglutide to act effectively while being administered less frequently than previous versions, which is crucial for improving patient adherence and treatment efficacy [60, 632].

Absorption

Semaglutide is available in both injectable (Ozempic, Wegovy) and oral (Rybelsus) forms, each demonstrating distinctive absorption characteristics. For injectable semaglutide, subcutaneous administration results in a slow and gradual absorption profile from the injection site, leading to stable plasma drug levels throughout the week, with a bioavailability of approximately 89% [214]. The delayed absorption contributes to a steady state after 4–5 weeks of weekly dosing, which enhances patient compliance with the treatment regimen [45, 214].

Bioavailability refers to the proportion of a medication that successfully enters the bloodstream in an active form after it is administered. Not all of a drug dose is absorbed—some may break down, remain at the injection site, or be metabolised before reaching circulation. For injectable semaglutide, approximately 89% of the dose reaches the bloodstream. This means that if a person injects 1 mg, about 0.89 mg becomes available for the body to use, with only around 11% lost through natural biological processes. This level of absorption is considered very high for an injectable medication.

This high bioavailability has several important implications. First, it allows for reliable and predictable therapeutic effects, because nearly the entire administered dose enters systemic circulation. Second, it enables efficient dosing—smaller amounts of the drug produce strong clinical benefits. Third, because most of the medication is absorbed and semaglutide has a long half-life, the therapeutic effect remains stable throughout the week, making once-weekly dosing both practical and effective.

In contrast, the oral form of semaglutide (Rybelsus) has a bioavailability of only about 1%. Much of the dose is broken down in the stomach or lost during absorption, which is why oral formulations require significantly higher doses (e.g., 7–14 mg daily) compared with the very small weekly injectable doses (0.25–2.4 mg).

Put simply, 89% bioavailability means that almost all of the injected semaglutide is absorbed and usable by the body, which helps explain its strong clinical effect even at low weekly doses.

In contrast, oral semaglutide requires co-administration with an absorption enhancer, sodium N-(8-2-hydroxybenzoylamino) caprylate (SNAC). This enhancer facilitates better absorption across the gastrointestinal tract, although the bioavailability of oral semaglutide is notably low, around 1% [58, 218]. The absorption primarily occurs in the stomach and is sensitive to gastric conditions, necessitating administration on an empty stomach with a small volume of water, followed by fasting to maximize drug uptake [45, 101].

Half-Life

Half-life is a pharmacological term that refers to the amount of time it takes for the concentration of a drug in the bloodstream to decrease by 50%. Each medication has its own half-life, and this value determines how long the drug remains active in the body. For example, if a medication such as injectable semaglutide has a half-life of approximately seven days, this means that seven days after a dose is absorbed, only half of the drug remains in circulation. After another seven days, half of that remaining amount persists, and this pattern continues until the medication is gradually eliminated. Complete clearance requires several half-life cycles.

Half-life has significant clinical implications. It determines how frequently a drug must be taken. Medications with short half-lives require multiple daily doses to maintain therapeutic levels, while those with long half-lives—such as semaglutide—can be dosed as little as once per week. A longer half-life also creates steadier and more predictable drug levels in the body. This avoids sharp peaks and troughs, reduces side effects, and supports stable appetite and glucose control, which is particularly important in conditions like diabetes and obesity.

The long half-life of semaglutide also explains its slow onset and slow offset. Because it accumulates gradually in the body, several weeks may be needed to reach full therapeutic effect. Likewise, if side effects occur, they may take weeks to resolve. After stopping the medication, semaglutide may take four to six weeks to fully clear the system. This prolonged presence also influences dosing schedules: titration must be done slowly, typically increasing the dose every four weeks, to allow the body time to adjust.

Half-life is also important for safety considerations. Because semaglutide remains in the body for a long time, individuals planning pregnancy must discontinue it at least two months beforehand. Side effects, drug interactions, and considerations for surgical procedures—particularly those related to delayed gastric emptying—must also take the long half-life into account.

A simple way to understand half-life is to imagine a cup of water draining slowly through a small leak. A slow leak (long half-life) means the cup stays fuller for longer, while a fast leak (short half-life) empties quickly. Semaglutide's "slow leak" characteristics explain why it lasts a full week, provides smooth and consistent effects, is dosed only once weekly, and remains in the body long after treatment stops.

Semaglutide's pharmacokinetics are characterized by an exceptionally long half-life of approximately 165 hours (or about 7 days), allowing for the convenience of once-weekly dosing [16, 214]. This protracted half-life is advantageous for maintaining stable plasma concentrations that minimize fluctuations, thereby reducing the risks of drug-related side effects, such as nausea and hypoglycaemia [16] . Clinical studies have demonstrated that steady-state concentrations are achieved within 4–5 weeks, permitting gradual accumulation of the drug in therapeutic contexts [60, 214].

Metabolism

One of the important features of semaglutide's pharmacology is its metabolism. Unlike many drugs, semaglutide is not significantly metabolized by the cytochrome P450 (CYP450) enzyme system, leading to minimal drug-drug interactions [16, 214]; . The metabolism is primarily mediated through slow enzymatic degradation involving proteolytic cleavage and the beta-oxidation of its fatty acid side chain, which aligns with natural metabolic processes rather than traditional hepatic pathways [214, 633]. This reduces the need for dose adjustments in patients taking other medications, strengthening its position in polypharmacy scenarios typical in diabetic management [60].

Unlike many medications, semaglutide is not significantly metabolised by the cytochrome P450 (CYP450) enzyme system, which is one of the body's primary pathways for breaking down drugs. The CYP450 enzymes—particularly CYP3A4, CYP2D6, and CYP2C9—are responsible for metabolising a large proportion of prescription medications. When multiple drugs depend on the same CYP pathway, they can interfere with each other's metabolism. This may lead to reduced effectiveness, increased side effects, or dangerous accumulation of one or more medications in the bloodstream. Because semaglutide does *not* rely on CYP450 metabolism, it avoids this common cause of drug–drug interactions.

Instead, semaglutide is metabolised primarily through general proteolytic pathways—meaning it is broken down by enzymes that digest proteins throughout the body—and then cleared slowly by the kidneys and liver. This metabolic route does not compete with the pathways used by most other medications. As a result, semaglutide maintains stable, predictable blood levels even when taken alongside drugs that heavily use CYP450 enzymes. It also means that medications that inhibit or induce CYP450 activity (such as certain antibiotics, antifungals, antiepileptics, or herbal products like St. John's wort) have little or no effect on semaglutide's concentration or therapeutic impact.

This unique metabolic profile gives semaglutide a major safety advantage. Patients with complex medication regimens—for example, those with diabetes, cardiovascular disease, or multiple chronic conditions—are often at high risk for drug interactions. Since semaglutide bypasses the CYP450 system, clinicians can prescribe it with greater confidence that it will not destabilise other treatments. This reduces the need for frequent medication adjustments and makes semaglutide easier to integrate into personalised diabetes or obesity management plans.

Another important implication is its consistent pharmacokinetics across diverse patient populations. Foods, supplements, or genetic variations that influence CYP450 enzyme activity do not significantly alter semaglutide's metabolism. This contributes to its reliable once-weekly dosing and predictable clinical response. However, while CYP-related interactions are minimal, semaglutide's effects on gastric emptying can still influence the absorption of certain oral medications. Therefore, timing and monitoring remain important in specific cases—particularly with drugs requiring rapid or precise absorption, such as oral contraceptives or fast-acting pain medications.

Elimination

Elimination of semaglutide occurs through both renal and hepatic pathways, with very little unchanged drug appearing in urine. Studies reveal that only about 3.1% of the administered dose is excreted as intact semaglutide, indicating extensive breakdown into peptide fragments that are then cleared by the kidneys [16, 60]. Furthermore, the fatty acid components undergo hepatic metabolism, contributing to elimination via both urine and faeces [60]. Importantly, no dose modifications are necessary for patients with mild to moderate renal or hepatic impairment, although caution is advised in end-stage renal disease due to the lack of sufficient study data [60].

Renal and hepatic pathways are the two major routes the body uses to process and eliminate medications, toxins, and metabolic waste. Understanding them helps explain how drugs like semaglutide are cleared from the system and why certain medical conditions can affect medication safety.

Hepatic Pathway (Liver Clearance)

The hepatic pathway refers to drug processing and breakdown that occurs in the liver. The liver is the body's main chemical processing centre, responsible for:

- Metabolising drugs into inactive or more easily excreted forms
- Detoxifying chemicals
- Producing enzymes used to break down medications

Medications cleared via the hepatic pathway may be:

1. Metabolised by liver enzymes

Most commonly by the cytochrome P450 (CYP450) enzyme system. Some drugs are broken down quickly, others slowly—this depends on genetics, liver function, alcohol, other medications, and overall health.

2. Inactivated or modified

The liver may convert a drug into:

- A less active form
- A more active metabolite
- A water-soluble form for excretion through urine or bile

3. Excreted into bile

Drugs processed by the liver may leave the body through bile and be removed in faeces.

Why this matters

If a drug relies heavily on the hepatic pathway:

- Liver disease can slow clearance → higher drug levels
- Drug–drug interactions are more common
- Alcohol or herbal supplements may alter metabolism

Semaglutide, by contrast, uses minimal CYP450 hepatic metabolism, reducing the risk of interactions.

Renal Pathway (Kidney Clearance)

The renal pathway refers to drug elimination through the kidneys. The kidneys filter blood, removing:

- Excess salts
- Metabolites (broken-down drug components)
- Water-soluble drugs

Drugs cleared via the renal pathway may be:

1. Filtered directly into urine

If the drug is small and water-soluble, the kidneys filter it easily.

2. Secreted into the renal tubules

Some drugs bypass filtration and are actively transported into the urine.

3. Reabsorbed or eliminated depending on pH

Urine acidity can influence how quickly certain drugs are excreted.

Why this matters

If a drug significantly uses the renal pathway:

- Kidney impairment slows drug clearance, increasing the risk of toxicity.
- Dose adjustments are often required in chronic kidney disease (CKD).

Semaglutide's renal clearance is limited to the removal of its broken-down peptides; the drug itself is not significantly excreted unchanged through the kidneys. This is why semaglutide can be used even in moderate renal impairment.

How This Applies to Semaglutide

Semaglutide is processed through general proteolytic pathways (protein breakdown throughout the body), not heavily through liver CYP enzymes. Its fragments are then cleared partly through:

- Renal pathways → filtered and excreted
- Hepatic pathways → metabolised and eliminated

Because neither pathway is dominant, semaglutide avoids:

- High drug–drug interaction risk (CYP450 involvement minimal)
- The need for large dose adjustments in most liver or kidney conditions

Clinical Relevance of Pharmacokinetics

Semaglutide's pharmacokinetic properties are directly linked to its clinical efficacy. The stable and prolonged release helps maintain consistent glycaemic control, thereby reducing the incidence of adverse effects commonly associated with rapid fluctuations in blood glucose levels. Moreover, the convenience of once-weekly dosing not only bolsters patient adherence but also simplifies the management process for healthcare providers [101, 633]. Additionally, the low risk of drug interactions owing to its metabolic profile makes semaglutide particularly beneficial for patients managing diabetes alongside multiple comorbidities [60, 633]. Overall, semaglutide exemplifies how tailored pharmacokinetics can enhance therapeutic outcomes in chronic diseases like type 2 diabetes.

Interactions

Interactions with Oral Medications (Due to Delayed Gastric Emptying)

The interactions between oral medications and semaglutide, particularly due to its effect of delaying gastric emptying, raise concerns regarding how these medications may function under such altered gastrointestinal conditions. This response synthesizes various studies that elucidate the impact of semaglutide on the pharmacokinetics of oral medications, particularly about the timing of action, peak concentration, and the overall therapeutic effect.

The mechanism by which semaglutide affects gastric emptying has been well-documented. Specifically, it induces a slowdown in gastric emptying which can result in altered absorption rates for numerous oral medications. Dahl et al. demonstrated that the administration of semaglutide leads to delayed gastric emptying without significantly altering the total absorption of certain medications; for example, while paracetamol showed unchanged total absorption over five hours, a more gradual absorption pattern was observed compared to a placebo [634]. This slowing effect can crucially impact medications that rely on timely absorption to achieve effective therapeutic outcomes.

One class of medications that may experience notable interactions due to delayed gastric emptying is oral contraceptives. It has been indicated that the absorption of ethinylestradiol and progestins can be affected when co-administered with GLP-1 receptor agonists like semaglutide. Although data specifically regarding semaglutide and its interactions with contraceptives are limited, there is evidence suggesting that GLP-1 receptor agonists may alter the absorption of these medications, thus highlighting the need for backup contraception during the initiation of therapy with such agents [635].

Antibiotics, such as azithromycin, could also experience a delay in reaching peak concentrations, although the clinical significance of this effect may vary depending on the severity of the infection being treated [636]. Fast-acting pain medications, particularly non-steroidal anti-inflammatory drugs (NSAIDs) and opiates such as codeine, may have their onset of action prolonged due to this delayed gastric motility as well [634].

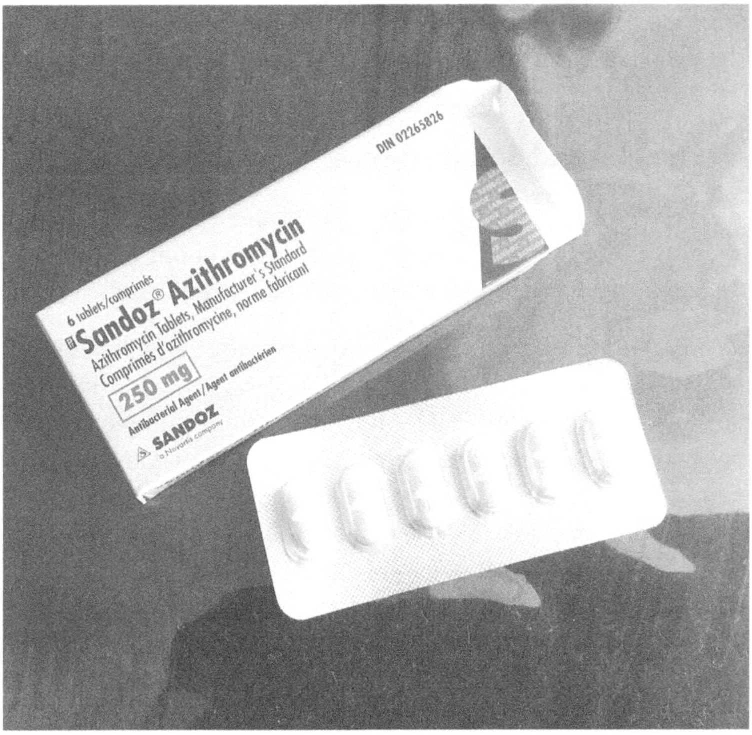

Figure 33: 250 mg Azithromycin tablets. Anonymous1941, CC BY-SA 4.0, via Wikimedia Commons.

Levothyroxine represents another medication that may require special consideration. Studies have shown that absorption of levothyroxine can be significantly impacted by food and other gastrointestinal factors, often suggesting that it should be taken on an empty stomach [637, 638]. The delay in gastric emptying caused by semaglutide may exacerbate this issue, posing challenges for patients who rely on strict timing for the administration of this medication. Clinicians are advised to recommend taking levothyroxine at times distinct from semaglutide to ameliorate potential absorption issues [637].

Medications requiring precise timing can also be influenced by altered gastric emptying. For example, Parkinson's disease medications like levodopa and antiepileptics, including carbamazepine and lamotrigine, can experience clinically relevant delays that might affect symptomatic control [636]. Similarly, immunosuppressants like tacrolimus may pose risks if absorbed irregularly due to this altered pharmacokinetic profile [635].

While most medications maintain their total absorption when used concomitantly with semaglutide, the critical aspect of timing must be closely monitored. Delays may not be clinically meaningful for all medications, yet for those with narrow therapeutic windows, vigilance is required. Thus, understanding the nuances of how semaglutide influences gastric emptying presents an important consideration for clinicians managing treatment regimens involving various oral medications.

Interactions with Insulin and Sulfonylureas

When semaglutide is co-administered with other hypoglycaemic agents, particularly insulin and sulfonylureas, the risk of hypoglycaemia can increase substantially [639, 640]. Therefore, it is crucial to adjust the dosages of these agents when initiating semaglutide therapy.

Interactions with Insulin: The combination of insulin with semaglutide can pose a risk of hypoglycaemia. This issue may be exacerbated by the appetite-suppressing effects of semaglutide, which can lead to decreased food intake and consequently lower glucose levels. Clinical recommendations suggest a reduction of basal insulin by 10–20% when initiating semaglutide therapy to mitigate this risk, and continuous glucose monitoring is essential for appropriate glycaemic management [641]. For patients using bolus insulin, significant dose adjustments may be necessary if appetite diminishes [642]. This adjustment is supported by the understanding that semaglutide not only lowers blood glucose levels but also reduces caloric intake, which can make existing insulin doses overly aggressive and potentially lead to hypoglycaemia [640].

Interactions with Sulfonylureas: The risk of hypoglycaemia increases when semaglutide is combined with sulfonylureas such as glimepiride and gliclazide. Sulfonylureas stimulate insulin secretion from the pancreas regardless of blood glucose levels, which can predispose patients to hypoglycaemic events if not properly managed [643]. Therefore, it is recommended to reduce sulfonylurea doses by approximately 50% upon starting semaglutide and to consider discontinuing their use if hypoglycaemic episodes occur. Additional caution is recommended for older adults or those with irregular meal patterns, as they may have an increased risk of hypoglycaemia [641, 644].

Interactions with Meglitinides: Meglitinides, such as repaglinide and nateglinide, function similarly to sulfonylureas by promoting insulin secretion [645]. Therefore, combining them with semaglutide can also elevate the risk of hypoglycaemia. It is imperative for healthcare providers to monitor for potential interactions that could lead to adverse effects, particularly in populations that may be more susceptible, such as older adults [644, 646].

Meglitinides are a class of oral medications used to manage type 2 diabetes by stimulating a rapid, short-acting release of insulin from the pancreas. Although they work through a mechanism similar to sulfonylureas, meglitinides have a faster onset and much shorter duration of action, which reduces the risk of prolonged hypoglycaemia. Their quick effect makes them especially useful for controlling spikes in blood glucose after meals (postprandial hyperglycaemia).

Meglitinides are considered insulin secretagogues—they prompt the pancreatic β-cells to release insulin. The two main medications in this class are repaglinide (Prandin / NovoNorm) and nateglinide (Starlix). They are typically taken shortly before meals, often two to four times per day, depending on how often a person eats.

These medications act by binding to a receptor on pancreatic β-cells that is related to, but distinct from, the sulfonylurea receptor. This binding closes potassium channels, causes cell depolarisation, and opens calcium channels, which triggers rapid insulin release. Because their effect is short-lived, insulin secretion returns to baseline within a few hours. This meal-dependent dosing provides flexibility and reduces the risk of sustained hypoglycaemia compared with longer-acting secretagogues.

Meglitinides offer several advantages: they effectively lower post-meal glucose levels, are flexible in timing (doses can be skipped if meals are skipped), carry a lower risk of prolonged low blood sugar, and can be used in patients who cannot tolerate sulfonylureas, including those with sulfa allergies. However, they also have limitations. Hypoglycaemia can still occur, especially if meals are delayed or skipped. Weight gain is possible because increased insulin promotes fat storage. Their short duration requires multiple daily doses, which may be inconvenient, and they do not help with fasting glucose control. Over time, as pancreatic β-cells lose function, these medications may become less effective.

People who may benefit from meglitinides include those with high postprandial glucose, individuals with irregular meal schedules, those unable to take sulfonylureas, or patients needing additional therapy alongside metformin. However, when semaglutide is introduced, meglitinides can significantly increase hypoglycaemia risk, as semaglutide suppresses appetite and reduces food intake while meglitinides continue stimulating insulin regardless of how much a person eats. Therefore, meglitinide doses typically need to be reduced or discontinued when starting semaglutide.

Meglitinides are rapid-acting, short-duration insulin-releasing medications that help control post-meal blood sugar in type 2 diabetes. While they offer dosing flexibility and quick action, their need for frequent dosing, potential for hypoglycaemia, and association with weight gain have led to declining use in favour of modern therapies like semaglutide. Nevertheless, they remain a useful option for specific clinical scenarios requiring targeted postprandial glucose control.

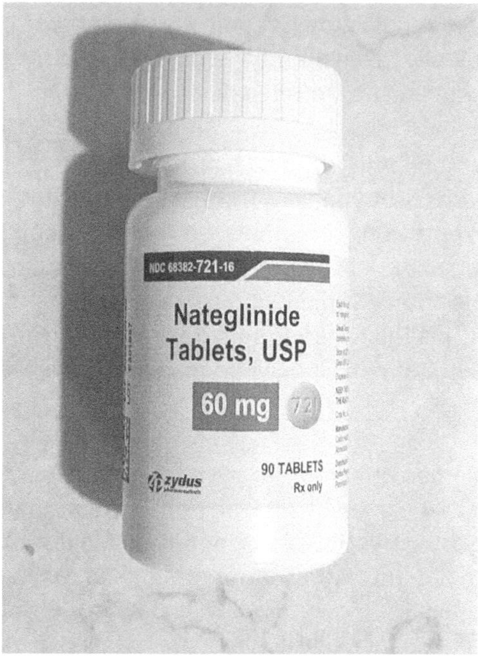

Figure 34: A bottle of generic Nateglinide 60 mg tablets, manufactured by Zydus. Grendelkhan, CC BY-SA 4.0, via Wikimedia Commons.

While semaglutide is a well-tolerated drug that minimizes hypoglycaemia risks in isolation, its interactions with insulin, sulfonylureas, and meglitinides necessitate careful dosage adjustments and ongoing monitoring. The recommendation to reduce the doses of these concurrent medications underscores the importance of personalized diabetes management to ensure patient safety and effective glycaemic control [643, 646].

Interactions with CNS-Active Medications (Rare and Mostly GI-Related)

Interactions between semaglutide, a glucagon-like peptide-1 receptor agonist, and central nervous system (CNS)-active medications are an important area of investigation, particularly regarding their gastrointestinal and metabolic effects rather than direct pharmacokinetic interactions. Semaglutide does not undergo metabolism via the CYP450 pathways, thereby decreasing the likelihood of standard drug-drug interactions that are mediated through these enzymes [647]. However, indirect interactions can occur due to shared side effects and their influence on gastrointestinal functions.

CNS-active medications are drugs that act on the central nervous system (CNS)—the brain and spinal cord—to influence mood, cognition, perception, or neurological function. These medicines can affect how a person thinks, feels, behaves, or physically responds to stimuli. They include a broad range of therapeutic classes prescribed for mental health conditions, neurological disorders, chronic pain, sleep disturbances, and behavioural regulation.

Major categories of CNS-active medications include antidepressants (such as SSRIs like sertraline and fluoxetine, SNRIs like venlafaxine and duloxetine, and older drugs such as TCAs and MAOIs), antipsychotics used for schizophrenia, bipolar disorder, and severe mood disorders (e.g., quetiapine, olanzapine, risperidone, aripiprazole), and anxiolytics or sedatives such as benzodiazepines, zolpidem, and buspirone. Mood stabilisers—including lithium, valproate, carbamazepine, and lamotrigine—are common in bipolar disorder, while stimulants like methylphenidate, amphetamine salts, and modafinil are used for ADHD and some sleep conditions. Anti-epileptic medications (gabapentin, pregabalin, levetiracetam, topiramate) treat seizures and sometimes neuropathic pain, and opioid analgesics such as morphine, oxycodone, and fentanyl are used for acute and chronic pain.

Understanding these medications is important when prescribing semaglutide, not because of direct metabolic interactions—semaglutide does *not* interfere with CNS drugs at the receptor or CYP450 metabolism level—but because of indirect effects. Semaglutide slows gastric emptying, which can alter how oral CNS medications are absorbed, affecting the timing or consistency of their therapeutic levels. This is particularly relevant for medicines with narrow therapeutic ranges such as lithium or for antidepressants where stable blood concentrations are important. Overlapping side effects also matter: nausea, dizziness, or sedation may be more pronounced when semaglutide is combined with opioids, benzodiazepines, antipsychotics, or other sedatives.

Additionally, many CNS medications contribute to weight gain—especially antipsychotics and some antidepressants—while semaglutide tends to produce weight loss and improve metabolic markers. This can be beneficial but may require monitoring in patients with complex psychiatric or metabolic profiles. Finally, although semaglutide has shown neutral or mildly positive effects on mood, rapid weight loss or hormonal changes may impact emotional stability in sensitive individuals, making clinical observation essential.

Overall, CNS-active medications influence the brain and neurological function, and while semaglutide does not directly interact with them pharmacologically, clinicians should consider delayed gastric emptying, overlapping side effects, and changes in weight or metabolism when these therapies are used together.

First, examining the relationship between semaglutide and antidepressant medications such as SSRIs and SNRIs reveals a generally safe profile, although caution should be exercised. Both semaglutide and these classes of antidepressants can induce nausea. This overlapping side effect may exacerbate gastrointestinal discomfort, underscoring the need for patient monitoring when these medications are co-prescribed [648]. Additionally, the appetite-modulating effects of SSRIs, which often increase appetite, could contrast with semaglutide's appetite suppression, contributing to variable outcomes in weight management and nutritional status [649].

In the context of antipsychotics, there are no direct pharmacological interactions established, but the metabolic benefits of semaglutide are noteworthy. Antipsychotics are commonly associated with weight gain and metabolic syndrome; semaglutide has shown effectiveness in mitigating these side effects, making its co-administration potentially beneficial for counteracting antipsychotic-induced weight gain [46, 650]. However, no direct drug interaction has been established.

When considering benzodiazepines and other sedatives, delayed gastric emptying caused by semaglutide may moderately impact the onset of action of orally administered CNS medications, although the degree of this effect is typically minor [651]. Clinicians should be aware of this possibility when prescribing.

Stimulant medications used for ADHD, such as methylphenidate, present a distinct concern. Since both agents suppress appetite, their concurrent use could raise the risk of under-eating and inadequate nutrition, potentially leading to unintended weight loss [652]. This highlights the importance of monitoring patients for signs of nutritional deficits when these classes of medications are prescribed together.

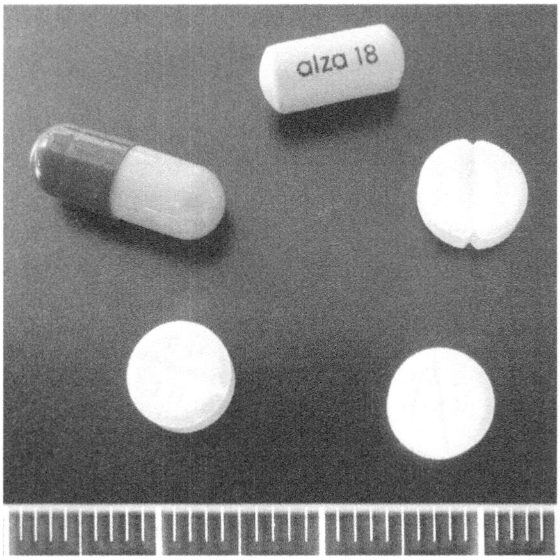

Figure 35: Various formulations of methylphenidate marketed in Germany. Clockwise from top: Concerta 18 mg (osmotic pump), Medikinet 30 mg, Methylphenidat TAD 10 mg, Ritalin 10 mg (immediate release tablets), Medikinet retard 30 mg (modified release capsule). Alfie↑↓©, CC BY-SA 3.0, via Wikimedia Commons.

For managing gastrointestinal adverse effects, anti-nausea medications like ondansetron can be helpful, though caution is warranted. For instance, metoclopramide, while effective for alleviating nausea, might counteract semaglutide's mechanism by increasing gastric motility, thus affecting its rate of absorption and overall efficacy [647].

Overall, the findings underscore the absence of significant pharmacokinetic interactions between CNS-active medications and semaglutide. Most observed effects are minor, primarily related to gastrointestinal disruptions, appetite changes, or the timing of drug absorption. Regular monitoring is recommended, especially during the initiation or dosage adjustment of semaglutide therapy.

Special Considerations in Renal or Hepatic Impairment

Semaglutide's pharmacological profile indicates that semaglutide is generally safe and well-tolerated in patients with renal and hepatic impairments. Importantly, the drug is minimally cleared by the kidneys and is not significantly affected by hepatic metabolism, reducing the need for dose adjustments even in patients with advanced kidney or liver disease [16].

In patients with chronic kidney disease (CKD), studies have shown that the pharmacokinetics of semaglutide remain stable across varying stages, including mild to severe CKD, and even in end-stage renal disease, albeit with caution [653]. The main clinical concern in such populations is not the accumulation of the drug, but rather the potential for dehydration induced by gastrointestinal adverse effects such as nausea, vomiting, and diarrhea, which can lead to acute kidney injury or worsen existing CKD [230]. The FLOW trial provides evidence of semaglutide's renal benefits, illustrating its ability to reduce albuminuria and slow CKD progression [654]. Consequently, it is recommended that patients start with low doses and titrate slowly while maintaining hydration and closely monitoring for any gastrointestinal side effects.

Similarly, in patients with hepatic impairment, semaglutide does not require dosage modifications, as its pharmacokinetic profile is largely unaffected by liver function [16, 653]. Studies indicate that semaglutide may improve liver health by reducing liver fat and inflammation, thereby benefiting patients with non-alcoholic fatty liver disease (NAFLD) and metabolic liver disease [369, 654]. Notably, routine monitoring of liver enzymes and cautious management in cases of decompensated cirrhosis is advisable, as individuals with advanced liver disease may be more susceptible to the metabolic disruptions and gastrointestinal symptoms associated with the drug [16, 655].

The interaction of renal and hepatic impairment is particularly concerning since these conditions often coexist in patients with diabetes and obesity. This demographic requires the utmost vigilance as the cumulative risks posed by gastrointestinal side effects can significantly destabilize their health status (Barritt et al., 2022). Patients exhibiting warning signs such as persistent vomiting, reduced urine output, or severe abdominal pain should be evaluated for acute medical intervention [16]. Encouraging adequate hydration of 1.5–2.0 L/day, unless fluid-restricted, is essential, alongside a review of concomitant medications that may elevate the risk of dehydration [230].

> Semaglutide presents a dual benefit for patients with both renal and hepatic impairments, offering significant metabolic and cardiovascular advantages when administered with proper clinical oversight. With proactive monitoring and a focused approach to managing gastrointestinal risks, semaglutide can be integrated safely into therapeutic regimens for these high-risk populations.

Polypharmacy in Older Adults

Polypharmacy, defined as the simultaneous use of five or more medications, is a prevalent issue among older adults. This phenomenon is largely attributed to the increasing incidence of chronic health conditions prevalent in aging populations, such as diabetes, hypertension, cardiovascular diseases, arthritis, and cognitive disorders [656-658]. The complexity of managing these multiple conditions often results in diverse medications prescribed by multiple healthcare providers, leading to situations where the prescribing of new medications may not adequately consider existing pharmacotherapy. This circumstance complicates medication management and exacerbates the risk of adverse events and interactions [656, 659].

As older adults undergo age-related physiological changes, they become more susceptible to the potential dangers associated with polypharmacy. Common risks associated with polypharmacy in this demographic include increased side effects and toxicities, drug-drug interactions, and cognitive impairments, which can collectively diminish overall health status and increase hospitalization rates [658-660]. The presence of multiple medications greatly elevates the likelihood of adverse drug events, particularly in older populations where functional reserve is already diminished [657, 661]. Additionally, drug interactions can manifest as compounding effects that disproportionately influence health outcomes in older individuals. For instance, combining medications for hypertension and diabetes can lead to heightened risks of hypotension and hypoglycaemia, respectively, which are particularly concerning in frail patients [657-659].

When considering the introduction of semaglutide into an older adult's medication regimen, clinicians must carefully weigh the implications of existing polypharmacy. Although semaglutide is associated with minimal direct drug interactions, its addition can exacerbate complications related to polypharmacy due to adverse gastrointestinal side effects, such as nausea and potential dehydration, which are particularly problematic for those on diuretics or with compromised renal function [662-664]. Moreover, semaglutide's appetite-suppressing effects could lead to unintended weight loss and malnutrition, especially in patients already at risk due to multimorbidity and polypharmacy [664, 665].

The assessment and management of older patients starting on semaglutide should include a thorough medication review, considering the necessity of existing prescriptions coupled with the potential for drug-drug interactions. This process, known as "deprescribing," aims to reduce the medication burden and target medications that provide tangible health benefits while minimizing harmful side effects [659, 666]. Gradual titration of semaglutide and close monitoring can aid in identifying adverse reactions early and adjusting treatment protocols as needed [656, 659]. This is particularly relevant when managing blood glucose levels, as hypoglycaemia may occur with concurrent use of insulin or sulfonylureas [662, 663].

While semaglutide presents substantial benefits for managing diabetes in older adults, its integration into a polypharmacy context necessitates vigilant scrutiny. The potential for increased adverse effects and complications underscores the importance of comprehensive management strategies—such as regular medication reviews, tailored dose adjustments, and consideration of individual patient characteristics—to ensure patient safety and optimize therapeutic outcomes related to semaglutide use.

Chapter 11

Comparison With Other GLP-1 and GIP/GLP-1 Medications

The rapid expansion of incretin-based therapies has transformed the modern management of type 2 diabetes, obesity, and cardiometabolic disease. What began with early GLP-1 receptor agonists has evolved into a diverse therapeutic class that now includes long-acting weekly GLP-1 analogues, dual-hormone agents such as tirzepatide, and emerging multi-incretin compounds currently in development. As these options increase, clinicians and patients face a more complex decision-making landscape—one that requires careful evaluation of efficacy, safety, tolerability, cardiovascular outcomes, dosing flexibility, cost, and access.

This chapter situates semaglutide within that broader therapeutic context. Semaglutide has become a benchmark medication due to its potent effects on glycaemic control, weight reduction, and cardiometabolic risk. However, other GLP-1 receptor agonists such as liraglutide, dulaglutide, and exenatide continue to play valuable roles in specific clinical scenarios, particularly when cost, tolerability, or dosing preferences influence treatment choice. Meanwhile, tirzepatide—through its dual GIP/GLP-1 receptor activation—offers even greater metabolic potency and is reshaping expectations regarding non-surgical weight loss and diabetes control.

By comparing mechanisms of action, clinical outcomes, practical considerations, and emerging evidence, this chapter provides a comprehensive framework to support informed prescribing and personalised treatment planning. It also looks forward to next-generation therapies—such as cagrilintide combinations, retatrutide, and oral multi-incretins—that may further redefine standards of care in the coming decade.

GLP-1 RA Class Overview

GLP-1 receptor agonists (GLP-1 RAs)—the majority of which are injectable—mimics the physiological effects of glucagon-like peptide-1 (GLP-1), a gut-derived hormone released post-prandial that plays a vital role in appetite regulation, glucose homeostasis, and metabolic processes [667, 668]. The actions of GLP-1 RAs contribute to beneficial outcomes in both glucose regulation and weight management, leading to their widespread acceptance in clinical practice.

Mechanisms of Action

Improvement of Blood Glucose Regulation: GLP-1 RAs exert a multifaceted effect on glycaemic control. They enhance glucose-dependent insulin secretion, reduce glucagon release, and lower blood glucose levels without inciting significant hypoglycaemia—particularly when not used concurrently with insulin or sulfonylureas [331, 669]. Metabolic studies confirm these effects, highlighting GLP-1's role in augmenting insulin responses during hyperglycaemia [18].

Slowing Gastric Emptying: Another critical action of GLP-1 RAs is the retardation of gastric emptying. This pharmacodynamic effect leads to improved postprandial glucose control through modifications in digestive transit, thereby enhancing feelings of satiety which can subsequently result in calorie intake reduction [79, 670].

Reduction of Appetite and Cravings: Central nervous system effects, particularly within the hypothalamus, dictate that GLP-1 receptor activation reduces hunger sensations and food cravings. This central regulation supports better management of eating behaviours and portion control [162, 671]. Clinical trials have corroborated these findings by demonstrating significant decreases in both hunger and food-related impulses with GLP-1 RA treatment [670, 672].

Promotion of Weight Loss: All GLP-1 RAs are associated with weight loss, although the magnitude of this effect can vary widely among different agents, influenced by their pharmacokinetic profiles and dosing regimens. Semaglutide, for instance, shows the most pronounced weight loss efficacy in clinical settings [139, 673].

Cardiovascular Protection: GLP-1 RAs also confer substantial cardiovascular benefits. Evidence from large-scale outcomes trials indicates that these medications lower the risk of major adverse cardiovascular events (MACE), including myocardial infarction and stroke, particularly in high-risk populations [165, 674]. Semaglutide and liraglutide have firmly established their cardioprotective roles, contributing to reduced cardiovascular mortality [331, 670].

Efficacy and Variability Among GLP-1 RAs

Among the different GLP-1 receptor agonists, there are notable distinctions in efficacy and side effects. For example, semaglutide has emerged as the most effective agent for significant weight loss and cardiometabolic improvements compared to others like dulaglutide and liraglutide [18, 673]. In a comparative analysis, semaglutide (Wegovy) is associated with greater weight loss percentages compared to older agents such as exenatide or lixisenatide, which demonstrate more modest effects [167, 670].

Moreover, the side effect profiles of GLP-1 RAs generally include gastrointestinal disturbances such as nausea and diarrhea, which are more pronounced in short-acting agents [375, 671]. Over time, patients typically develop a tolerance to these effects, allowing for sustained use and optimization of therapeutic outcomes [675].

Clinical Positioning

In modern diabetes management, GLP-1 RAs are increasingly becoming the preferred first-line add-on therapy to metformin for patients with type 2 diabetes, notably benefiting those with concurrent obesity, cardiovascular disease, or chronic kidney disease risk. This strategic positioning underscores their dual efficacy in controlling blood glucose and supporting weight management, thus vital in comprehensive treatment protocols [669, 676]. Additionally, ongoing research and emerging agents, such as dual GIP/GLP-1 agonists like tirzepatide, further expand therapeutic options by targeting broader metabolic pathways [669, 673].

GLP-1 receptor agonists represent a major advancement in diabetes care, combining significant metabolic benefits with a favourable safety profile, thus improving patient outcomes in both diabetes and obesity management.

Semaglutide Vs Liraglutide, Dulaglutide, Exenatide, Etc.

Glucagon-like peptide-1 receptor agonists (GLP-1 RAs) represent a significant class of medications for the management of Type 2 diabetes (T2D) and obesity. It is widely recognized that while they share a fundamental mechanism—mimicking the action of the endogenous hormone GLP-1 to enhance glucose control and suppress appetite—they exhibit notable differences in potency, dosing regimens, weight loss effectiveness, cardiovascular advantages, and side effect profiles.

Semaglutide (Ozempic, Wegovy, Rybelsus) is currently the most potent GLP-1 RA. It offers both weekly injections (0.25–2.4 mg) and a daily oral formulation. Semaglutide has shown superior efficacy in reducing HbA1c levels, with reductions typically ranging from ~1.5% to 1.8% [677]. Its weight loss profile is also remarkable, with patients achieving an average weight loss of approximately 15% at higher doses, often surpassing 20% in some cases [677]. This agent has been associated with substantial cardiovascular benefits, highlighted in trials such as SUSTAIN-6 and SELECT, which demonstrate cardiovascular risk reduction (Husain et al., 2019; Sinha et al., 2023). Moreover, semaglutide has been shown to improve outcomes related to non-alcoholic fatty liver disease (NAFLD) and insulin resistance, further solidifying its status as the benchmark in GLP-1 therapy [677].

Liraglutide (Victoza, Saxenda) follows as a significant GLP-1 RA, being primarily administered via daily injection (0.6–3.0 mg). It has a proven track record for cardiovascular protection, supported by the LEADER trial, which confirms its beneficial effects on heart health [132, 678]. Nevertheless, liraglutide is less potent than semaglutide, achieving HbA1c reductions around 1.0% to 1.2% and facilitating weight loss of approximately 5% to 8% at the highest doses [679]. Its daily dosing regimen can be less favourable in promoting patient adherence compared to weekly options like semaglutide [680].

Dulaglutide (Trulicity) is another well-tolerated GLP-1 RA, administered as a weekly injection (0.75–4.5 mg). While it also demonstrates cardiovascular benefits established in the REWIND trial [678], it is not as potent, with HbA1c reductions typically around 1.0% to 1.3% and weight loss between 2% and 4% [680, 681]. It is particularly useful in elderly patients who require gentler glycaemic control or when gastrointestinal tolerability is a primary concern [677].

Exenatide (Byetta, Bydureon BCise), the pioneer of GLP-1 RAs, is less commonly used today due to its inferior efficacy compared to newer agents. It is available in both a twice-daily (Byetta) and a once-weekly (Bydureon) formulation, yet its weight loss effect is limited to about 1–3% [679]. Additionally, there is a higher incidence of gastrointestinal side effects such as nausea with this agent, and it lacks demonstrated cardiovascular benefits in older formulations [132, 678].

The discontinued agent albiglutide (Tanzeum/Eperzan) had a modest efficacy in HbA1c reduction and weight loss but was withdrawn primarily due to commercial reasons rather than safety concerns [677].

In terms of pharmacological innovation, newer dual or multi-agonists like Tirzepatide (Mounjaro), which concurrently targets GLP-1 and GIP receptors, are gaining attention. This agent has shown even greater HbA1c reductions (up to 2.0–2.3%) and weight loss achievements (15–22% on average) compared to semaglutide, leading to its rapid adoption in clinical practice [677]. Furthermore, the combination of semaglutide with other agents, such as cagrilintide in the trial CagriSema, suggests potential for enhanced weight loss outcomes approaching those seen in bariatric surgery [677].

While all GLP-1 receptor agonists fundamentally aim to manage diabetes and promote weight loss, they markedly differ in their effectiveness, dosage, and associated benefits. Semaglutide continues to emerge as the leader within this class, setting a high benchmark for both weight loss and glycaemic control, although alternatives like liraglutide and dulaglutide retain clinical relevance for specific patient needs.

Table 15: Head-to-Head Comparison Summary.

Medication	Dosing	HbA1c Reduction	Weight Loss	CV Benefit	Notes
Semaglutide	Weekly or daily oral	★★★★☆	★★★★★	Yes	Most potent GLP-1 RA
Liraglutide	Daily	★★★☆☆	★★★☆☆	Yes	Good but requires daily injections
Dulaglutide	Weekly	★★★☆☆	★★☆☆☆	Yes	Easy to use, gentler
Exenatide	Twice daily / weekly	★★☆☆☆	★☆☆☆☆	Mixed	Older agent, more nausea

Tirzepatide	Weekly	★★★★★	★★★★★+	Yes	Outperforms semaglutide for many patients

Semaglutide generally outperforms other GLP-1 receptor agonists because of its stronger effects on appetite suppression and reward-pathway regulation. Its long half-life of about one week provides stable, consistent drug levels with fewer peaks and troughs, which enhances both effectiveness and tolerability. Many patients also experience better gastrointestinal tolerance compared with older agents. In addition, semaglutide has demonstrated superior outcomes in reducing visceral and liver fat, producing greater overall weight loss, and offering robust cardiovascular risk-reduction benefits supported by large clinical trials.

However, there are situations where other GLP-1 receptor agonists may be preferred. Liraglutide can be a suitable option for patients who prefer or require daily dosing, or for those who struggle with the weekly injection profile of semaglutide. Dulaglutide may be better tolerated in older adults or in individuals who require slower, gentler titration with fewer gastrointestinal side effects. Exenatide remains useful in cost-sensitive settings or when targeting specific post-meal glucose patterns. Although semaglutide is often the most potent choice, the broader GLP-1 RA class still provides important alternatives tailored to individual patient needs.

Semaglutide Vs Tirzepatide (Mounjaro/Zepbound)

Semaglutide and tirzepatide represent two of the most advanced pharmacotherapeutic options for managing obesity and type 2 diabetes mellitus (T2DM). Semaglutide functions as a GLP-1 receptor agonist, while tirzepatide acts as a dual GIP/GLP-1 receptor agonist. The dual mechanism of tirzepatide has been shown to provide enhanced effects in terms of both weight loss and glycaemic control compared to the monotherapy provided by semaglutide.

In terms of their mechanisms of action, semaglutide primarily mimics the action of the glucagon-like peptide-1 (GLP-1), which aids in reducing appetite, enhancing satiety, improving insulin secretion, and slowing gastric emptying [611]. Conversely, tirzepatide synergistically targets GLP-1 and glucose-dependent insulinotropic polypeptide (GIP) receptors, resulting in a more pronounced release of insulin post-meal and better fat metabolism, which significantly improves metabolic outcomes [612, 613, 682]. This compounded effect illustrates why tirzepatide is often seen as a more potent agent for the treatment of T2DM and obesity.

Regarding weight loss outcomes, extensive clinical trials have demonstrated that tirzepatide tends to exhibit superior efficacy compared to semaglutide. For instance, participants receiving higher doses of tirzepatide (10-15 mg) have achieved weight loss in the range of 15-22% of total body weight, with some cases exhibiting losses upwards of 30%, thus approaching the outcomes observed post-bariatric surgery [276, 683, 684]. In contrast, individuals on semaglutide 2.4 mg typically see about 15% weight loss [276, 683]. The comparative efficacy is further substantiated by findings from the SURPASS trials, where tirzepatide consistently outperformed semaglutide on several weight reduction metrics [3, 685].

When examining diabetic outcomes, tirzepatide has also shown superior performance in glycaemic control metrics compared to semaglutide. Specifically, head-to-head studies, such as the SURPASS-2 trial, have noted that tirzepatide achieves greater reductions in HbA1c levels than the semaglutide 1 mg dose, with patients on tirzepatide more frequently reaching normoglycemic thresholds [624, 686]. Additionally, tirzepatide has demonstrated improvements in insulin sensitivity that are greater per unit of weight lost compared to semaglutide [624, 682].

In terms of cardiometabolic benefits, both medications improve blood pressure and lipid profiles. However, semaglutide has more established cardiovascular outcomes data, partly due to trials like SUSTAIN-6, while ongoing studies are expected to elucidate tirzepatide's impact in this area [611, 684].

The side-effect profiles for both medications are similar, with gastrointestinal disturbances being the most common [113, 683]. However, tirzepatide may produce slightly more nausea, particularly at higher doses, which could affect patient tolerability [683]. Therefore, careful titration is recommended for both medications to alleviate potential intolerances.

Finally, the selection of a preferred medication often hinges on individual patient factors and specific health goals. Semaglutide may be more suitable for patients who prioritize established cardiovascular safety profiles or those who are sensitive to rapid weight loss [611, 684]. Conversely, tirzepatide may be favoured by patients aiming for maximum weight reduction or needing substantial HbA1c declines [614, 687].

While both semaglutide and tirzepatide provide substantial benefits for managing obesity and T2DM, tirzepatide's dual-action mechanism offers distinct advantages in weight loss and glycaemic control. Healthcare providers must consider patient-specific factors to effectively guide decision-making.

Benefits, Differences, Limitations, Cost

Benefits Compared with Other GLP-1 and GIP/GLP-1 Drugs

The assessment of semaglutide illustrates its efficacy compared to other GLP-1 receptor agonists such as liraglutide, dulaglutide, and exenatide, particularly regarding key outcomes such as HbA1c reduction, weight loss, and cardiovascular benefits. In numerous trials, semaglutide has shown a greater reduction in HbA1c levels compared to its counterparts, achieving reductions of approximately 1.45% compared to 1.12% for liraglutide and 1.20% for dulaglutide at standard doses [80, 87]. Notably, the SUSTAIN-6 trial demonstrated that semaglutide effectively reduced HbA1c and significantly decreased the incidence of major adverse cardiovascular events (MACE) in high-risk populations [92, 688].

In addition to glycaemic control, semaglutide has a significant impact on weight management. Clinical evidence indicates that semaglutide typically results in around a 15% body weight loss at higher doses, which is substantially more than the weight loss seen with liraglutide (1.8 mg) or dulaglutide (1.5 mg) [82, 87]. This enhanced efficacy in weight reduction makes semaglutide a preferred option when weight loss is a primary target along with significant HbA1c elevations or pre-existing cardiovascular conditions [87, 92].

Conversely, when semaglutide is compared to tirzepatide, a GIP/GLP-1 dual agonist, clinical evidence suggests that tirzepatide may provide superior results for HbA1c reduction and weight loss. Trials indicate that tirzepatide can achieve HbA1c reductions that are 0.3% to 0.5% lower than those seen with semaglutide, along with an average body weight reduction of approximately 20% at higher doses, compared to around 15% with semaglutide [92, 333]. While tirzepatide often displays superior numerical outcomes for glucose management and body weight, it is essential to recognize semaglutide's extensive evidence base, particularly concerning cardiovascular outcomes, which remains significant among GLP-1 receptor agonists, underscoring its clinical relevance [333, 688].

> Semaglutide demonstrates advantages over other GLP-1 receptor agonists in terms of HbA1c reduction and weight loss, as well as substantial evidence of cardiovascular safety. However, it's vital to consider the emerging competitiveness of tirzepatide in clinical practice. Semaglutide continues to provide a strong evidence base, especially regarding cardiovascular safety, which is a critical aspect in treating patients with type 2 diabetes.

Key Differences (Mechanism, Dosing, Effect Profile)

The mechanisms, dosing, and effect profiles of semaglutide, tirzepatide, and other glucagon-like peptide-1 receptor agonists (GLP-1 RAs) are essential areas of discussion in managing type 2 diabetes. By examining these elements, we can better understand the distinction and clinical implications of these therapeutic agents.

Mechanism of Action

Semaglutide and other GLP-1 RAs primarily function by activating GLP-1 receptors. This activation leads to several physiological effects: reducing appetite, delaying gastric emptying, enhancing insulin secretion, and suppressing glucagon levels, which collectively contributes to improved glycaemic control [20, 87]. The unique mechanism of tirzepatide, which targets both GLP-1 and glucose-dependent insulinotropic peptide (GIP) receptors, appears to magnify these effects. Tirzepatide not only promotes enhanced insulin secretion but also significantly assists in fat loss and appetite regulation, perceived to be superior to GLP-1 activation alone [611, 620]. This dual-action model suggests that tirzepatide may induce greater metabolic benefits compared to traditional GLP-1 RAs like semaglutide [3].

Dosing & Formulation

In terms of dosing, semaglutide is available in multiple formulations; it can be administered as a once-weekly injection (Ozempic/Wegovy) or a once-daily oral tablet (Rybelsus) [689]. Other GLP-1 RAs, such as liraglutide, typically require an injection every day, while dulaglutide is formulated for once-weekly injections, distinguished by its user-friendly dosing apparatus [680]. Tirzepatide is also offered as a once-weekly injection [569]. The variety in dosages and formulations may influence patient adherence and treatment outcomes across different populations with diabetes.

Effect Profile

The comparative efficacy of semaglutide over older GLP-1 RAs has been well-documented, showcasing its superior ability in lowering HbA1c levels, inducing weight loss, and yielding beneficial cardiovascular outcomes [20, 87]. As for tirzepatide, emerging studies indicate it may offer even greater decreases in HbA1c and weight compared to semaglutide, albeit with a similar burden of gastrointestinal side effects [3, 690]. Importantly, while the short-term data on tirzepatide's cardiovascular safety profile are still developing, it points to a comprehensive benefit horizon in managing type 2 diabetes compared to its predecessors [611, 691]. The effect size in weight reduction, particularly noted in cohorts with higher obesity prevalence, also suggests clinical advantages over both semaglutide and traditional treatments [690].

The differences in mechanisms, dosing, and effect profiles of semaglutide and tirzepatide indicate a transformative potential in diabetes management. Tirzepatide's dual receptor agonism may represent a paradigm shift in treatment approaches, promising better control of metabolic parameters and weight management compared to conventional GLP-1 RA therapies like semaglutide.

Limitations Across the Class

Incretin-based therapies, particularly GLP-1 receptor agonists (GLP-1 RAs), have become prevalent in the treatment of type 2 diabetes and obesity due to their effectiveness in managing glycaemic control and facilitating weight loss. However, these medications are not without limitations, which can affect patient adherence and overall efficacy across different patient populations.

Gastrointestinal (GI) Side Effects

One of the most notable limitations across all incretin-based drugs is the occurrence of gastrointestinal side effects, including nausea, vomiting, diarrhea, and constipation. These effects are often observed to be dose-dependent and particularly prominent at the initiation of therapy or during dose escalation. Studies have shown that gastrointestinal adverse events are common with GLP-1 RAs, and while they tend to diminish over time as patients adjust, they remain a significant barrier for many individuals [219, 492, 692]. Notably, the incidence of nausea has been reported to be higher during the dose-escalation phase, aligning with findings that suggest a gradual increase in tolerability over time [219].

Need for Injection and Patient Acceptance

The requirement for subcutaneous injection can be a deterrent for patients, particularly those averse to needles. This concern is widely applicable across all GLP-1 RAs except for oral semaglutide, which offers a non-injection alternative. The injection frequency varies between medications, with some requiring daily or bi-daily administration (such as liraglutide and exenatide), which can be burdensome for patients [95, 693]. Ease of use is better with once-weekly options like semaglutide and dulaglutide, yet the necessity of injections may still hinder treatment initiation and adherence for some patients [692]

Titration for Tolerance

Titration is especially critical for medications like semaglutide and tirzepatide, necessitating careful management to enhance GI tolerability. Rapid titration can exacerbate adverse GI effects like nausea, leading to treatment discontinuation in some cases [3, 395]. Studies show that adopting a slower dose escalation regimen may mitigate these adverse effects and improve overall patient outcomes [395]. This careful management is vital, particularly with potent medications such as tirzepatide, which has shown significant efficacy but also comes with increased reporting of GI side effects at higher doses [694, 695].

Contraindications and Safety Concerns

Finally, safety concerns and contraindications must be considered. There is a noted caution against using these agents in individuals with a personal or family history of medullary thyroid carcinoma (MTC) or multiple endocrine neoplasia syndrome type 2 (MEN2) due to the potential risk factors involved [219, 696]. Additionally, patients with a history of pancreatitis or severe GI motility disorders may require close monitoring or avoidance of incretin therapies altogether, compounding the complexity of choosing the right treatment option [3, 95]. Furthermore, monoclonal antibodies against GLP-1 receptors have shown varying effects on diabetic retinopathy; rapid HbA1c reductions can exacerbate pre-existing retinopathy, warranting caution in susceptible populations [40, 697].

Specific Incretin Analogues

When evaluating specific agents:

- **Semaglutide** exhibits strong efficacy but can cause significant nausea if titrated too quickly, and it carries concerns about exacerbating advanced retinopathy with rapid glucose control shifting [79, 136].
- **Liraglutide** provides lesser weight-loss benefits and often requires daily or twice-daily injections, potentially limiting its appeal compared to more potent alternatives [692].
- **Dulaglutide** is recognized for its user-friendly administration but may have milder impacts on weight loss relative to semaglutide [219, 692].
- **Tirzepatide** demonstrates high potency with significant benefits but also presents a higher GI burden at maximum doses while raising concerns for long-term safety outcomes data [694, 695].

Thus, while incretin-based drugs mark significant advancements in diabetes treatment, understanding their limitations—including GI side effects, injection requirements, the necessity for titration, contraindications, and specific drug profiles—remains essential for optimizing patient care.

Cost, Access, and Practical Considerations

The utilization and access to glucagon-like peptide-1 receptor agonists (GLP-1 RAs), including semaglutide, tirzepatide, and older formulations such as liraglutide and exenatide, are significantly influenced by cost, insurance coverage, and practical considerations related to patient needs and healthcare services.

Cost Considerations of GLP-1 RAs

Semaglutide pricing varies considerably based on healthcare systems and insurance coverage. Generally, semaglutide is considered expensive, especially when prescribed for obesity without public subsidies. In certain systems, it is more accessible for diabetes management due to subsidized reimbursements, which are not uniformly applicable for its obesity formulation, Wegovy. This pattern reflects broader trends where newer medications often have stricter access conditions and higher out-of-pocket costs associated with them compared to older medications like liraglutide, which typically have better coverage due to their longer presence in the market [233, 698, 699].

Older GLP-1 RAs like liraglutide and exenatide are often more cost-effective due to their established presence in the market, which allows for more favourable insurance coverage. These formulations might represent a reasonable alternative for patients who face financial barriers to accessing newer agents like semaglutide and tirzepatide. This situation can create a triage system where cost considerations, along with clinical efficacy and side effects, heavily influence the decision-making process regarding which GLP-1 RA to prescribe [699, 700].

Access to Medications

The eligibility for semaglutide and other GLP-1 RAs can vary widely across different indications and patient demographics, complicating access. While a large portion of the U.S. adult population may qualify for semaglutide based on obesity criteria, actual access is hampered by coverage limitations imposed by payers. Many patients who are eligible for obesity treatments may not have those indications adequately supported by insurance, pushing them to rely on older, often less effective or less innovative options [701, 702]. Furthermore, race and ethnicity can affect access, evidenced by disparities where minority populations report higher out-of-pocket costs and challenges in acquiring necessary medications. This underscores a systemic issue within healthcare practices that can perpetuate health inequities [702, 703].

Practical Considerations for Prescribing

Prescribing decisions regarding GLP-1 RAs are often influenced more by practical considerations than clinical guidelines alone. Factors such as self-administration requirements, patient preferences, and overall medication costs significantly influence both adherence and persistence with prescribed treatments. For instance, patients on stringent budgets might opt for older medications despite the potential benefits of newer agents, necessitating healthcare providers to navigate financial discussions thoroughly with their patients [699, 704]. Additionally, the negotiation between healthcare providers, patients, and insurance systems could lead to variability in agent selection, emphasizing the need for accessible cost data alongside clinical efficacy to guide treatment [698, 702].

While new GLP-1 RAs such as semaglutide and tirzepatide show great promise with superior efficacy profiles, their impact is tempered by substantial barriers to access driven by cost, insurance coverage, and practical considerations inherent in patient management. Ongoing evaluations of coverage policies are crucial to enhance patient access and improve treatment outcomes in the management of obesity and diabetes.

Putting It Together

Putting all of this together, semaglutide occupies a strong and well-defined niche within the GLP-1 and GIP/GLP-1 medication landscape. It offers an excellent balance of potency, safety, and breadth of evidence, while also providing flexibility through both weekly injectable and oral formulations. Because of its robust effects on weight, glycaemic control, visceral fat, cardiovascular outcomes, and liver health, semaglutide is often considered the first-line GLP-1 receptor agonist when meaningful weight loss and broad cardiometabolic improvement are the primary therapeutic goals.

Other GLP-1 RAs continue to play important roles in clinical practice. Liraglutide, dulaglutide, and exenatide may be preferable when cost or formulary access limits options, when patients require gentler titration due to gastrointestinal sensitivity, or when dosing preferences lean toward daily versus weekly administration. Their long-standing safety profiles and familiarity among clinicians also support their continued use in specific contexts.

Tirzepatide, as a dual GIP/GLP-1 agonist, may be chosen when the strongest possible weight loss and HbA1c reduction are required, particularly in individuals with severe obesity or more advanced type 2 diabetes. However, access, cost, and availability remain important determinants, and gastrointestinal effects may be more pronounced in some users.

Future Pipeline: Cagrilintide, Retatrutide, Oral Multi-Incretins

The future pipeline includes Cagrilintide, an amylin analogue in combination trials; Retatrutide, a triple agonist for weight loss and metabolic control currently in Phase 3 trials; and the emergence of Oral Multi-Incretins, which offer a more convenient administration method for future weight loss therapies.

Cagrilintide (Amylin Analogue / Amylin ± Calcitonin Receptor Agonist)

Cagrilintide, a long-acting analogue of amylin, presents a novel and promising approach in the management of obesity and metabolic disorders. It functions in synergy with GLP-1 receptor agonists, notably semaglutide, to enhance therapeutic efficacy through complementary mechanisms. The pharmacological interaction of cagrilintide centres around its action as an amylin receptor agonist, which, alongside some calcitonin receptor activation, contributes significantly to appetite regulation and modulation of gastric emptying. Clinical trials have demonstrated that treatment with cagrilintide results in notable weight loss, with reports indicating reductions ranging from 7.4% to 17.1% in various patient cohorts when combined with semaglutide [33, 503, 705].

The integration of cagrilintide with semaglutide, leading to the development of CagriSema, has been particularly noteworthy. Recent phase III trials have illustrated substantial weight loss outcomes, averaging reductions of approximately 20% to 22.7% over 68 weeks, with significant proportions of participants achieving weight losses of 20% or more [505, 508]. This combination appears to harness the strengths of both agents, whereby cagrilintide's effects on satiety and gastric emptying complement semaglutide's appetite-suppressing capabilities, leading to greater overall efficacy than either drug could provide alone [33, 505].

In addition to facilitating weight management, CagriSema has been associated with various metabolic improvements, including reductions in blood pressure and enhancements in lipid profiles and inflammatory markers such as C-reactive protein (CRP) [505, 508]. This multifaceted approach highlights the drug's potential for weight loss and its broader implications for metabolic health, particularly for individuals with conditions such as type 2 diabetes, where obesity is a significant risk factor.

The mechanism of action of cagrilintide primarily revolves around its ability to activate specific receptors in the brain and gastrointestinal tract, thereby regulating satiety and influencing food intake behaviours [503, 706]. Furthermore, evidence suggests that the effects of cagrilintide on appetite and energy expenditure may involve pathways linked to the extracellular signal-regulated kinase (ERK) signalling cascade, although further research is required to elucidate the complexities of these mechanisms fully [707, 708].

Overall, cagrilintide represents a significant advancement in the pharmacotherapeutic landscape for obesity treatment, primarily through its dual action as an amylin analogue and its strategic combination with GLP-1 receptor agonists. Ongoing studies are expected to further clarify its long-term efficacy, safety, and potential applications in the context of obesity and metabolic dysfunction [505, 508].

Retatrutide (Triple Agonist: GLP-1 / GIP / Glucagon Receptors)

Retatrutide, a novel tri-agonist targeting glucagon-like peptide 1 (GLP-1), glucose-dependent insulinotropic polypeptide (GIP), and glucagon receptors, represents a significant advancement in next-generation multi-hormone therapies. By engaging multiple metabolic pathways, retatrutide potentially provides a more robust therapeutic effect compared to single-pathway agents. In clinical trials, particularly Phase 2 studies, retatrutide has demonstrated impressive efficacy in both weight management and glycaemic control, signalling a potential "metabolic reset" for individuals with obesity and type 2 diabetes.

Retatrutide's tri-agonism is critical in its action. It activates GLP-1 and GIP, both of which play vital roles in insulin secretion and glucose metabolism while also influencing satiety and body weight regulation. The glucagon receptor agonism may counterbalance the effects of insulin, thereby increasing energy expenditure [709, 710]. Research indicates that participants in Phase 2 trials experienced weight reductions of up to 24.2% after 48 weeks, confirming its significant impact on obesity management [711, 712]. The ability of retatrutide to act on multiple receptors underlines its potential to induce substantial metabolic shifts that could lead to enhanced therapeutic outcomes [712].

In terms of glycaemic control, retatrutide has shown promising results in individuals with type 2 diabetes. Phase 2 trials reported reductions in HbA_1c levels averaging around 2 percentage points alongside notable weight loss, with reductions averaging around 17.5% over a span of 48 weeks [711, 713]. This efficacy is likely due to the coordinated action of GLP-1 and GIP in augmenting insulin secretion in a glucose-dependent manner while mitigating glucagon release, thus improving overall glycaemic control [714]. Such findings position retatrutide favourably among existing diabetes and obesity pharmacotherapies, offering a unique mechanism that capitalizes on the synergetic effects of tri-hormonal activation [715].

Continuing into Phase 3 clinical trials indicates a crucial step in the drug development pathway, essential for providing additional validation of retatrutide's efficacy and safety in broader populations [716, 717]. Preliminary data suggest not only significant weight loss but also improvements in cardiometabolic parameters, including reductions in blood pressure, lipids, and liver fat. For instance, retatrutide treatment correlated with a significant decrease in triglyceride levels and improvements in liver health metrics in both clinical and preclinical studies [709, 718].

Retatrutide exemplifies the evolution of diabetes and obesity treatments through its multifaceted agonistic action on GLP-1, GIP, and glucagon receptors. The promising early clinical results underscore its potential as a cornerstone in the management strategies for metabolic diseases, paving the way for more effective interventions backed by robust, tri-hormonal therapeutic approaches.

Oral Multi-Incretins and Other Novel Agents

The development of oral multi-incretins and other novel agents represents a significant advancement in pharmacotherapy for obesity and type 2 diabetes mellitus (T2DM). Traditional incretin therapies have primarily relied on injectable formulations, which can complicate patient adherence and management. In contrast, recent advancements focus on the creation of oral formulations, such as Orforglipron, an oral glucagon-like peptide-1 (GLP-1) receptor agonist designed to enhance convenience and improve metabolic outcomes [719]. Notably, Orforglipron demonstrates improved oral bioavailability compared to its injectable counterparts, facilitating dosing without the requirement for gastric emptying [719, 720].

The strategic aim behind dual and multi-receptor agonists, particularly combining GLP-1 with other hormonal pathways like glucose-dependent insulinotropic peptide (GIP) and glucagon, is to amplify the metabolic benefits associated with weight loss and glucose regulation. Research indicates that such dual agonist therapies can yield greater weight loss effects and improved metabolic control compared to monotherapies. For example, Retatrutide, a triple receptor agonist targeting GLP-1, GIP, and glucagon, has shown promising results, achieving weight loss that is competitive with surgical interventions [623, 721].

Mechanistically, these agents act on multiple gut hormone receptors, capitalizing on the intricate pathways that regulate appetite, energy expenditure, and glucose metabolism [504, 722]. This strategy aims for robust obesity management and seeks to mitigate risks commonly associated with surgical treatments. The convenience of daily oral administration could markedly enhance treatment adherence, addressing a critical barrier to effective obesity management [723].

Moreover, studies reveal that therapies including both peptide and non-peptide compounds are being investigated, with an emphasis on developing small-molecule drugs that can be taken orally [722, 724]. These oral therapies are expected to represent a transformative advance in patient-centred care, making diabetes and obesity management more accessible and efficient. For instance, Orforglipron is currently in late-stage clinical development, with potential FDA approval anticipated by early 2026 [623, 719].

Ongoing research into oral multi-incretins and multi-receptor agonists signifies a paradigm shift in obesity and diabetes treatment strategies. By combining hormonal signals and facilitating non-injectable options, these novel therapies may provide deeper metabolic benefits with greater patient compliance, aligning with contemporary healthcare goals of improving patient accessibility and outcomes.

Potential Benefits, Limitations and Uncertainties

Next-generation anti-obesity and metabolic therapies offer several potential advantages over current GLP-1 receptor agonists such as semaglutide. Early studies suggest that agents like retatrutide and the cagrilintide–semaglutide combination (CagriSema) may produce greater and faster weight loss than semaglutide alone. These emerging therapies work by targeting multiple hormonal pathways—GLP-1, GIP, glucagon, and amylin—allowing for a more comprehensive influence on appetite regulation, energy expenditure, fat metabolism, glucose control, lipid levels, and systemic inflammation. Another promising development is the creation of oral multi-incretin medications, which may significantly improve accessibility and adherence for individuals who prefer oral dosing over injections. Stronger early metabolic responses may also translate into better long-term maintenance, although more research is needed before firm conclusions can be drawn.

Despite the excitement surrounding these therapies, several uncertainties and limitations remain. More potent hormonal effects may bring increased side-effect risks, including gastrointestinal symptoms, hormonal disturbances, and changes in heart rate—as observed in some retatrutide trials. Long-term safety data are still lacking, and questions remain about cardiovascular outcomes, durability of weight loss, and the potential for weight regain once treatment stops. Regulatory approval is not guaranteed, and the cost of these next-generation agents may limit access for many patients. Equity considerations are important, as these therapies may initially be available only to those who can afford premium-priced medications. Furthermore, even with powerful pharmacological tools, sustained results will still depend on behavioural factors such as nutrition, physical activity, and hydration, especially for preserving lean mass and metabolic health.

Several key developments are worth monitoring as the pipeline advances. Phase 3 trials of CagriSema are underway, and early data show highly promising weight-loss outcomes. Retatrutide is also being evaluated in larger population studies and may emerge as the most potent nonsurgical metabolic therapy available if approved. Parallel research into oral multi-incretins and small-molecule GLP-1 receptor agonists aims to reduce reliance on injectable treatments and broaden patient uptake. Future studies must clarify long-term safety, the durability of metabolic improvements, effects on comorbidities such as cardiovascular disease,

NAFLD, and diabetes complications, and the real-world effectiveness of these novel interventions.

Taken together, these innovations point toward a major transformation in obesity and metabolic disease management. The field is moving from single-pathway treatments to multi-hormone agents capable of inducing deeper metabolic change—sometimes called metabolic "rewiring." Therapies such as cagrilintide, retatrutide, and oral multi-incretins could achieve levels of weight reduction and metabolic improvement that rival bariatric surgery, but with far less invasiveness. If proven safe, effective, and accessible, these next-generation medications may redefine standard of care for obesity, type 2 diabetes, fatty liver disease, and broader cardiometabolic disorders.

Chapter 12

The Patient Journey: A Practical Guide

Beginning semaglutide marks the start of a gradual, structured transformation—not only in weight and metabolic health, but also in daily habits, appetite patterns, and overall well-being. This chapter guides readers through what to expect at each stage of the journey, from the first month of adjustment to long-term maintenance beyond a year. Understanding the timeline of change helps set realistic expectations, reduce anxiety, and reinforce the importance of consistent self-monitoring and lifestyle habits.

Semaglutide works slowly and steadily, with its full benefits unfolding over months rather than weeks. Early changes in appetite and digestion pave the way for meaningful improvements in glucose control, liver health, mobility, cardiovascular risk, sleep, and overall functioning. By learning how the body responds during Month 1, Month 3, Month 6, and beyond, patients can better interpret their progress, recognise normal fluctuations, and stay engaged with treatment even during plateaus.

This chapter also provides practical strategies for monitoring symptoms, appetite, weight trends, and laboratory markers—empowering patients to recognise both scale and non-scale victories. It highlights the importance of clear communication with healthcare providers, realistic goal-setting, and thoughtful dose adjustments to maintain safety and maximise benefits. Above all, the patient journey with semaglutide is about combining medication with sustainable routines and supportive behaviours that contribute to long-term metabolic health.

What to Expect in Month 1, Month 3, Month 6, And Beyond

Semaglutide produces gradual, cumulative metabolic changes. Its long half-life, slow titration schedule, and progressive effects on appetite, glucose regulation, and body weight mean that the full impact unfolds over several months. Understanding this timeline helps patients set realistic expectations and stay motivated.

Month 1: Adjustment Phase ("Getting Used to It")

Dose: Usually 0.25 mg weekly (starter dose).

This dose is *not* intended for major weight loss or strong glucose control—its purpose is tolerability.

Getting to Know Semaglutide and Other GLP-1–Based Medications

What Patients Commonly Experience:

- Mild appetite reduction, especially in the evening.
- Earlier fullness—smaller meals feel adequate.
- Possible gastrointestinal effects:
  nausea, burping, constipation, or softer stools; often dose-dependent and temporary.
- Smoother glucose levels with fewer post-meal spikes.
- Small but noticeable weight changes (1–3 kg for many people).

Clinical focus during Month 1:

- Learning to eat slowly and stop early when full.
- Hydration and balanced electrolyte intake.
- Preventing or managing nausea (smaller portions, bland foods).
- Monitoring glucose if diabetic (risk of hypoglycaemia if combined with insulin or sulfonylureas).

Month 3: Therapeutic Phase ("The Benefits Become Obvious")

Dose: Typically 0.5–1.0 mg weekly for diabetes; 1.0–1.7 mg for weight management.

What Patients Commonly Experience:

- Stronger appetite suppression.
- Meaningful, steady weight loss, often 5–10% of body weight.
- Lower HbA1c and fasting glucose with greater stability.
- Reduced cravings, especially for sugar and high-fat foods.
- More energy and improved mobility due to early weight reduction.
- Decreasing visceral fat, which improves blood pressure and liver function.

Clinical improvements typically seen by Month 3:

- HbA1c reduction by ~1.0–1.5%.
- Lower triglycerides.
- Reduced ALT/AST in people with fatty liver.
- Better blood pressure control.

This is often the time when patients say, "I'm finally in control of my appetite."

Month 6: Peak Effect Phase ("Metabolic Reset")

Dose: Often 1.0–2.4 mg weekly, depending on indication.

What Patients Commonly Experience:

- Significant weight loss, typically 10–15% of starting weight.
- Dramatic reductions in waist circumference and visceral fat.
- Much easier glycaemic control, sometimes near-remission in type 2 diabetes.
- Better sleep, reduced snoring or improvement in sleep apnoea.
- Improved joint pain, mobility, and exercise tolerance.
- Lower inflammation (CRP and liver markers drop).
- Reduced insulin resistance, which helps metabolic flexibility.

Clinical milestones by Month 6:

- Many patients qualify for medication reduction (insulin, sulfonylureas, or antihypertensives).
- Kidney markers (albuminuria) may improve.
- Cardiovascular risk factors substantially shift downward.

By Month 6, most metabolic benefits—blood pressure, cholesterol, liver fat, insulin resistance—are well established.

Month 12 and Beyond: Maintenance and Long-Term Transformation

Dose: Maintained at the patient's optimal tolerated level.

What Patients Commonly Experience:

- Sustained weight loss, often 15–20% or more.
- Stable appetite control, less preoccupation with food.
- Improved relationship with eating, reduced emotional/impulsive eating.
- Better long-term glycaemic control and lower risk of diabetes complications.
- Continued improvements in fitness and mobility, often allowing more exercise.

- Enhanced quality of life—confidence, mood, and daily functioning.

Long-term clinical benefits:

- Reduced risk of cardiovascular events (heart attack, stroke).
- Slowing of kidney disease progression.
- Reduced progression of diabetic retinopathy (with appropriate monitoring).
- Reduced fat in the liver (NAFLD/NASH improvement).

What stabilises long-term:

- Weight typically plateaus.
- Appetite remains regulated, though slightly stronger than at peak effect.
- Behavioural habits determine maintenance success.

Table 16: Summary: How the Journey Progresses.

Time Period	What's Happening	Expected Benefits
Month 1	Body adapts to drug; minimal metabolic impact	Mild appetite change, small weight loss
Month 3	Therapeutic levels reached	5–10% weight loss, improved glucose and lipids
Month 6	Peak metabolic impact	10–15%+ weight loss, major cardiometabolic improvements
12+ Months	Maintenance phase	Long-term disease modification, stable weight control

Monitoring Progress (Blood Tests, Symptoms, Weight, Appetite)

Monitoring progress while taking semaglutide is essential for ensuring safety, tracking effectiveness, and guiding appropriate dose adjustments. Because semaglutide influences several interconnected metabolic pathways—including glucose control, appetite regulation, gastric emptying, and inflammation—monitoring must be comprehensive and ongoing. Four key areas are typically assessed: blood tests, symptoms, weight, and appetite patterns.

1. Blood Tests: What to Monitor and Why

Although semaglutide itself does not require routine blood testing for safety, regular laboratory monitoring helps assess metabolic improvements and detect any emerging issues. Core tests usually include HbA1c, which reflects average blood glucose over three months and is especially important for individuals with diabetes or pre-diabetes. Fasting glucose or continuous glucose monitoring (CGM) is useful early in therapy and during insulin or sulfonylurea dose adjustments to avoid hypoglycaemia. Kidney function tests (eGFR, creatinine) are important for anyone with vomiting, diarrhoea, or dehydration, and for those with chronic kidney disease. Liver enzymes (ALT, AST) are often checked to monitor improvement in fatty-liver conditions. Lipid profiles help track reductions in triglycerides and LDL cholesterol. Additional tests—such as electrolytes, TSH, or vitamin B12—may be ordered in specific circumstances.

2. Symptom Monitoring: Understanding the Body's Response

Tracking symptoms helps identify side effects early and ensures safe progression through dose titration. Gastrointestinal symptoms such as nausea, vomiting, bloating, early fullness, constipation, or diarrhoea are the most common. Patients should observe whether symptoms improve after dose increases and whether particular foods or eating patterns worsen them. Red-flag symptoms—persistent vomiting, inability to tolerate fluids, or severe abdominal pain—require medical review. Monitoring energy, mood, and signs of low blood sugar (especially in those using insulin or sulfonylureas) is also important. Symptoms such as shaking, sweating, dizziness, or confusion may indicate the need to adjust other diabetes medications.

3. Weight Monitoring: Patterns and Expectations

Weight should ideally be measured weekly or fortnightly under consistent conditions. In the first month, most people see modest reductions due to appetite suppression. By three months, weight loss often reaches 5–10% of starting body weight. Between six and twelve months, the rate typically slows as metabolism adapts and the body reaches a new, lower "set point." Plateaus are normal and reflect changes in energy expenditure and stabilising eating patterns. For this reason, progress should be evaluated over longer intervals (months rather than weeks).

4. Appetite Monitoring: Hunger Cues and "Food Noise"

Changes in appetite are one of the clearest indicators that semaglutide is working. Many individuals experience less hunger between meals, feel full after smaller portions, snack less frequently, and notice fewer intrusive food thoughts ("food noise"). Keeping track of hunger levels, portion sizes, cravings, and triggers helps clinicians assess whether the dose is appropriate and whether behavioural strategies are supporting long-term success. Appetite monitoring also highlights emerging habits that can sustain weight maintenance even as biological factors change over time.

Monitoring progress helps answer key questions:

- Is weight decreasing at a healthy, sustainable pace?
- Are GI symptoms manageable?
- Is metabolic health improving (HbA1c, lipids, liver fat)?
- Is appetite appropriately reduced?
- Is the current dose effective?
- Are there signs of intolerance or dehydration?
- Is additional support (exercise, nutrition, behavioural counselling) needed?

Table 17: A typical monitoring framework.

Parameter	Month 1	Month 3	Month 6	Ongoing
Symptoms	Weekly	Weekly	Monthly	Monthly
Weight	Weekly	Weekly	Every 2 weeks	Every 2–4 weeks
HbA1c	—	✓	✓	Every 6 months
Lipids	—	Optionally	✓	Annually
Liver enzymes	—	✓ (NAFLD)	✓	As needed
Appetite	Weekly	Weekly	Monthly	Monthly

Monitoring progress on semaglutide involves assessing metabolic markers, physical changes, appetite regulation, and symptom patterns. This multidimensional approach ensures safe dose escalation, early detection of side effects, and reinforcement of long-term weight-management habits.

Setting Realistic Goals

Setting realistic goals is a vital part of the patient journey with semaglutide. Because the medication works gradually, influences multiple biological systems, and relies on behavioural changes to maximise results, clear expectations help patients stay motivated and avoid frustration. Realistic goal-setting also encourages individuals to recognise meaningful improvements in health and well-being—not just changes on the scale. Ultimately, semaglutide works best when combined with supportive habits such as balanced nutrition, physical activity, and consistent self-monitoring.

Realistic goals matter because many people begin semaglutide hoping for dramatic or rapid weight loss. While it is one of the most effective weight-management medications available, progress occurs in phases and varies from person to person. Setting appropriate expectations prevents discouragement during slower periods, promotes long-term adherence, and shifts the focus toward overall health rather than purely weight outcomes. Semaglutide is most effective when patients understand that weight loss is gradual and that the formation of new habits is essential.

A key part of realistic goal-setting is understanding typical weight-loss trajectories. In the first month, most people experience modest reductions—often 1–3 kg—mainly from appetite changes. By three months, many achieve a 5–10% reduction in starting body weight, with continued progress over six to twelve months often reaching 10–20%. Beyond the first year, the body typically settles into a new lower metabolic "set point," and weight loss naturally slows or plateaus. These patterns help shape achievable goals and reassure patients that plateaus are normal. Importantly, even 5–10% weight loss significantly improves metabolic health.

Because weight outcomes are influenced by biology, behavioural goals are often more effective and empowering than outcome-focused goals alone. Behavioural goals might include eating more slowly, stopping when comfortably full, drinking adequate water, increasing daily movement, including protein at each meal, incorporating resistance training, or reducing emotional eating. These actions build sustainable habits that support long-term success regardless of medication use.

Patients should also track "non-scale victories," which often appear before major weight loss. These may include improved blood glucose, lower HbA1c, reduced triglycerides or LDL cholesterol, improved liver enzymes, lower blood pressure, reduced cravings, better sleep, improved mobility, less joint pain, reduced reflux, greater energy, or enhanced mood stability. Recognising these benefits reinforces motivation and highlights the broader health impact of treatment.

Goal-setting should be personalised based on the individual's health profile. For people with diabetes, goals may focus on reducing HbA1c, lowering insulin requirements, or improving insulin resistance. Those with severe obesity may emphasise improved mobility, reduced sleep apnoea symptoms, or gradual long-term weight reduction. Individuals with PCOS may track improvements in cycle regularity or cravings, while older adults may prioritise muscle preservation and functional strength. Tailoring goals ensures they remain relevant, achievable, and health-centred.

During plateau phases, goals should shift away from scale changes and toward maintaining consistent habits. This may involve reinforcing protein intake, increasing strength training, improving sleep and stress management, preventing "portion creep," and supporting the new metabolic set point. Plateaus are a normal part of the process and signal that the body is adapting—not that progress has stalled permanently.

Finally, long-term maintenance requires planning. Semaglutide treats a chronic, relapsing condition, and long-term management may include continuing healthy habits, monitoring weight weekly, addressing early signs of regain, considering lower maintenance doses, or transitioning to alternative therapies if needed. The aim is not temporary dieting but the development of sustainable lifestyle changes that protect the progress made during treatment.

Realistic goal-setting means understanding expected weight-loss patterns, focusing on behaviours over outcomes, celebrating non-scale improvements, personalising goals, preparing for plateaus, and planning for long-term maintenance. This approach enhances satisfaction, supports adherence, and promotes durable, health-driven results with semaglutide.

The following are three case study scenarios that demonstrate how setting realistic goals supports success during semaglutide therapy.

<u>**Case Study 1: "Lisa – The Early Plateau"**</u>

Profile:
Age 42 • BMI 36 • Works full-time • History of emotional eating • No diabetes but has high triglycerides and NAFLD

Initial Expectations:
Lisa started semaglutide hoping to lose "20 kg in three months." She had previously attempted many crash diets and expected rapid results.

Month 1:
Lisa lost 2.5 kg—within the expected early range—but felt discouraged, believing it wasn't "enough." Her clinician reframed her goals, explaining typical trajectories and highlighting non-scale victories:

- Reduced cravings
- Less evening snacking
- Improved sleep
- Lower morning appetite
- Improved ALT levels
  These improvements reassured her that the medication was working as intended.

Month 3:
She reached 7% total body weight loss (about 7 kg). However, weight loss slowed in weeks 10–12, and she experienced a plateau. The team helped her set behavioural goals instead of pushing for unrealistic weekly losses:

- Include protein at each meal
- Continue walking 5 days per week
- Eat slowly and stop at comfortable fullness
  These goals helped stabilise her progress, maintain motivation, and prevent rebound eating.

Outcome:
By focusing on realistic expectations and behaviour change, Lisa continued losing weight steadily and regained confidence. She learned that early plateaus are normal and that health gains extend beyond the scale.

Case Study 2: "Mark – Focusing on Functional Goals, Not Just Weight"

Profile:
Age 58 • BMI 32 • Type 2 diabetes • On metformin • Knee osteoarthritis • Sedentary lifestyle

Initial Expectations:
Mark hoped to lose weight quickly to "fix his knees and get off diabetes medication." He believed semaglutide alone would solve both problems without additional lifestyle changes.

Month 1:
Mark lost only 1 kg, which frustrated him. However, his clinician helped him identify important non-scale victories:

- Lower fasting glucose
- HbA1c drop from 7.4% to 6.9%
- Less daytime hunger
- Improved blood pressure
- Able to walk 10 minutes without knee pain
  These changes formed the basis of new, realistic goals.

New Goals:
Instead of aiming solely for rapid weight loss, Mark set personalised, functional goals:

- Walk 15–20 minutes daily without pain
- Incorporate resistance band exercises twice weekly
- Reduce emotional eating during stressful workdays
- Aim for gradual weight loss of 5–10% over 6 months

Month 6:
Mark achieved 8% weight loss, significantly reduced knee pain, and improved glucose control. He still used metformin but avoided needing insulin. His biggest victory was functional: climbing stairs comfortably for the first time in years.

Outcome:
By shifting his goals toward mobility, diabetes control, and strength, Mark achieved sustainable progress instead of becoming discouraged by slower-than-expected early weight loss.

Case Study 3: "Sara – Using Behavioural Goals During a Long-Term Plateau"

Profile:
Age 33 • BMI 41 • PCOS • Severe cravings and irregular eating patterns • Works night shifts

Initial Expectations:
Sara expected extreme weight loss because her friend lost 15% in six months. She aimed for the same, despite her irregular schedule and metabolic challenges from PCOS.

Months 1–3:
Sara lost 5% of her body weight—within expected range—but less than she hoped. Her cravings and cycle regularity improved, which her clinician emphasised as key metabolic wins.

Months 4–6:
Her weight plateaued for nearly eight weeks. Frustrated, she considered stopping the medication. Instead, the care team set behavioural and metabolic goals:

- Increase daily protein to 1.2 g/kg
- Add two resistance-training sessions weekly
- Track hunger cues during night shifts
- Maintain regular meal timing
- Continue sleep hygiene strategies
  She also tracked non-scale victories: improved cycle regularity, reduced acne, and less fatigue.

Months 7–12:
Once her habits stabilised, her plateau ended, and she achieved 12% weight loss overall. Her menstrual cycles became consistent for the first time in years, a major win related to insulin sensitivity improvements.

Outcome:
By reframing her expectations and focusing on behaviours rather than speed, Sara stayed committed long enough to experience significant metabolic and hormonal improvements.

Across all three case studies, several consistent principles emerge. Setting realistic expectations plays a central role in maintaining motivation, especially because semaglutide works gradually and weight loss naturally fluctuates over time. When patients understand what typical progress looks like, they are less likely to feel discouraged during slower phases or plateaus.

The cases also highlight that behavioural goals—such as eating more slowly, staying hydrated, prioritising protein intake, and incorporating regular movement—are more sustainable and within the patient's control than focusing solely on the number on the scale. These habits reinforce the medication's effects and contribute to long-term success.

Equally important are the non-scale victories that signal genuine metabolic improvements. Better glucose regulation, reduced hunger, improved mobility, enhanced sleep quality, and greater hormonal stability often appear before significant weight changes. Recognising these benefits helps patients appreciate the broader health gains achieved through treatment.

The scenarios further emphasise that plateaus are a predictable and normal part of the journey, not an indication of failure. During these periods, maintaining consistent habits and shifting focus to strength, energy, and overall well-being becomes essential.

Finally, personalised goal-setting—tailored to each individual's medical conditions, lifestyle, and specific barriers—supports better adherence and outcomes. Taken together, these principles demonstrate that semaglutide is most effective when paired with sustainable behavioural changes, rather than being relied on as a standalone solution.

Managing Plateaus

Weight-loss plateaus are a normal and expected phase during semaglutide therapy. While semaglutide is highly effective at reducing appetite and improving metabolic health, the body naturally adapts over time. As weight decreases, energy requirements fall, metabolic efficiency increases, and appetite-regulating hormones begin to stabilize, often leading to a slowing or temporary halt in weight loss, especially after the first 3–6 months of therapy [725-728]. These plateaus are primarily biological, not behavioural, and recognizing this helps prevent discouragement and supports long-term engagement in treatment [728, 729].

Biological Basis and Set Point

Plateaus typically indicate that the body is settling into a new metabolic "set point"—a protective mechanism rather than a sign that semaglutide has stopped working [728, 729]. Even during plateaus, patients often continue to experience significant health improvements, such as reduced visceral fat, better glycaemic control, improved liver function, lower blood pressure, and decreased inflammation [725, 726, 729, 730]. Emphasizing these non-scale benefits reassures patients that progress continues beneath the surface [725, 729, 730].

Managing Plateaus: Lifestyle and Behavioural Strategies

Effective management of plateaus involves reinforcing healthy habits. Reviewing eating patterns—such as portion sizes, meal timing, and speed of eating—can reveal small behavioural drifts that are correctable. Increasing protein intake, improving meal structure, and reducing grazing between meals support satiety and minimize unintentional caloric increases [728]. Hydration, fibre intake, and bowel regularity should also be assessed, as slowed digestion or constipation can affect appetite and weight trends [726].

Physical activity is especially important during plateaus. Adding or increasing resistance training helps build lean mass, which boosts resting metabolic rate and supports long-term weight maintenance. Moderate aerobic exercise—such as brisk walking, cycling, or swimming—further enhances cardiovascular health and fat oxidation. Even small increases in daily movement can help resume gradual progress [728, 731].

Dose Optimization and Clinical Review

For some, behavioural and lifestyle adjustments may not fully overcome a plateau. In these cases, dose optimization should be considered. If the patient has not reached their maintenance dose, cautious upward titration of semaglutide may restore appetite control and further weight loss [728]. Conversely, if side effects like nausea or reduced intake have led to inconsistent eating, adjusting meal timing or temporarily pausing dose escalation can be helpful. Clinical review ensures decisions are tailored to the patient's tolerability, goals, and metabolic profile [727, 728].

Reframing Plateaus

Ultimately, plateaus should be reframed as a normal stage of weight loss physiology, not as failure. Consistency and focus on long-term habits—structured dietary patterns, adequate protein, regular movement, proper hydration, and ongoing monitoring—help most individuals move through plateau phases and maintain progress toward healthier weight and metabolic outcomes [728, 729].

Communicating with Your GP/Endocrinologist

Effective communication with your GP or endocrinologist is essential for safe, successful, and long-term semaglutide treatment. Because this medication influences multiple metabolic systems—including appetite regulation, glucose control, gastric motility, and weight—it requires shared decision-making and regular review. Open, proactive communication ensures that treatment remains safe, tailored to your needs, and aligned with both medical goals and personal expectations.

Semaglutide is not a "set and forget" therapy; your clinician relies on accurate information about your symptoms, progress, and lifestyle to guide decisions. Providing clear updates allows your doctor to adjust the dose safely, recognise early signs of side effects, prevent complications such as dehydration or hypoglycaemia, coordinate semaglutide with your other medications, and support longer-term behaviour and nutrition strategies. Good communication also helps plan for maintenance phases or future transitions in therapy.

At each review appointment, it helps to discuss weight and appetite changes, such as weekly fluctuations, shifts in hunger or cravings, and changes in portion sizes. These cues assist your clinician in determining whether the current dose is appropriate. You should also describe any side effects—including nausea, bloating, constipation, diarrhoea, dizziness, or fatigue—as this enables your doctor to adjust titration, recommend dietary approaches, or pause treatment if needed. Notify your clinician of any new prescriptions, supplements, or changes in other diabetes medications, as this is crucial to avoid medication interactions and prevent hypoglycaemia. For patients with diabetes, sharing blood glucose trends, hypoglycaemic episodes, or CGM reports helps guide safe adjustments to insulin or sulfonylurea therapy.

Some situations require contacting your clinician between scheduled appointments. These include persistent vomiting, inability to keep fluids down, signs of dehydration, severe abdominal pain, repeated low blood sugar, unexpected rapid weight loss, chest discomfort, or new pregnancy. Early communication can prevent small issues from escalating into medical problems.

Preparing for appointments by keeping a symptom diary, weight or appetite logs, a list of questions, and recent glucose readings (if relevant) allows for more productive, efficient consultations. Asking targeted questions—such as whether your progress is typical, whether doses should be adjusted, whether blood tests are needed, or how to manage specific symptoms—helps clarify expectations and supports confident participation in treatment decisions.

Honesty is vital. Patients sometimes hesitate to report missed doses, emotional eating, temporary treatment pauses, alcohol use, financial strain, or fears about weight regain. Being open about these challenges allows your healthcare provider to offer solutions, adjust goals, and connect you with additional support when needed. Your clinician may also coordinate care with other professionals such as a dietitian, exercise physiologist, psychologist, bariatric specialist, or liver/kidney specialist, ensuring an integrated approach—particularly for complex conditions like diabetes, NAFLD, PCOS, or cardiovascular disease.

Finally, semaglutide is a long-term therapy for a chronic condition. Communicating about broader plans—such as maintenance dosing, managing plateaus, travel, future pregnancy, or potential transition to other medications—helps align treatment with your long-term health and lifestyle.

When to Increase, Hold, or Decrease the Dose

The management of semaglutide dosing is a crucial aspect of treatment, particularly due to the drug's long half-life and its effects on the gut–brain axis. Understanding when to increase, hold, or decrease the dose requires careful consideration of various factors, including appetite control, weight loss responses, and side-effect profiles [225, 228, 732].

When to Increase the Dose

Increasing the semaglutide dose is typically recommended when patients demonstrate a tolerable response to the current dosage, generally after four-week intervals. Such increases can be indicated if patients experience mild gastrointestinal side effects like short-lived nausea or appetite suppression that are manageable [35, 732]. A higher dose is also warranted if appetite control is not sufficient—illustrated by signs such as a swift return of hunger or increased snacking despite consistent behavioural efforts. Clinical guidelines suggest optimizing to therapeutic doses—approximately 1.0-2.4 mg for weight management or 0.5-1.0 mg for diabetes—especially when weight loss stagnates prior to achieving expected goals [35, 228].

When to Hold the Dose

Conversely, holding the dose is prudent when gastrointestinal symptoms are still prevalent, including moderate to severe nausea, constipation, or changes in bowel habits. This stagnation in dosage adjustment allows the body additional time to acclimate [35, 225]. Maintaining the current dose is also advisable when patients experience a steady pace of weight loss or good appetite control, indicating effective use of the drug even at lower dosages [225, 228]. External life factors, such as stress or travel, can also necessitate a pause in dose increases to preserve stability during treatment [225] .

When to Decrease the Dose

A dose reduction is essential when adverse effects become pronounced or interfere with daily living. Notably, signs such as severe nausea, persistent vomiting, or debilitating gastrointestinal distress necessitate immediate attention to prevent dehydration and preserve patient quality of life [35, 225]. Moreover, weight loss rates exceeding 1 kg weekly or the emergence of signs indicative of muscle wasting or malnutrition might necessitate a dosage modification [225, 228]. In the context of diabetes management, lower doses can be considered if patients develop hypoglycaemia from simultaneous insulin use [35, 732].

When to Pause the Dose Entirely

Temporarily pausing semaglutide is critical during acute incidents, such as gastrointestinal illnesses or significant dehydration. The medication should also be discontinued prior to surgeries involving anaesthesia, given its potential to delay gastric emptying [225, 331]. A pause is imperative if adverse conditions like pancreatitis arise, and if pregnancy is confirmed, continued use of the drug is contraindicated [225]. Additionally, when a pause in treatment extends beyond 5-6 weeks, it is advisable to restart at a lower dose to mitigate overwhelming gastric responses [225, 228].

Titration of semaglutide should be carefully monitored and adjusted based on a multi-faceted assessment focusing on side effects, appetite control, and weight maintenance to ensure patient safety and treatment efficacy.

Chapter 13

Ethical, Social, and Economic Issues

As semaglutide continues to transform the landscape of obesity and metabolic disease treatment, its influence now extends far beyond the boundaries of clinical practice. The medication has become a cultural touchpoint—shaping public discourse, social media narratives, patient expectations, and even global pharmaceutical markets. While the science behind GLP-1 therapy is grounded in decades of metabolic research, the social environment surrounding these medications is far more complex. Misinformation, shifting attitudes about weight and health, ethical dilemmas, and widespread supply pressures all intersect to create new challenges for patients, clinicians, policymakers, and health systems.

This chapter explores these broader social and systemic impacts. It examines how public perceptions of obesity are changing, how stigma and body-image pressures are evolving in the era of medicalised weight loss, and how health-care systems worldwide are adapting—or struggling—to meet unprecedented demand. It also addresses the rise of misinformation on social media, the ethical issues associated with non-medical or cosmetic use, and the growing concern around compounded and counterfeit versions of GLP-1 medications.

By understanding the cultural, ethical, and structural forces shaping the semaglutide boom, clinicians and readers can better appreciate the lived experience of patients navigating treatment—while recognising the responsibilities and challenges facing society as these therapies become increasingly mainstream.

Access, Cost, and Insurance/PBS Coverage (Australia-Specific)

Semaglutide is widely available for diabetes and weight management, but access, cost, and insurance coverage vary dramatically worldwide. The U.S. has the highest prices and limited insurance coverage, while countries with regulated healthcare systems (e.g., UK, France, Australia) offer lower costs and broader reimbursement. Global shortages and off-label demand for weight loss have strained supply everywhere.

Global Access

- United States: Approved since 2017 for diabetes and 2021 for weight loss. Extremely high demand, especially off-label, has caused shortages.

- Canada: Approved in 2018, widely available, lower prices due to regulation, and covered by most provincial/private insurance for diabetes.
- European Union: EMA approved in 2018. Access varies by country, but pricing is negotiated nationally, keeping costs lower. Some countries (e.g., Germany) faced shortages and considered export bans.
- United Kingdom: Available through NHS for diabetes patients; weight-loss coverage is more limited.
- Australia: Ozempic subsidized under the PBS for diabetes only. Wegovy not yet PBS-listed for weight loss [733].
- Emerging markets: China and India are seeing rapid growth, with generics expected sooner due to patent variations [734].

One of the most notable global issues with semaglutide is the enormous variation in cost between countries. Prices differ widely based on national health policies, government pricing regulations, patent protections, and whether a country provides public subsidies or insurance coverage for the medication. These structural factors create large disparities in affordability and access across different health systems.

In the United States, semaglutide is among the most expensive in the world. A one-month supply of Ozempic is listed at approximately US $936, while the weight-loss formulation, Wegovy, carries a list price of around US $1,349 per month. These high costs reflect the U.S. market's limited price regulation and heavy reliance on private insurance coverage, leaving many patients with substantial out-of-pocket expenses.

In contrast, many European countries—and several other high- and middle-income regions—have far lower regulated prices. In some European markets, Ozempic may cost only US $83–$100 per month due to government-controlled pricing and national reimbursement systems. These lower prices make semaglutide far more accessible, although they do not necessarily guarantee coverage for weight-management indications.

In several countries, stricter regulatory controls or high demand have contributed to shortages and limited availability. These supply constraints can make access unpredictable, even in places where semaglutide is technically approved and reimbursed.

Looking ahead, patent expiries expected from around 2026 onward will likely change the landscape significantly. As patents lapse in various global regions, the market will open to generic or biosimilar versions of semaglutide. This shift has the potential to dramatically reduce prices, improve supply stability, and expand access worldwide—particularly in countries where the current cost puts treatment out of reach for many patients.

Table 18: Cost Comparison (Indicative as at December 2025).

Country	Monthly Ozempic Price	Monthly Wegovy Price	Notes
United States	$936	$1,349	Highest globally; limited insurance coverage
Japan	$169	N/A	Regulated pricing, much lower than U.S.
France	$83	N/A	Among the lowest prices
Germany	~$328	~$328	Controlled pricing, reimbursement available
Russia	$47–65 (generics)	N/A	Compulsory licensing allowed early generics
Australia	~$130–150	Not PBS-listed	Subsidized for diabetes only

Insurance, public subsidies, and reimbursement for semaglutide differ dramatically between countries, leading to wide variations in affordability and access. What a patient ultimately pays depends heavily on their healthcare system, local pricing regulations, and whether their insurer recognises obesity as a condition eligible for medication coverage.

In the United States, coverage is inconsistent. Many employer-sponsored private insurance plans offer at least partial reimbursement for GLP-1 medications used for weight loss, but this coverage is far from universal. Some insurers exclude obesity drugs entirely, while others require strict eligibility criteria or prior authorisation. Public programs such as Medicare and many Medicaid plans typically do not cover GLP-1 medications prescribed solely for weight management, leaving many patients with high out-of-pocket costs.

Across Europe, pricing regulation and national health systems generally make semaglutide more affordable. In most countries, Ozempic is reimbursed for type 2 diabetes, though coverage for obesity varies widely. Some countries offer partial subsidy for Wegovy under strict clinical criteria, while others provide no reimbursement for weight-loss indications at all.

In lower- and middle-income nations, access is often limited by price, supply shortages, or delays in regulatory approval. However, approval and market expansion in regions such as India, China, and other parts of Asia suggest that availability may improve over time. Until regulatory frameworks and pricing agreements mature, semaglutide in these regions often remains a private, out-of-pocket expense for weight management.

Because of these global variations, semaglutide is still largely a "private-pay" medication for obesity in many countries, with affordability and access heavily influenced by economic factors and national policy decisions.

Global access to semaglutide is shaped by several major challenges—most notably limited supply, affordability issues, and questions about long-term sustainability for both individuals and health systems. These challenges affect countries differently, but together they highlight the need for careful planning as demand for GLP-1 medications continues to rise.

Supply shortages have been reported even in wealthy nations with well-developed healthcare systems. Rapidly increasing demand for GLP-1 medications has outpaced manufacturing capacity, resulting in intermittent shortages that can last months. These disruptions limit continuity of care and may force patients to pause treatment, potentially leading to weight regain or worsening metabolic control.

Cost remains a major barrier worldwide. In countries where semaglutide is priced at a premium—such as the United States—access is often determined by the ability to pay. This creates significant inequity, as people who could benefit most may be unable to afford ongoing therapy. Even in regions with lower prices, lack of public insurance coverage for obesity treatment means many patients still face substantial out-of-pocket expenses.

Affordability challenges are likely to persist until generic or biosimilar semaglutide becomes available after patent expiry in many regions beginning around 2026. Until then, high private costs will continue to limit access, especially for long-term therapy, which is essential for sustained metabolic benefits.

Public health systems face their own obstacles. Funding widespread access to chronic weight-management medications is expensive, particularly given the lifelong nature of obesity and associated comorbidities. Governments must balance the potential long-term healthcare savings from improved metabolic health with the immediate budget impact of subsidising these therapies.

For patients and clinicians, this means access and affordability depend heavily on national reimbursement policies. In countries with strong public drug coverage, semaglutide may be accessible and affordable for approved indications. In regions where insurance is limited or where semaglutide remains private-pay, individuals must consider long-term financial commitment before starting therapy.

For policymakers, rising demand for GLP-1 medications will require strategic planning. Ensuring equitable access, supporting sustainable healthcare budgets, and preparing for the arrival of generics are key priorities. Once biosimilar alternatives enter the market, costs may fall and global access may expand, creating a more equitable landscape for metabolic health treatments worldwide.

Compounded Weight-Loss Drugs

These medications, often unofficial versions of FDA-approved drugs such as semaglutide, tirzepatide, and liraglutide, are being produced and sold through compounding pharmacies and online platforms [735]. The surge in demand for rapid weight-loss solutions, combined with drug shortages and high costs, has driven patients toward these alternatives. However, compounded drugs lack the rigorous testing, oversight, and quality standards of FDA-approved formulations, creating significant risks for consumers and health-care systems [735].

Drug compounding involves mixing or altering ingredients to tailor medications to patient needs. Under U.S. law, compounding is permitted only in specific circumstances, such as when FDA-approved drugs are unavailable due to shortages [735]. Yet, the shortage of GLP-1 drugs since 2022 has opened regulatory loopholes, allowing pharmacies to replicate brand-name drugs. Even after the FDA declared the shortages resolved, some compounders continued production, leading to legal disputes between the FDA and compounding associations. This conflict has created uncertainty for patients who rely on these drugs for weight management and diabetes care [735].

The risks associated with compounded GLP-1 agonists are considerable. Unlike FDA-approved drugs, compounded versions are not clinically tested for safety or efficacy. Reports of adverse events have already surfaced, with hundreds of cases linked to compounded semaglutide and tirzepatide [735]. Differences in formulations, such as the use of salt forms or the addition of ingredients like vitamin B12 or NAD, can alter absorption, distribution, and therapeutic outcomes. Non-standard labelling and inconsistent dosing further increase the likelihood of errors, while inadequate sterility standards raise the risk of contamination and infection [735].

Online pharmacies have amplified the problem by offering easy access to compounded weight-loss drugs, often without prescriptions [735]. These platforms frequently misbrand or adulterate products, disguising them as legitimate medications. Their popularity stems from affordability and convenience, particularly for patients whose insurance does not cover FDA-approved weight-loss drugs. Vulnerable populations, including those with limited financial resources, are disproportionately affected, as they are more likely to turn to cheaper compounded alternatives despite the risks [735].

Several critical factors drive this trend: the demand for quick-fix solutions, weak regulatory frameworks, lack of transparency in ingredients, affordability concerns, and the exploitation of online marketplaces [735]. Marginalized groups are especially at risk, as compounded drugs are marketed at lower prices, worsening health outcomes in already vulnerable communities. The lack of insurance coverage for weight-loss medications further pushes patients toward unsafe alternatives [735].

To address these challenges, the article proposes a multi-pronged strategy. Regulatory oversight must be strengthened by clarifying FDA guidelines, increasing inspections of compounding facilities, and mandating adverse event reporting. Quality control should be improved through prohibiting unauthorized ingredient variations, requiring third-party testing, and enforcing sterility standards. Online and telehealth sales need stricter monitoring, with limits on misleading advertising and oversight of telehealth clinics prescribing compounded drugs [735]. Health-care providers should be educated to recognize adverse effects and guide patients toward FDA-approved alternatives and financial assistance programs. Finally, consumer protection requires transparency, including mandatory disclosures, accredited pharmacy databases, and public awareness campaigns about the risks of compounded medications [735].

Compounded weight-loss drugs have emerged as a dangerous substitute for FDA-approved therapies, driven by shortages, affordability issues, and online accessibility. Their inconsistent formulations and inadequate oversight pose serious safety risks. The article emphasizes that stronger regulation, improved quality control, provider education, and consumer awareness are essential to ensure compounded medications remain safe and ethical options only when truly necessary.

Supply Shortages and Global Demand

Supply shortages of semaglutide and other GLP-1–based medications have become a major global challenge. The sharp rise in demand for both diabetes and weight management has outpaced production capacity, resulting in ongoing disruptions and limited availability in many regions [736-740].

Drivers of Demand and Shortages

The global surge in demand is driven by semaglutide's dual indications for diabetes and obesity, its superior weight-loss efficacy, increased public awareness (including social and mainstream media), and growing recognition of obesity as a chronic, treatable disease [736-739]. Additional cardiometabolic benefits, such as cardiovascular and liver improvements, have further increased uptake [738, 741, 742]. In some markets, demand has increased several-fold within a short period [738-740].

Shortages result from a combination of manufacturing, clinical, and regulatory pressures. Production of peptide-based medications is complex and relies on specialized facilities that cannot be rapidly scaled [736, 739]. Regulatory bodies in the US, UK, and Australia have prioritized diabetes care, limiting access for weight-loss patients and further straining supply chains, especially with the introduction of Wegovy [736, 737, 739].

Regional Impact and Consequences

Shortages have affected countries differently. In the US, Ozempic and Wegovy have faced persistent supply gaps, with pharmacies limiting dispensing or requiring prior authorization [736, 738]. Across Europe and the UK, regulators have urged prioritization for diabetes, and Wegovy rollouts have been staggered [736, 737]. Australia and Canada have experienced recurring shortages, with authorities instructing clinicians to reserve supply for diabetes [736, 739]. In lower- and middle-income countries, access is further limited by high cost, regulatory delays, and restricted supply [738].

The impact extends beyond inconvenience: people with diabetes risk destabilized blood glucose and complications, while weight-loss patients face treatment interruptions, weight regain, and psychological distress. Shortages also fuel stockpiling, pharmacy shopping, and diversion into grey markets [737, 738, 743-745].

Responses and Outlook

Manufacturers are investing in new production facilities and expanding capacity [739]. Governments and regulators have introduced measures to prioritize diabetes care, stagger launches, and discourage inappropriate prescribing [736, 739]. The entry of competing drugs (e.g., tirzepatide) and future generics/biosimilars (post-2026) may improve supply and affordability [746]. However, intermittent shortages—especially of Ozempic—are likely to persist until manufacturing expansions and regulatory changes take full effect [736, 737, 739].

Semaglutide For Non-Medical/Cosmetic Weight Loss—Ethical Dilemmas

While semaglutide is effective for obesity and metabolic disease, its cosmetic use in healthy-weight individuals raises significant ethical, medical, and societal concerns. The use of semaglutide for cosmetic weight loss—meaning in people without obesity, metabolic disease, or other clinical indications—has become a global concern. Semaglutide is an evidence-based treatment for obesity, type 2 diabetes, and cardiometabolic risk reduction, but its growing popularity among individuals within a healthy weight range introduces complex ethical, medical, and societal dilemmas, including patient safety, equitable access, resource allocation, cultural pressures, and the medicalization of normal body-weight variation [728, 729, 747].

Semaglutide is clinically indicated for adults with obesity (BMI ≥30), overweight with comorbidities (BMI ≥27 with conditions like diabetes or sleep apnoea), or type 2 diabetes [728, 729]. Use outside these parameters, such as for aesthetic enhancement or social media-driven goals, diverts medication from those with genuine medical need and raises ethical questions about the appropriateness of prescribing a potent metabolic drug for non-medical purposes, especially amid global supply shortages [747].

Semaglutide is not a benign appetite suppressant; it is a potent hormonal therapy with risks including gastrointestinal distress, gallbladder disease, pancreatitis, dehydration, and potential exacerbation of eating disorders [747]. In healthy-weight individuals, the potential harms outweigh any cosmetic benefit, violating the ethical principle of "do no harm." Discontinuation often leads to weight regain, and long-term safety in normal-weight populations is unknown [728, 748].

Cosmetic use of semaglutide contributes to the medicalization of normal body-weight diversity, driven by social media trends and cultural beauty ideals. This can reinforce body dissatisfaction and disordered eating, pathologizing normal variations in size and promoting medication use for conformity rather than health [728].

Many seeking semaglutide for cosmetic reasons may not understand its intended long-term use or the likelihood of weight regain after stopping. Risks are heightened when obtained through unregulated sources, where proper counselling is lacking. Cosmetic use also reflects privilege, as the drug is expensive and often not subsidized, potentially reducing access for those with medical need and exacerbating health inequities [728, 747].

The demand for cosmetic use has fuelled unsafe compounded or counterfeit products, which may cause dosing errors, contamination, and hospitalizations [728]. This underscores broader public health risks when medical therapies are used for non-medical purposes.

Impact on Healthcare Systems

Semaglutide, a glucagon-like peptide-1 (GLP-1) receptor agonist, has emerged as a transformative agent in the management of obesity and type 2 diabetes, significantly impacting healthcare systems on multiple fronts. The drug's ability to induce weight loss comparable to bariatric surgery, along with its cardiometabolic benefits, compels health systems to reassess their chronic disease management strategies and financial frameworks.

1. Reduced Burden of Chronic Disease (Long-Term Potential)

The clinical benefits associated with semaglutide are profound, particularly concerning obesity and cardiometabolic disorders. Studies indicate that modest weight loss (5-10%) can yield improvements in a range of health metrics including blood pressure and insulin sensitivity, while higher reductions (15-20%) can drastically reduce the risk of severe health outcomes such as diabetes and cardiovascular diseases [749, 750]. However, achieving long-term benefits relies on factors such as sustained patient access and adherence rates, which fluctuate considerably across different socioeconomic strata [226, 749]. Notably, equitable access is critical to mitigate unintended consequences of such therapeutics in creating or exacerbating health inequities, especially for those in lower-income brackets who are less likely to afford long-term treatment [226, 749].

2. Cost Pressures on National Health Systems

Semaglutide's high cost presents significant challenges for public health budgets globally. For countries with publicly funded healthcare systems, like Australia and Canada, the long-term financial implications of subsidizing this treatment for obesity can be considerable [751, 752]. Health authorities are confronted with the dilemma of balancing immediate fiscal burdens against the projected long-term healthcare savings from reduced incidence and management of chronic diseases [752]. Current healthcare policies in some regions limit coverage based on the severity of obesity or the presence of diabetes, creating disparities in treatment accessibility and complicating the ethical landscape of healthcare funding [751, 752].

3. Inequities in Access and Outcomes

The accessibility of semaglutide is heavily influenced by socioeconomic factors, with stark disparities in out-of-pocket costs leading to inequitable treatment access [226, 749]. Wealthier individuals are more likely to leverage the benefits of semaglutide due to their ability to afford it, potentially worsening health disparities among populations with higher rates of obesity and metabolic disease who cannot afford sustained therapy [749, 753]. This introduces ethical concerns about the just allocation of healthcare resources, particularly when the medication has significant public health benefits [749, 753].

4. Pressure on Pharmaceutical Supply Chains

The rapid adoption of semaglutide has strained global pharmaceutical supply chains, leading to shortages that disrupt diabetes management and force clinical adjustments, such as switching patients to alternative treatments [749]. Such supply issues necessitate that healthcare systems allocate resources towards effective stock management and emergency planning to mitigate treatment interruptions and ensure patient safety [754]. The resultant instability can lead to increased patient reliance on unregulated alternatives, thereby heightening the risk of adverse health consequences [749, 754].

5. Shifts in Clinical Practice and Workforce Demands

The introduction of semaglutide is reshaping clinical practices concerning obesity and diabetes management. Increased demand for comprehensive care from various health professionals—ranging from general practitioners to dietitians—reflects a growing recognition of the importance of multidisciplinary support [749, 755]. This shift necessitates an expansion of workforce capabilities surrounding metabolic health while emphasizing the need for ongoing education concerning medication management and lifestyle modifications [226, 755].

6. Ethical and Policy Challenges

Healthcare ethics surrounding the prescription and funding of semaglutide remain contentious. Questions arise about the subsidization of obesity medications given the lifestyle factors contributing to obesity's prevalence as a public health issue [753, 754]. The prioritization of limited resources—whether they should go towards managing diabetes or treating obesity—poses ethical dilemmas for policymakers [754, 756].

7. Increased Demand for Preventive Health Services

As therapeutic interventions such as semaglutide yield better health outcomes, the resultant shift in patient health profiles raises new demands on preventive health services [160, 754]. A decrease in chronic disease incidence may pivot resource allocation towards preventive care, highlighting the need for healthcare systems to be flexible and proactive in adapting their service delivery models to support this transition [753, 754].

8. Preparing for Next-Generation Therapies

Semaglutide is paving the way for more advanced therapies in the obesity landscape, including new agents promising even greater efficacy [226, 749]. Healthcare systems need to prepare for an escalating demand for these therapies, alongside the complexities of reimbursement and regulatory assessments [754, 755]. Proactive planning will be crucial to ensure that next-generation obesity pharmacotherapy can be effectively integrated into routine care.

> The deployment of semaglutide signals profound shifts within healthcare systems, offering substantial opportunities for improved health outcomes while simultaneously challenging existing frameworks regarding cost, access, and resource management. The trajectory towards a model that incorporates pharmacotherapy into chronic disease management necessitates thoughtful re-evaluation of ethical, financial, and operational paradigms within health systems globally.

Stigma, Body Image, and Public Attitudes

The rapid rise of semaglutide as a treatment for obesity and diabetes has not only transformed clinical approaches but has also initiated complex discussions surrounding cultural perceptions of weight, health, and identity. Glucagon-like peptide-1 (GLP-1) therapies, including semaglutide, provide significant health benefits, revealing biological and neurohormonal underpinnings of obesity that counter long-standing stigmas associating obesity with a lack of willpower. This shift towards understanding obesity as a chronic medical condition diminishes self-blame among individuals affected by obesity, while simultaneously exposing them to scepticism from proponents of conventional, lifestyle-based methods of weight management [757, 758].

For many years, societal discourse framed obesity predominantly as a personal failure, downplaying the complex interplay of genetic, biological, and environmental factors that contribute to this condition. The scientific recognition of these factors challenges outdated notions of weight control and encourages societal empathy towards individuals living with obesity. Puhl and Liu's [759]analysis underscores that recognizing obesity as a disease can foster more compassionate healthcare practices, yet public opinion remains mixed, particularly concerning the appropriateness of semaglutide for non-severe obesity. Such dilemmas illustrate the broader cultural conflicts regarding weight control, where rapid advancements in medical treatment collide with entrenched beliefs regarding personal responsibility and effort.

Alongside these advancements, a new form of stigma has emerged, often termed "Ozempic shaming," where individuals utilizing semaglutide face accusations of taking shortcuts or engaging in cheating rather than pursuing traditional methods of weight loss [760]. This stigma is compounded by pre-existing societal biases against those with higher body weights, which can deter individuals from seeking necessary medical treatment for fear of judgment [761]. The psychological repercussions of this stigma can be profound, as it influences individuals' perceptions of their own health and affects their willingness to engage with healthcare systems [762, 763].

Moreover, the cultural narrative surrounding semaglutide use often perpetuates unrealistic body standards, complicating societal perceptions of weight loss and body image. On platforms like social media, dramatized testimonials focusing on physical transformations can create distorted expectations about what health means through weight loss. These narratives can lead to feelings of inadequacy among individuals whose results differ from those portrayed online, signifying the need for comprehensive psychological support during the treatment process to help navigate these complex emotional landscapes [760].

The debate over "who deserves" semaglutide also poses ethical questions about access to treatment. While there is substantial support for its use in cases of severe obesity or diabetes, critiques often arise regarding its application for mild weight loss or cosmetic purposes. Such distinctions fuel moral debates around healthcare access and highlight socioeconomic disparities, as semaglutide may be prohibitively expensive for many individuals, limiting accessibility to privileged populations [764].

Thus, while semaglutide represents a significant advancement in the medical treatment of obesity, its cultural implications are multifaceted. It challenges outdated narratives about weight and health, potentially reduces stigma by reinforcing obesity as a chronic condition, yet risks complicating the emotional and societal landscape for individuals seeking treatment and the broader context of healthcare provision. Understanding these dynamics is crucial for effective clinical practice and promoting compassionate, inclusive care that respects the complexities surrounding obesity and the individuals affected by it.

Misinformation on Social Media

The rise of misinformation surrounding semaglutide, particularly within social media platforms, has significant implications for public health, public perception, and treatment outcomes. This misinformation often becomes entrenched within discussions about health and wellness, particularly as semaglutide garners attention for its applications in managing obesity and diabetes. The convergence of social media dynamics and health narratives creates an environment ripe for distortion, wherein medically effective treatments are misrepresented, and critical information regarding their use is oversimplified or misconstrued.

Social media serves as a powerful tool for amplifying health-related misinformation due to its structure and the nature of content consumption. Social media algorithms prioritize engagement metrics, often appearing to prefer sensational storytelling and quick-fix narratives over nuanced, scientifically accurate information. For instance, a systematic literature review highlighted a correlation between social media exposure and an increased likelihood of consuming health misinformation [765]. The platform's reward system for eye-catching content facilitates the circulation of misleading before-and-after images related to semaglutide without critical context regarding its usage, side effects, and the necessity of medical supervision [112]. Furthermore, influencers, many of whom may have financial incentives, often promote semaglutide as a miracle solution, thereby creating unrealistic expectations about its efficacy and safety [253].

A prevalent theme in misinformation about semaglutide is the misconception that it leads to rapid weight loss, which can mislead consumers into bypassing healthy lifestyle changes that are instrumental for effective weight management [766]. Clinical evidence suggests that sustainable weight loss with semaglutide occurs gradually, often over months, rather than the instantaneous results that social media claims might suggest [767]. Moreover, influencers on these platforms sometimes imply that the drug is necessary for everyone, neglecting individual differences in biological responses, which perpetuates a one-size-fits-all narrative [112, 766]. At the opposite extreme, some discussions amplify fears surrounding semaglutide, such as claims of severe gastrointestinal side effects or psychiatric effects, which are not fully substantiated by evidence [768].

This misinformation carries tangible consequences that can jeopardize public health. Such unfounded claims increase the likelihood of unsafe practices, as individuals might resort to purchasing semaglutide from unregulated sources or using incorrect formulations that can be either ineffective or hazardous [768]. The stigma surrounding legitimate users of semaglutide, often termed "Ozempic shaming," emerges as a societal backlash against individuals seeking treatment for their medical conditions, further complicating health-seeking behaviours and fostering emotional distress [766]. Moreover, misinformation can strain the supply of these essential medications, particularly for patients with diabetes who rely on them for legitimate medical purposes, complicating their access to necessary treatments [765].

Recognizing reliable and authoritative information in the face of rampant misinformation is therefore essential, involving educational initiatives that underscore evidence-based practices. Regulatory bodies and healthcare providers must engage more actively in correcting misconceptions by promoting reputable sources and addressing the misinformation narrative directly [253]. Patients need guidance to navigate the deluge of information they encounter on social media, emphasizing the crucial role that healthcare professionals play in this evolving landscape [112].

The intersection of semaglutide with social media influencers and misinformation constructs a challenging environment that compromises the integrity of medical information and public health. Addressing this misinformation requires a multifaceted approach, encompassing education, robust healthcare communication, and community awareness campaigns aimed at fostering critical evaluation of health information disseminated through social media channels.

Chapter 14

Scientific Evidence and Landmark Studies

Semaglutide's emergence as one of the most impactful metabolic therapies of the modern era did not happen by accident—it is the result of a deep and expanding body of scientific evidence. Over the past decade, a series of rigorous clinical trial programs has transformed the understanding of obesity, diabetes, and cardiometabolic disease. These landmark studies—STEP, SUSTAIN, PIONEER, and SELECT—have collectively demonstrated that semaglutide is far more than a weight-loss agent. It is a therapy capable of altering disease trajectories, reducing cardiovascular risk, improving quality of life, and reshaping how chronic metabolic conditions are managed around the world. This chapter synthesises the pivotal research underpinning semaglutide's clinical use, examines what the data truly shows across diverse populations, and highlights how trial findings translate into real-world outcomes and modern clinical guidelines. Through this evidence, semaglutide's place as a cornerstone therapy in obesity and diabetes care becomes unmistakably clear.

Seminal Trials: STEP, SUSTAIN, PIONEER, SELECT

Semaglutide has garnered attention as a pivotal metabolic therapy, supported by extensive clinical evidence from major trial programs—STEP, SUSTAIN, PIONEER, and SELECT. Each of these trials has elucidated different aspects of semaglutide's effects on weight management, glycaemic control, and cardiovascular health.

The STEP trials were specifically designed to assess the impact of high-dose semaglutide (2.4 mg weekly) on obesity and weight management. Participants across these studies demonstrated significant weight loss, often achieving reductions exceeding 15% in some studies, as highlighted in STEP 1 and STEP 2, which included both individuals with obesity and those with type 2 diabetes. These consistent results highlight semaglutide's position as an effective non-surgical weight-loss therapy. STEP 4 uniquely identified the challenges associated with drug cessation, where individuals experienced weight regain, underscoring the chronic nature of obesity management [71, 769]. The improvement in cardiometabolic markers and quality of life further solidifies semaglutide's reputation in managing obesity [71].

The STEP program (STEP 1–8) evaluated high-dose 2.4 mg semaglutide in adults with overweight or obesity, with or without diabetes. These trials established semaglutide as the most effective medical therapy for chronic weight management to date.

Key Findings

- Average weight loss: 10–15% of body weight in most trials Some participants lost up to 20%.
- Significant reductions in:
    - waist circumference
    - blood pressure
    - HbA1c
    - triglycerides
    - liver fat
- Improved quality of life and physical functioning.
- Effects seen as early as 4–8 weeks, with plateau around 9–12 months.

Notable STEP Results

- **STEP 1:** Non-diabetic adults lost ~14.9% body weight vs 2.4% with placebo.
- **STEP 2:** Adults with type 2 diabetes lost ~9.6% vs 3.4% with placebo.
- **STEP 4:** Demonstrated rebound weight gain after stopping the drug.
- **STEP 8:** Compared semaglutide to liraglutide—semaglutide produced nearly double the weight loss.

Conversely, the SUSTAIN trials explored the efficacy of subcutaneous semaglutide (0.5–1.0 mg) specifically for type 2 diabetes management. These trials reported substantial reductions in HbA1c levels and modest weight loss without an increased risk of hypoglycaemia [1, 18]. The pivotal SUSTAIN-6 trial notably demonstrated a 26% reduction in major cardiovascular events, affirming semaglutide's dual role in managing diabetes and providing cardiovascular protection [1, 280]. This cardiovascular benefit is critical, positioning semaglutide among the leading GLP-1 receptor agonists for diabetes treatment.

The SUSTAIN program (SUSTAIN 1–10) evaluated once-weekly injectable semaglutide for glucose control.

Key Findings

- Strong reductions in HbA1c (1.2–1.8%)

- Significant weight loss (4–6 kg on average)
- Lower risk of hypoglycaemia compared with insulin or sulfonylureas
- Improved cardiovascular and kidney markers

Notable Trial: SUSTAIN-6

- A cardiovascular outcomes trial (CVOT)
- Found a 26% reduction in major adverse cardiovascular events (MACE)
  (heart attack, stroke, or CV death)
- Demonstrated renal protective effects, particularly reduced albuminuria

In addition to injectable forms, the PIONEER trials have evaluated the efficacy of oral semaglutide—the first oral GLP-1 receptor agonist. Results from these studies have shown significant reductions in HbA1c and comparable efficacy against established oral diabetes medications like sitagliptin, thus expanding treatment options for patients who prefer oral medications [151, 169, 769]. Oral semaglutide demonstrated an average weight reduction similar to its injectable counterpart, highlighting its potent effect across different modalities. The medication was well tolerated, maintaining a safety profile consistent with that of other GLP-1 receptor agonists [770].

The PIONEER program (PIONEER 1–12) evaluated the world's first oral GLP-1 receptor agonist.

Key Findings

- HbA1c reductions comparable to injectable semaglutide (~1.0–1.4% depending on dose)
- Weight loss of 2–4 kg
- Superior glucose control compared with many oral agents:
    - DPP-4 inhibitors
    - SGLT2 inhibitors
    - some basal insulins
- Best results at the 14 mg daily dose
- Similar safety profile to injectable GLP-1s (nausea, decreased appetite)

The SELECT trial represents a groundbreaking advancement by establishing that treating obesity directly with semaglutide can significantly reduce cardiovascular risks, evidenced by a 20% reduction in major cardiac events among participants without diabetes. This trial has crucial implications for clinical practices and guidelines, demonstrating that targeted obesity therapy can influence not just weight but also long-term cardiovascular health [71, 771].

The SELECT trial (2023) is one of the most important obesity trials ever conducted.

Participants

- 17,500 adults
- BMI ≥ 27
- Established cardiovascular disease
- No diabetes
- Semaglutide 2.4 mg weekly vs placebo, over ~3–5 years

Key Findings

- 20% reduction in major cardiovascular events (MACE) (heart attack, stroke, CV death)
- Significant weight loss (~10% long term)
- Improvements in:
    - blood pressure
    - CRP (inflammation)
    - lipid profile
    - kidney markers
- Showed cardioprotective effects beyond glucose control

Table 19: Seminal Trials Summary (STEP, SUSTAIN, PIONEER, SELECT)

Trial Program	Primary Use	Dosage	Population	Key Outcomes
STEP	Weight loss (Wegovy)	2.4 mg weekly	Obesity ± diabetes	10–20% weight loss
SUSTAIN	Diabetes (Ozempic)	0.5–1 mg weekly	T2DM	HbA1c ↓, weight ↓, CV benefits
PIONEER	Oral diabetes therapy	3–14 mg daily	T2DM	First oral GLP-1, strong glycaemic control
SELECT	CV risk reduction	2.4 mg weekly	BMI ≥27 + CVD, no diabetes	20% reduction in CV events

Overall, the cumulative evidence from the STEP, SUSTAIN, PIONEER, and SELECT trials convincingly illustrates that semaglutide is more than a weight-loss aid; it is a transformative metabolic therapy that enhances glycaemic control, mitigates obesity, safeguards cardiovascular health, and alters the trajectory of chronic metabolic diseases [18, 769, 772].

What the Data Actually Shows

The data regarding semaglutide, particularly through its various clinical trials—STEP, SUSTAIN, PIONEER, and SELECT—highlights its multifaceted therapeutic effects not only on weight loss but also on glycaemic control, cardiovascular risk, and overall metabolic health. Thus, semaglutide is recognized not merely as a weight-loss medication but as a comprehensive treatment that addresses several health markers critical for managing obesity and related comorbidities.

1. Semaglutide Produces Large, Sustained Weight Loss (STEP Trials)

The STEP trials have produced compelling evidence that semaglutide, when administered at the obesity dosing of 2.4 mg, leads to substantial weight loss ranging from 10% to 15%, with some participants achieving losses of up to 20% of their body weight. Improvements have been noted in waist circumference, liver fat, blood pressure, and lipid levels, corroborating the idea that semaglutide significantly enhances several health metrics beyond mere weight reduction [105, 278, 773]. Furthermore, quality of life improvements have been reported, particularly regarding mobility and physical function, thus addressing not only physical health but also psychosocial aspects [105, 278, 774]. Notably, the trials indicate that while significant weight loss can be achieved, a plateau typically occurs after 9–12 months, and cessation of the drug leads to weight regain, emphasizing obesity's chronic nature that requires long-term management [79, 99, 105].

2. It Dramatically Improves Glucose Control and Metabolic Health (SUSTAIN Trials)

The SUSTAIN trials explore the effects of semaglutide on glycaemic control in individuals with type 2 diabetes. Consistently, semaglutide dosages of 0.5 to 1.0 mg result in reductions of HbA1c by approximately 1.5% to 1.8%, as well as a body weight loss of about 4–6 kg [18, 99]. Compared to traditional diabetes medications, semaglutide exhibits superior efficacy with a significantly lower risk of hypoglycaemia [18, 769]. Landmark trials, such as SUSTAIN-6, reveal that semaglutide reduces major cardiovascular events (MACE) by 26%, underscoring its role in enhancing cardiovascular health beyond mere glucose control, which is a vital consideration for individuals at high cardiovascular risk [79, 775].

3. Oral Semaglutide Works Nearly as Well as Injectable Forms (PIONEER Trials)

The PIONEER trials have demonstrated that oral semaglutide (Rybelsus) can effectively manage blood glucose levels and induce weight loss, yielding HbA1c reductions of 1.0% to 1.4% and weight losses of 2–4 kg. This oral formulation is particularly noteworthy as it provides a viable alternative for individuals who may be reluctant to use injectable therapies [18, 99, 776]. The findings also illustrate that oral semaglutide outcompetes other oral agents such as DPP-4 inhibitors and is associated with improved patient satisfaction due to its convenience [263, 770, 777].

4. Semaglutide Reduces Cardiovascular Events Even in People WITHOUT Diabetes (SELECT Trial)

The SELECT trial emphasizes semaglutide's transformative potential in treating obesity as a cardiometabolic risk factor, finding that it leads to a 20% reduction in cardiovascular incidents such as heart attacks and strokes among participants, including those without diabetes [77, 775]. Furthermore, semaglutide has shown effectiveness in lowering inflammation and improving various cardiovascular risk factors independent of diabetes status, reinforcing the concept that obesity should be treated as a significant risk condition rather than a simple weight issue [278, 771].

5. What the Totality of Evidence Shows

When collating the evidence across the STEP, SUSTAIN, PIONEER, and SELECT trials, several significant conclusions arise:

1. **Consistent Effectiveness Across Populations**: Semaglutide demonstrates efficacy in diverse patient groups, including those with obesity, diabetes, and high cardiovascular risk [105, 775].
2. **Clinical Significance of Weight Loss**: Even modest weight loss (5-10%) leads to substantial improvements in health markers such as blood pressure and insulin sensitivity, thus reinforcing the clinical impact of treatment [79, 278, 769].
3. **Broad Health Benefits**: Data supports additional therapeutic effects on cardiovascular health, kidney function, inflammation, and fatty liver disease—indicating that the benefits of semaglutide extend significantly beyond weight control [79, 263, 770].
4. **Need for Ongoing Treatment**: Evidence confirms that sustained benefits are contingent upon continued therapy; discontinuing semaglutide results in weight regain and loss of metabolic improvements [18, 99, 105].
5. **Established Safety Profile**: The side effects primarily include gastrointestinal issues, which are dose-dependent and generally manageable, corroborating the drug's tolerability [769, 773].

The collective findings from these pivotal trials substantiate semaglutide's status as a groundbreaking therapy in the management of obesity and related metabolic disorders. It produces exceptional weight-loss results, improves glycaemic control and cardiovascular health, and extends its accessibility through both oral and injectable forms. The necessity for continuous treatment echoes the concept that obesity is a chronic disease requiring long-term strategies for effective management.

Differences Between Diabetes-Dose Vs Obesity-Dose Outcomes

Semaglutide produces meaningful benefits at both diabetes doses (0.25–1.0 mg weekly or 3–14 mg oral) and obesity doses (up to 2.4 mg weekly). However, the therapeutic goals, magnitude of outcomes, and patient responses differ substantially. These differences exist because the drug acts on multiple metabolic pathways, and higher doses produce stronger effects on appetite, weight, and cardiometabolic health.

1. Dose Differences: What Is "Diabetes Dose" vs "Obesity Dose"?

Table 20: Dose differences.

Indication	Formulation	Typical Dose	Goal
Type 2 diabetes (Ozempic)	Injectable	**0.5 mg or 1.0 mg weekly** Higher dose *up to 2.0 mg* now approved in some regions	Improve glycaemic control
Type 2 diabetes (Rybelsus)	Oral	**7 mg or 14 mg daily**	Glycaemic control
Obesity (Wegovy)	Injectable	**2.4 mg weekly**	Chronic weight management, cardiometabolic risk reduction

The 2.4 mg dose provides a far stronger appetite-suppressing and weight-reducing effect.

2. Weight-Loss Outcomes: The Bigger the Dose, the Bigger the Effect

The outcomes achieved with semaglutide depend heavily on the dose used and the condition being treated. At diabetes-level dosing (0.5–1 mg weekly), as studied in the SUSTAIN and PIONEER programs, typical weight loss ranges from about 4–6 kg, or roughly 4–6% of total body weight. Some individuals lose more, but weight loss at these doses is generally modest. This is partly because people with type 2 diabetes often face additional metabolic challenges: insulin resistance slows fat loss, and many diabetes medications—such as insulin or sulfonylureas—counteract semaglutide's weight-lowering effects by promoting weight gain.

In contrast, obesity-level dosing (2.4 mg weekly), evaluated in the STEP trials, produces far more substantial results. Average weight loss typically falls between 10–15% of body weight, with some participants achieving reductions of up to 20%. These outcomes are comparable to those seen with certain types of bariatric surgery, underscoring the potency of higher-dose semaglutide for chronic weight management.

The difference between diabetes-dose and obesity-dose outcomes comes down to both dose intensity and biology. Higher doses provide stronger signalling to the brain's appetite regulatory centres, resulting in greater suppression of hunger, reduced food cravings, and diminished reward responses to highly palatable foods. Meanwhile, individuals with type 2 diabetes often face metabolic barriers—such as elevated insulin levels, reduced metabolic flexibility, and medication-related weight gain—that make significant weight loss more difficult. Thus, while semaglutide is effective across both groups, the magnitude of change varies depending on dose, metabolic health, and clinical context.

3. Glycaemic Outcomes: Diabetes Doses Are Optimised for Glucose Control

Diabetes-dose semaglutide, as demonstrated in the SUSTAIN and PIONEER trials, produces significant improvements in glycaemic control. Across these studies, HbA1c typically falls by 1.0–1.8%, with many patients achieving an HbA1c below 7%. These doses also reduce the need for exogenous insulin, lower the risk of hypoglycaemia compared with sulfonylureas or insulin, and provide a strong cardioprotective profile. The primary therapeutic effect at this dose is glucose regulation, with weight loss occurring as a secondary benefit.

In contrast, obesity-dose semaglutide (2.4 mg weekly), evaluated in non-diabetic populations in the STEP program, produces much smaller direct effects on HbA1c—typically a reduction of 0.3–0.5%. Instead of lowering glucose through pancreatic or incretin mechanisms, the obesity dose primarily enhances insulin sensitivity, reduces fasting glucose modestly, and stabilises post-meal glucose excursions. Most of its metabolic benefits arise indirectly through substantial weight loss rather than through a direct glucose-lowering effect.

> The diabetes dose of semaglutide delivers stronger and more targeted improvements in glycaemic control, whereas the obesity dose produces far more robust weight-reduction outcomes. Both dosing strategies enhance metabolic health, but they work through different dominant mechanisms: glucose regulation at lower doses and significant weight loss at higher doses.

4. Cardiovascular Outcomes: Beneficial at Both Doses, but SELECT Is Groundbreaking

At diabetes doses, semaglutide has demonstrated powerful cardiovascular protection. In the SUSTAIN-6 trial, weekly doses of 0.5–1 mg led to a 26% reduction in major adverse cardiovascular events (MACE), including meaningful reductions in the risk of stroke and myocardial infarction. The trial also showed that semaglutide slowed the progression of kidney disease, reinforcing its role as a cardiometabolic therapy rather than just a glucose-lowering agent.

At obesity-focused doses, the SELECT trial evaluated semaglutide 2.4 mg weekly in adults with overweight or obesity who did not have diabetes. Results showed a 20% reduction in MACE, accompanied by improvements in systemic inflammation (measured by CRP), blood pressure, and lipid profiles. This finding is groundbreaking: it confirms that treating obesity itself—

independent of diabetes—reduces cardiovascular risk. The benefits arise largely from substantial weight reduction and associated metabolic improvements.

Together, these trials demonstrate that semaglutide provides cardiovascular protection across different populations, with diabetes-dose regimens enhancing glucose-driven cardiometabolic pathways, and obesity-dose regimens improving cardiac outcomes through weight loss, inflammation reduction, and improved cardiometabolic function.

5. Appetite, Cravings, and Quality of Life: Significantly Stronger Effects at Obesity Dose

The behavioural effects of semaglutide differ significantly depending on whether it is used at diabetes doses (0.5–1 mg) or at the higher obesity dose (2.4 mg). At diabetes-level dosing, appetite suppression tends to be moderate, with noticeable but milder reductions in cravings, hunger cues, and everyday "food noise." Emotional eating may improve, but the changes are typically subtle. Functional improvements—such as mobility, energy levels, or reductions in joint pain—do occur, though they are generally modest because the degree of weight loss is smaller.

At the obesity dose, these behavioural and functional effects become far more pronounced. Appetite suppression is strong, cravings decline dramatically, and many people report a striking reduction in food-related thoughts and mental preoccupation with eating. Emotional eating often improves substantially, as the higher dose more powerfully affects reward pathways and satiety signalling. Functional gains are also more significant at 2.4 mg, with many individuals experiencing better mobility, reduced joint pain, improved sleep quality, and easing of conditions such as sleep apnoea. These larger behavioural shifts at the obesity dose support greater and more sustained lifestyle change, forming an essential part of long-term weight-management success.

Table 21: Appetite, Cravings, and Quality of Life Summary.

Effect	Diabetes Dose	Obesity Dose
Appetite suppression	Moderate	Strong
Reduction in cravings	Moderate	Strong–very strong
Food "noise" reduction	Mild–moderate	Strong
Improvement in emotional eating	Present	More pronounced
Functional improvements	Mild	Often major (mobility, joint pain, sleep apnoea)

People at 2.4 mg typically report much stronger behavioural shifts, which help sustain long-term lifestyle changes.

6. Side Effects: Higher Doses = Higher GI Burden

Side-effect profiles differ noticeably between diabetes-dose and obesity-dose semaglutide, largely because higher doses have stronger effects on gastric emptying and appetite pathways. At the diabetes dose of 0.5–1 mg, most people experience only mild to moderate gastrointestinal symptoms such as nausea or transient constipation. These effects usually settle within days or weeks as the body adapts, and many patients find the medication well tolerated after the initial adjustment period.

At the obesity dose of 2.4 mg, side effects tend to be more pronounced. People commonly report stronger nausea, occasional vomiting, marked early satiety, and more frequent bowel changes, including constipation or diarrhoea. Because appetite suppression is greater at this dose, there is also an increased risk of dehydration—especially if food or fluid intake drops sharply. These side effects are not unexpected, but they require careful management through hydration, adequate dietary protein, fibre intake, and pacing the dose schedule.

For these reasons, a slow and deliberate titration schedule is essential when escalating to higher doses of semaglutide. Gradual increases give the gastrointestinal system time to adjust and significantly improve tolerability, reducing the likelihood of treatment interruption and supporting better long-term outcomes.

7. Long-Term Maintenance: Different Strategies Needed

The diabetes-dose range of semaglutide (0.5–1 mg weekly) is typically used as an ongoing part of glucose-management therapy. At these doses, most patients experience modest but meaningful weight loss before their weight stabilises. In contrast, the obesity-dose formulation (2.4 mg weekly) produces a more substantial weight-loss response, with progress generally continuing for 9 to 12 months before reaching a plateau. However, evidence from STEP 4 and other studies shows that if treatment is stopped, weight regain is very common, often reversing much of the progress achieved. Because obesity is a chronic, relapsing condition, long-term therapy—including ongoing medication, lifestyle strategies, or both—is usually required to maintain the benefits gained from the 2.4 mg dose.

The management of diabetes and obesity reveals several critical differences in goals, weight loss expectations, glycaemic control efficacy, side effects, long-term strategies, and cardiovascular benefits. By examining these facets, we can clarify how these conditions are approached differently and identify effective treatment strategies backed by recent literature.

1. **Goal**: The primary objective for diabetes management is glucose control, particularly achieving optimal glycaemic levels to reduce complications associated with diabetes. Research indicates that for obese individuals with type 2 diabetes, additional goals include achieving weight reduction and improving cardiometabolic health [778]. Diabetes care focuses on metabolic parameters such as HbA1c levels, while obesity treatments are more holistic, aiming for lifestyle changes that include dietary and physical activity adjustments [779].

2. **Weight Loss**: For diabetes management, a weight loss of approximately 5-10% is often deemed sufficient to yield improvements in glycemia and metabolic health [778, 780]. In contrast, obesity management may necessitate a more substantial reduction of 10-20% in body weight to significantly impact cardiometabolic markers, including blood pressure and lipid profiles [781]. Notably, studies such as those by Gregg et al. [782] reported that more extensive weight loss correlates with better cardiovascular outcomes and diabetes management.

3. **Glycaemic Control**: The evidence suggests that glycaemic control is markedly stronger with interventions aimed specifically at managing diabetes [783]. For instance, medications like GLP-1 receptor agonists, while beneficial for weight loss, are significantly effective in controlling blood sugar levels in diabetic populations [784]. Additionally, bariatric surgery shows considerable enhancements in glycaemic control primarily in diabetic patients versus non-diabetic individuals [785].

4. **Side Effect Profile**: The side effect profile for pharmacological interventions can be higher when doses are adjusted for obesity compared to those managed with diabetes-specific doses. For example, while optimizing doses for weight loss may lead to increased gastrointestinal side effects and potential discontinuation, diabetes medications such as liraglutide appear to maintain a favourable safety profile at appropriate doses aimed at glycaemic improvement [783, 784].

5. **Long-Term Use**: Chronic use of treatments is required for both conditions. However, managing obesity typically requires additional behavioural support due to the behavioural aspects of weight management and psychological barriers associated with lifestyle changes [779, 786]. Evidence shows that sustained lifestyle interventions significantly improve outcomes in obesity compared to pharmacotherapy alone [787].

6. **Cardiovascular Benefit**: Both treatment pathways have demonstrated cardiovascular benefits, which are especially pronounced in those receiving treatment for diabetes. The SELECT trial extended the cardiovascular benefit evidence for diabetic medications to non-diabetic populations, indicating a significant overlap in therapeutic effects [582, 788]. Studies consistently affirm that weight loss, regardless of method, can lead to marked reductions in cardiovascular risk factors, underscoring the interrelationship between managing obesity and diabetes [789].

> While diabetes and obesity management share overlapping concerns regarding metabolic health and cardiovascular outcomes, they fundamentally diverge in therapeutic goals, treatment intensity, and the necessary support systems for long-term efficacy. Both domains benefit from interdisciplinary approaches that integrate behavioural and pharmacological strategies to enhance patient outcomes.

Place In Clinical Guidelines

Semaglutide, a glucagon-like peptide-1 (GLP-1) analogue, increasingly plays a significant role in international clinical guidelines addressing type 2 diabetes and obesity. Recent evidence from pivotal clinical trials—SUSTAIN, STEP, PIONEER, and SELECT—demonstrates its comprehensive benefits, including glycaemic control, weight reduction, and cardiovascular risk mitigation. This synthesis explores semaglutide's place in guidelines for diabetes, obesity, cardiovascular prevention, and chronic kidney disease.

Type 2 Diabetes Guidelines: Semaglutide has gained recognition as a second-line treatment option for type 2 diabetes, typically prescribed after lifestyle modifications and metformin. In some high-risk cases, it is considered first-line therapy. The American Diabetes Association (ADA) and the European Association for the Study of Diabetes (EASD) recommend semaglutide in situations where HbA1c levels exceed therapeutic targets despite metformin use, when weight reduction is necessary, or when patients present with established cardiovascular disease (CVD) or high atherosclerotic cardiovascular disease (ASCVD) risk. Evidence from the SUSTAIN-6 trial highlighted cardiovascular benefits associated with semaglutide usage, demonstrating significant reductions in cardiovascular events for individuals with type 2 diabetes [79].

The Australian Diabetes Society similarly supports these recommendations, advocating for the preferential use of GLP-1 receptor agonists (RAs) like semaglutide when weight loss is a treatment objective, particularly for individuals with diabetes and cardiovascular complications [71]. The robust data from these trials ensure that semaglutide is viewed as a critical component in managing type 2 diabetes, aligning with guidance recommending earlier initiation of interventions based on patient profiles and risk factors [84].

Obesity & Weight-Management Guidelines: The STEP program has established semaglutide (specifically dosed at 2.4 mg for weight loss) as a leading pharmacotherapeutic agent for chronic weight management. The American Association of Clinical Endocrinology (AACE), Endocrine Society, and Obesity Society guidelines emphasize the classification of obesity as a chronic condition necessitating ongoing treatment. Here, semaglutide is advocated as a first-line pharmacotherapy option for individuals possessing a body mass index (BMI) of 30 or greater, or 27 or higher in those with weight-related comorbidities [105].

Clinical findings illustrate that semaglutide achieves an average weight reduction of approximately 15% to 20%, comparable to outcomes from certain bariatric surgical procedures, validating its position as an effective pharmacological intervention [278]. Analyses of the STEP trials further attested to health improvements in cardiovascular risk factors and potential reductions in comorbidity medication use among patients undergoing semaglutide treatment [279].

Cardiovascular Prevention Guidelines: Following the SELECT trial, cardiovascular societies have integrated semaglutide into treatment regimens aimed at preventing cardiovascular events, even among patients who are overweight or obese but do not have diabetes. The trial findings suggest a 20% reduction in major adverse cardiovascular events (MACE) with semaglutide administration in broader populations, which could influence future cardiology guidelines to encompass semaglutide as a standard treatment for secondary cardiovascular prevention [773]. Consequently, experts foresee a paradigm shift in cardiometabolic prevention approaches, emphasizing the need to treat obesity proactively.

Kidney Disease Guidelines: GLP-1 receptor agonists, including semaglutide, are increasingly recognized in managing type 2 diabetes, particularly for patients with chronic kidney disease. While SGLT2 inhibitors maintain first-line status for diabetic kidney disease, semaglutide is being recommended as an adjunct therapy due to its cardiovascular protective effects, weight reduction capabilities, and significant reduction in albuminuria [790].

Clinical Guideline Trends: The consensus across various guidelines indicates an increased emphasis on the early initiation of semaglutide treatment in patients with type 2 diabetes, particularly when concerns about weight or cardiovascular risk are present. Furthermore, the evolving understanding of obesity as a medical condition necessitating routine treatment signifies that semaglutide is likely to remain pivotal in chronic disease management frameworks as emerging long-term data continue to support its efficacy and safety [71, 322].

Table 22: Summary - Where Semaglutide Fits in Modern Guidelines.

Clinical Area	Guideline Position
Type 2 Diabetes	Preferred second-line; first-line if ASCVD or weight loss needed
Obesity	First-line pharmacotherapy for eligible BMI groups
Cardiovascular Disease	Emerging role in secondary prevention (SELECT)
CKD in Diabetes	Recommended adjunct to SGLT2 inhibitors
Primary Care	Key agent for metabolic syndrome and weight-related comorbidities

The mounting evidence surrounding semaglutide underscores its multifaceted applications across diabetes, obesity management, cardiovascular health, and chronic kidney disease. These findings catalyse a shift towards more integrated therapeutic strategies that embrace comprehensive patient health and long-term outcomes.

Semaglutide has moved from an optional therapy to a core, guideline-backed treatment across multiple specialties—reflecting its broad metabolic, cardiovascular, and weight-management benefits.

Meta-Analyses and Real-World Evidence

Randomized Controlled Trials (RCTs), such as those encompassed in the STEP, SUSTAIN, PIONEER, and SELECT series, provide foundational evidence regarding the efficacy and safety of semaglutide. These trials have shown semaglutide to be an effective agent for weight loss, glycaemic control, and improvements in cardiometabolic outcomes across diverse patient populations. Specifically, data indicates that semaglutide has the potential to produce an average weight reduction of approximately 10-15% in obese patients receiving a higher dose (2.4 mg), while patients with diabetes may achieve a weight loss of around 4-6% with lower doses (0.5-1 mg) [228, 333, 791].

The efficacy of semaglutide has been corroborated by multiple meta-analyses published since 2019, which collectively highlight a consistent pattern of favourable outcomes. For instance, semaglutide has been shown to provide superior weight loss compared to other agents such as liraglutide and SGLT2 inhibitors [333, 791, 792]. A dose–response relationship is evident, with higher doses yielding greater weight reductions [94, 793]. Furthermore, significant reductions in HbA1c ranging from 1.0% to 1.8% have been observed in diabetic populations, with patients achieving HbA1c levels below 7% at higher rates than those on alternative medications [133, 219, 794].

In terms of cardiovascular risk, meta-analyses have affirmed that GLP-1 receptor agonists such as semaglutide not only reduce major adverse cardiovascular events (MACE) but also lower the rates of myocardial infarction and stroke, while contributing to a decline in cardiovascular mortality [213, 214]. These findings solidify semaglutide's position as a leading GLP-1 therapy regarding cardioprotective outcomes.

However, safety profiles for semaglutide also warrant attention. The most commonly reported adverse effects are gastrointestinal, including nausea, vomiting, diarrhea, and constipation, which have been shown to be comparable to other GLP-1 therapies, especially with careful dose titration [795, 796]. Such patterns in tolerability and adherence are critical, with real-world data offering additional insights into patient experiences outside controlled trial environments.

Real-world evidence (RWE) plays an essential role in understanding the real-world performance of semaglutide. These studies utilize broader population datasets and capture diverse patient experiences, including older adults and individuals with multiple comorbidities often excluded from rigid clinical trials [600, 797]. Observational studies have shown that while weight loss in real-world settings tends to be similar or slightly less than in clinical trials—averaging 10-12% at 12 months with the higher 2.4 mg semaglutide for weight loss and 4-6% with diabetes management—these outcomes remain clinically meaningful [223, 600].

Moreover, RWE highlights the barriers to treatment, such as high discontinuation rates when costs are prohibitively expensive or when there are supply challenges. Studies have indicated that up to 30-50% of patients may discontinue treatment within the first year due to these issues [333, 797]. Discontinuation is usually associated with weight regain, reiterating the necessity for sustained patient access to maintain treatment benefits [214, 223].

Meta-analyses and real-world evidence complement RCTs on semaglutide, providing a comprehensive understanding of its effects on weight, glycaemic control, and overall metabolic health. Clinical practice and health policy can benefit significantly from these combined insights, framing semaglutide as an effective first-line therapy for obesity, type 2 diabetes, and cardiovascular risk management [213, 798].

Limitations of the Current Evidence Base

The current evidence base surrounding semaglutide, a glucagon-like peptide-1 receptor agonist, suggests notable efficacy in weight management and diabetes treatment. However, there are substantial limitations that clinicians must consider when interpreting these findings, particularly regarding generalizability, long-term outcomes, and safety.

Limited Long-Term Data for Obesity Treatment: Current research, particularly the STEP trials, predominantly ranges in duration from 68 weeks to two years, which is insufficient for a condition as chronic as obesity. Findings indicate mean weight regain post-treatment, with participants regaining approximately two-thirds of their weight within one year after discontinuation of semaglutide [109]. This observation raises vital questions about the sustainability of weight loss and the physiological impact of long-term appetite suppression, as earlier studies suggest weight loss stabilization occurs only for a few months before plateauing or regaining occurs [103]. Additionally, optimal maintenance dosing strategies for long-term therapy remain elusive, illustrating the necessity for extended follow-up studies to evaluate weight trajectories and effective cessation protocols [103].

Most STEP trials lasted 68 weeks, with only a few extending to two years. Obesity is a lifelong, relapsing condition, so questions remain about:

- durability of weight loss beyond 2–3 years
- the long-term physiological effects of chronic appetite suppression

- how weight trajectories behave over multiple cycles of starting, stopping, and restarting treatment
- optimal maintenance dosing for lifelong therapy

SELECT provided multi-year cardiovascular data but did not track long-term weight regain after discontinuation.

Lack of Data on Diverse Populations: Many clinical trials involving semaglutide have inadequately represented diverse subgroups, including older adults, adolescents, and individuals with severe obesity or mental illness [3]. Such underrepresentation restricts the applicability of results, as these populations might exhibit distinct responses to treatment. Notably, individuals with severe obesity or a history of eating disorders may react differently to treatment paradigms, which could influence efficacy and safety profiles [799]. A failure to include these diverse populations in clinical trials may mislead clinicians regarding generalizability and effectiveness in broader, real-world contexts [3].

Many trials underrepresent important groups, including:

- older adults (>75 years)
- adolescents and children (data emerging but limited)
- people with severe mental illness
- minority ethnic groups
- individuals with severe obesity (BMI >50), who may respond differently
- those with eating disorders or a history of disordered eating

This limits how broadly results can be applied in real-world settings.

Limited Evidence in Normal-Weight or Mild Overweight Individuals: Research primarily focuses on individuals with a BMI of 27 or higher, leaving a significant gap in knowledge about those with lower BMI values who could benefit from interventions. The absence of substantial data addressing the effects of semaglutide in non-obese individuals reflects a critical limitation, particularly as off-label uses could arise without clear guidelines [68, 800]. This lack of evidence hinders informed clinical decision-making for patients who fall into these categories, making it difficult to ascertain safety and efficacy under those circumstances.

Trials were intentionally designed for people with:

- BMI ≥30, or
- BMI ≥27 with comorbidities

There is minimal data on:

- people with BMI <27

- cosmetic or non-medical use
- metabolic consequences of appetite suppression in normal-weight individuals

This leaves clinicians with little evidence to guide inappropriate or off-label use.

Stopping Rules and Long-Term Safety Uncertainties: The trials typically involve strict conditions, such as gradual titration and close monitoring, which do not necessarily replicate real-world scenarios where patients may stop abruptly or deviate from prescribed dosing regimens [81, 226]. Reports indicate that real-world utilization shows higher discontinuation rates and poor adherence to recommended titration schedules, compounding uncertainty regarding real-life safety and long-term effectiveness outcomes [801]. Such behavioural variances are crucial for understanding treatment sustainability and must be closely examined in future studies.

Most semaglutide data comes from participants who:

- titrated slowly
- were monitored closely
- did not discontinue suddenly

Real-world patients often:

- stop abruptly
- restart irregularly
- escalate doses outside recommended schedules
- combine with supplements or drugs not studied in trials

We lack data on how these real-world behaviours affect safety and outcomes.

Mechanisms Behind Weight Plateau and Regain: While studies show that participants often plateau in weight loss after 9 to 12 months, the mechanisms responsible for reestablishing a new set-point weight remain poorly understood [15]. The divergence in patient experiences regarding weight loss efficacy highlights the urgent need for research into behavioural interventions that may mitigate plateauing effects and enhance long-term success [227]. Understanding these mechanisms would significantly aid in personalizing treatment approaches.

Trials document that:

- weight loss plateaus around 9–12 months
- stopping the medication leads to substantial regain

But the mechanisms are not fully understood:

- How does the body establish a new "set point"?
- Why do some patients continue losing weight beyond 12 months while others plateau early?
- Can behavioural interventions modify plateau timing or severity?

These unanswered questions limit tailored treatment planning.

Cardiovascular Benefit Evidence in High-Risk Groups: The SELECT trial indicated a notable cardiovascular protective effect in participants with established cardiovascular disease, but extrapolating these benefits to younger or lower-risk groups remains speculative [802]. The variations seen in populations suggest a need for caution when generalizing cardiovascular safety profiles, as benefits may not extend similarly to those without pre-existing conditions [413].

SELECT demonstrated a 20% reduction in MACE, but:

- participants had established cardiovascular disease
- applicability to younger or lower-risk patients is unknown
- benefits may differ in those without underlying inflammation or atherosclerosis

Extrapolating SELECT to general population use requires caution.

Effects on Lean Mass, Bone Density, and Frailty: Data indicate that significant weight loss from semaglutide may also result in reductions in lean mass, which is particularly concerning for older adults vulnerable to sarcopenia [88]. Furthermore, long-term impacts on bone density and frailty are inadequately characterized, necessitating an integrated approach to patient management that includes nutritional support and resistance training to protect against adverse outcomes [105].

Semaglutide induces significant weight loss, but:

- up to 25–40% of weight lost may be lean mass (varies across studies)
- long-term effects on sarcopenia, particularly in older adults, are unknown

- no robust long-term data on bone mineral density

This highlights the need for integrated nutrition and resistance training support.

Limited Comparative Evidence with Newer Agents: The emergence of other multi-incretin therapies, such as tirzepatide, has not been extensively compared to semaglutide in head-to-head trials, leaving gaps in understanding relative efficacy, sustainability, and tolerability [803, 804]. As these newer treatments demonstrate potential for comparable or enhanced outcomes, it complicates the assessment of semaglutide's role in future treatment paradigms [805].

Tirzepatide, retatrutide, and CagriSema show equal or greater weight-loss effects. However:

- few head-to-head trials exist
- long-term comparative outcomes (CV risk, sustainability, tolerability) are still emerging

This makes it difficult to predict semaglutide's future place in therapy.

Evidence Gaps in Mental Health Outcomes: Existing trials have not adequately addressed the psychological ramifications of weight loss treatment, particularly in populations with pre-existing mental health conditions [806, 807]. Emotional and social implications of rapid body changes, as well as the connections between GLP-1 therapies and mental health trajectories, require additional investigation to guide comprehensive treatment approaches that consider both physical and psychological health [808].

Although many patients report improved mood due to weight loss:

- trials did not focus on people with depression, anxiety, PTSD, or eating disorders
- social and emotional effects of rapid body changes are understudied
- the relationship between GLP-1 therapy and compulsive eating, addiction pathways, or reward circuits needs more research

A fuller understanding of psychological outcomes is still developing.

Data on Real-World Adherence and Effectiveness

The discrepancy in adherence and discontinuation rates between clinical trials and real-world practices highlights a critical limitation in understanding true treatment effectiveness [755]. Variations arise from differing socioeconomic backgrounds and the associated challenges in maintaining a treatment regimen, indicating that clinical trial outcomes may not accurately reflect real-world results [809]. Expanded research into these dynamics will provide valuable insights into the actual patient experiences and challenges encountered in broad applications of semaglutide.

Real-world data shows:

- higher discontinuation rates than in trials
- larger variability in weight outcomes
- more frequent intolerability leading to dose holds or reductions
- differing results across socioeconomic groups

This suggests trial outcomes may not fully translate to everyday clinical practice.

While the evidence base for semaglutide is substantial, numerous limitations warrant careful consideration in clinical practice. Continued research is essential to fill these gaps, particularly those concerning long-term outcomes, diverse population representation, real-world adherence, and mechanisms underlying treatment responses.

Chapter 15

Future Directions

Next-Generation Incretin Therapies

Next-generation incretin therapies are poised to transform the treatment landscape for obesity, diabetes, and cardiometabolic diseases through innovative pharmacological approaches that diverge from traditional GLP-1 receptor agonism. Semaglutide has emerged as a landmark agent, offering significant benefits in weight management and glycaemic control among individuals with type 2 diabetes (T2D) and obesity. However, recent developments have introduced multi-hormone agents such as tirzepatide, retatrutide, CagriSema, and investigational oral incretin therapies that demonstrate potential for enhanced metabolic effects, setting the stage for a paradigm shift in clinical practice over the next decade.

The term "next-generation" incretins captures the evolution from isolated GLP-1 receptor modulation towards therapies that integrate multiple hormonal pathways involved in metabolic regulation. Traditional incretin therapy primarily focused on GLP-1, known for its effects on appetite suppression, glycaemic control, and gastric emptying. However, emerging insights reveal the significance of additional targets such as GIP, glucagon, and amylin. GLP-1 contributes to appetite reduction and insulin secretion, while GIP enhances insulin sensitivity and regulates fat storage, and glucagon plays a role in increasing energy expenditure [504, 722]. The integration of these mechanisms into drug design allows next-generation therapies to achieve superior outcomes in weight loss and glycaemic control compared to GLP-1 monotherapy [721].

Next-generation incretin therapies are reshaping the landscape of obesity and metabolic disease treatment. While first-generation agents such as semaglutide target a single hormonal pathway (the GLP-1 receptor), next-generation drugs activate multiple appetite- and metabolism-regulating receptors simultaneously. By combining GLP-1 activity with additional pathways—including GIP, glucagon, and amylin—these therapies produce synergistic effects that go far beyond what a single-agonist medication can achieve. Their mechanisms target not only appetite and food reward but also metabolic rate, fat oxidation, and energy balance, allowing for greater weight loss, improved glycaemic control, and broader cardiometabolic benefits.

One of the defining advantages of these emerging agents is their multi-agonist design. All next-generation incretins still stimulate the GLP-1 receptor, producing the well-known benefits of reduced appetite, slower gastric emptying, and improved insulin secretion. However, they add powerful new mechanisms. Drugs that also activate the GIP receptor, such as tirzepatide and retatrutide, enhance insulin responsiveness, improve fat metabolism, and appear to reduce GLP-1-related nausea—allowing for higher dosing and stronger therapeutic effects. Triple agonists like retatrutide include glucagon receptor activity as well, which boosts thermogenesis, increases resting energy expenditure, and accelerates fat loss. This carefully controlled glucagon stimulation works only because it is paired with GLP-1 and GIP signalling, creating a balanced metabolic response.

Other next-generation approaches involve pairing GLP-1 agonists with amylin analogues, as seen in CagriSema (cagrilintide + semaglutide). Amylin regulates satiety, meal size, and gastric emptying, making it a strong complement to GLP-1. Together, these molecules produce more profound appetite suppression, reduce reward-driven eating, and significantly decrease liver fat. Early data suggest that these combinations outperform semaglutide alone and may approach the metabolic impact of bariatric surgery.

A further innovation is the development of small-molecule oral incretin therapies. Unlike peptide-based injectables, small-molecule drugs can survive digestion and be absorbed like traditional tablets. These therapies aim to provide weekly or even daily oral dosing with effects comparable to injectable GLP-1s or dual agonists. If successful, they could dramatically expand global access by reducing manufacturing complexity and cost.

Across all next-generation incretin therapies, the unifying theme is synergy—multiple hormonal pathways acting together to produce stronger, faster, and more durable metabolic improvements. These agents enhance central appetite regulation, improve peripheral insulin sensitivity, increase fat oxidation, and maintain metabolic rate during weight loss, addressing many of the limitations of first-generation GLP-1 monotherapies like semaglutide. By doing so, they represent the next major leap toward more comprehensive, effective, and sustainable treatment of obesity, diabetes, and related cardiometabolic diseases.

Tirzepatide represents a pioneering dual agonist for both GIP and GLP-1, offering an enhanced therapeutic profile. Clinical studies demonstrate that tirzepatide therapy results in weight reductions of 15–22% at elevated doses and HbA1c reductions of approximately 2.0–2.5%, surpassing the efficacy seen with semaglutide [724, 810]. These results are attributed to the synergistic effects of dual receptor activation, which not only leads to improved appetite suppression but also enhances fat oxidation and energy expenditure [3] . Comparisons with semaglutide highlight tirzepatide's superior outcomes in head-to-head clinical trials, reflecting its position as a promising treatment option for individuals with T2D and obesity [811].

Retatrutide, structured as a triple agonist targeting GLP-1, GIP, and glucagon, is currently undergoing Phase 3 trials after demonstrating remarkable efficacy in Phase 2. Participants in these studies achieved weight losses of up to 24%, with some individuals recording reductions of 30–32%—approaching outcomes typically attributed to bariatric surgery [623, 709]. The comprehensive engagement of multiple hormone pathways positions retatrutide to markedly enhance metabolic health by optimizing appetite regulation, improving glycaemic control, and maximizing energy expenditure [812].

CagriSema, a combination of semaglutide and cagrilintide (an amylin analogue), illustrates the potential of multi-hormonal approaches by leveraging the distinct mechanisms of GLP-1 and amylin to enhance satiety and stabilize postprandial glucose levels. Early trials report weight loss of approximately 15–20%, alongside favourable tolerability profiles, especially for individuals who experience gastrointestinal side effects from traditional GLP-1 therapies [3, 813].

The development of oral investigational incretin therapies marks significant progress in accessible treatment options. Investigational oral agents such as orforglipron and danuglipron push the boundaries of incretin therapy by providing alternative administration routes, effectively overcoming barriers related to injections and broadening patient access [814, 815]. These oral agents have demonstrated favourable weight reduction outcomes, indicating their potential effectiveness in routine management and preventive strategies [816].

Considering the advancements in incretin therapies, next-generation agents cater to the growing need for personalized treatment pathways. These therapies specifically address diverse patient needs, including those who might suffer intolerable side effects from conventional therapies or require more aggressive intervention for severe metabolic conditions. Furthermore, the potential for these innovations to provide a foundational shift toward preventive strategies in cardiometabolic health underscores their importance in the broader healthcare landscape [810, 817].

Next-generation incretin therapies represent significant progress in the medical management of obesity, diabetes, and related cardiometabolic disorders. By harnessing the synergies between various hormonal pathways, agents like tirzepatide, retatrutide, and CagriSema promise greater efficacy in weight loss and metabolic control while enhancing patient tolerance. As these therapies undergo further clinical testing and refinement, they signal a future where pharmacological interventions could rival surgical outcomes in effectiveness and accessibility.

Semaglutide For Addiction, Alzheimer's Disease, Fertility, PCOS—Current Research Status

Semaglutide, a glucagon-like peptide-1 (GLP-1) receptor agonist, has garnered considerable attention for various therapeutic applications beyond its original indication for type 2 diabetes mellitus (T2DM). Current research suggests its potential in addressing addiction, Alzheimer's disease, fertility issues particularly in polycystic ovary syndrome (PCOS), as well as metabolic disorders associated with both PCOS and obesity. Each of these applications can be supported by robust scholarly references, demonstrating the multifaceted nature of semaglutide.

Semaglutide in Addiction

Recent investigations into the neurobiological effects of GLP-1 suggest that semaglutide and similar compounds could play a role in the treatment of addiction. Semaglutide is thought to influence dopaminergic pathways which are critical for addiction behaviours [161]. Additionally, studies have indicated that GLP-1 receptor agonists can reduce drug-seeking behaviour and cravings in rodent models, supporting their potential therapeutic application in managing substance use disorders [183]. The modulation of appetite through central GLP-1 receptors may extend to the management of addictive behaviours demonstrated by decreased food intake, which is associated with a reduction in the rewarding aspects of various substances [818].

GLP-1 receptors are present in brain reward circuits (e.g. ventral tegmental area, nucleus accumbens). Animal studies show that GLP-1 agonists can reduce intake of alcohol, opioids, and stimulants and blunt drug-seeking behaviours [819].

Human data so far

- Early phase and pilot studies (mostly with liraglutide and exenatide; some emerging with semaglutide) suggest:
    - Reduced alcohol craving and intake in people with alcohol use disorder.
    - Possible benefits on nicotine and other substance use, but data are very limited [819].

Current status

- No regulatory approval anywhere for *addiction treatment*.
- Research is still small-scale and early-phase; optimal dose, target populations, and long-term safety are unknown.
- At this point it's a research topic, not a standard therapy. Off-label use should only occur in clinical trials or under specialist supervision.

Semaglutide and Alzheimer's Disease

The emerging role of GLP-1 analogues including semaglutide in neurodegenerative conditions like Alzheimer's disease is promising. GLP-1 receptors not only regulate insulin secretion but also exhibit neuroprotective effects that may mitigate cognitive decline [138]. Research indicates that activating GLP-1 receptors can lead to enhanced synaptic plasticity and neurogenesis, suggesting a potential avenue for intervention in Alzheimer's [820]. Studies are exploring the mechanistic pathways through which semaglutide may decrease amyloid-beta accumulation—a hallmark of Alzheimer's pathology. While advanced preclinical data supports these hypotheses, clinical trials specifically targeting Alzheimer's treatment using semaglutide are still needed.

Type 2 diabetes and obesity increase risk of dementia. GLP-1 RAs may:

- Improve insulin signalling in the brain
- Reduce inflammation and oxidative stress
- Protect neurons and synapses in animal models of Alzheimer's and Parkinson's disease [821]

Clinical trials

- Multiple phase 2/3 trials are underway with semaglutide in early Alzheimer's disease, focusing on cognitive decline and brain imaging markers. [821]
- Earlier human work with other GLP-1s (liraglutide, exenatide) in small Parkinson's and Alzheimer's cohorts showed signals of benefit, but results are mixed and not definitive.

Current status

- As of now, no proven disease-modifying effect in humans.
- No approvals for Alzheimer's or other dementias.
- Until large trials report, use is experimental only.

Semaglutide in Fertility and PCOS

PCOS is one area where semaglutide shows significant potential, particularly in improving fertility outcomes. Obesity and insulin resistance, common in PCOS patients, are often associated with lower fertility rates [822]. Preclinical studies have indicated that semaglutide can reduce hyperinsulinemia and mitigate the symptoms of inflammation in models of PCOS, suggesting its utility in restoring reproductive function in these patients [183]. Clinical trials are underway to assess the efficacy of semaglutide to improve ovulatory function and pregnancy rates in overweight women with PCOS, with preliminary findings showing positive trends in metabolic and reproductive parameters [62, 823].

Semaglutide in Fertility

- Semaglutide itself is **not proven to increase fertility directly**, but weight loss and improved insulin resistance can restore ovulation and cycles in some people with obesity, PCOS, or insulin resistance [824].
- In women with obesity/PCOS, GLP-1 therapy (mostly liraglutide so far) plus lifestyle has been associated with:
    - Improved menstrual regularity
    - Better ovulation rates
    - Better metabolic profile (insulin, glucose, lipids) [825]

Key caution

- Semaglutide is not recommended in pregnancy and usually needs to be stopped at least 2 months before trying to conceive, because of its long half-life and lack of definitive safety data [826].
- There's no strong evidence that it harms fertility itself, but the main issue is what happens if you conceive while on the drug.

Pregnancy and "Ozempic babies"

- Human pregnancy data are still limited; animal studies show foetal harm at high doses, so regulators advise avoiding use during pregnancy [826].
- Case reports of "Ozempic babies" likely reflect:
  - Improved fertility after weight loss/insulin-resistance improvement
  - Reduced contraceptive effectiveness in some contexts (e.g. with tirzepatide and oral contraceptives) plus nausea/vomiting affecting pill absorption, rather than a direct fertility-boosting effect.

Current status

- Semaglutide is contraindicated in pregnancy and should be stopped before planned conception.
- Any use around fertility should be under specialist care with clear pre-conception planning.

Semaglutide and PCOS (Polycystic Ovary Syndrome)
Why it might help

PCOS is strongly linked with:

- Insulin resistance
- Central/visceral obesity
- Irregular or absent ovulation

GLP-1 agonists can:

- Reduce weight (particularly visceral fat)
- Improve insulin resistance
- Lower androgens indirectly via metabolic improvements [825]

Evidence so far

- Most data are with liraglutide, but early studies and clinical experience are extending to semaglutide:
  - Weight loss and improved insulin sensitivity in women with PCOS and obesity.
  - Better menstrual regularity and sometimes improved fertility when combined with lifestyle/metformin [825].
- Guidelines (e.g. Australian and international PCOS guidance) now mention GLP-1 RAs as potential weight-management options in adults with PCOS who meet obesity criteria and

haven't responded to lifestyle alone—but emphasise that evidence for *reproductive* outcomes is still limited [825].

Current status

- Semaglutide is not specifically licensed for PCOS, but can be used off-label mainly to treat:
  - Obesity
  - Metabolic complications
- Any fertility benefit is indirect (via weight and insulin changes), not an approved indication.
- Not recommended if actively trying to conceive; needs washout before pregnancy attempts.

Semaglutide and Metabolic Disorders

In addition to its impact on PCOS and fertility, semaglutide is being explored for its broader implications in weight management and metabolic health. Numerous studies indicate that semaglutide significantly reduces body weight in individuals with obesity [827], which is particularly salient given the association between obesity and several endocrine disorders including PCOS. Additionally, semaglutide's role in reducing ectopic fat deposition further supports its application in treating obesity-related metabolic syndromes [820]. The weight loss experienced by patients taking semaglutide might also improve insulin sensitivity and other parameters associated with metabolic health, thereby enhancing quality of life and reducing healthcare burdens related to obesity [823].

The accumulating evidence from preclinical and clinical studies presents semaglutide as a promising multi-dimensional therapeutic agent transcending its initial indication for T2DM. With specific implications in addiction treatment, potential cognitive benefits in Alzheimer's disease, improvements in fertility for women with PCOS, and significant impacts on obesity and metabolic health, semaglutide's versatility signifies a notable advancement in pharmacotherapy for these complex conditions. The trajectory of ongoing research will be critical in establishing definitive clinical guidelines and optimizing treatment protocols using this innovative GLP-1 receptor agonist.

Combination Therapies (GLP-1 + GIP + Glucagon Agonists)

Combination therapies that consist of triple agonists targeting GLP-1 (glucagon-like peptide-1), GIP (glucose-dependent insulinotropic polypeptide), and glucagon are emerging as a novel approach in the management of metabolic disorders, particularly obesity and type 2 diabetes. These therapies aim to leverage the synergistic effects of multiple hormonal pathways to optimize metabolic function, improve glucose control, and facilitate significant weight loss beyond what is achievable with existing monotherapies like semaglutide or tirzepatide alone.

The Three Hormone Targets in Brief

GLP-1, GIP, and glucagon play distinct yet interrelated roles in metabolic regulation. GLP-1 primarily reduces appetite, slows gastric emptying, and enhances insulin secretion while lowering glucagon levels, thus improving overall glycaemic control [828]. In clinical settings, GLP-1 receptor agonists have demonstrated efficacy in reducing hunger and promoting glycaemic control, though weight loss effects typically plateau around 10-15% in most patients [811].

GLP-1, GIP, and glucagon are three hormones produced in the gut or pancreas that play distinct but interconnected roles in regulating appetite, blood glucose, energy balance, and fat metabolism. Medications like semaglutide, tirzepatide, and retatrutide work by mimicking one or more of these hormones to improve metabolic health.

1. GLP-1 (Glucagon-Like Peptide-1)

Where it comes from:

Released from the intestine after eating.

Main functions:

- Enhances insulin secretion when blood glucose is high
- Suppresses glucagon (reducing glucose release from the liver)
- Slows gastric emptying → you feel full sooner
- Reduces appetite through gut–brain signalling
- Improves satiety and reduces food cravings

What GLP-1–based drugs achieve:

- Strong appetite suppression
- Reduced calorie intake
- Improved blood glucose control
- Weight loss (moderate to significant)

Examples of GLP-1 agonists:

Semaglutide, liraglutide, dulaglutide, exenatide.

GLP-1 = "Stop eating and store energy safely."

2. GIP (Glucose-Dependent Insulinotropic Polypeptide)

Where it comes from:

Released from the upper small intestine after eating, especially when consuming fats and carbohydrates.

Main functions:

- Stimulates insulin release in a glucose-dependent way
- Enhances fat metabolism and may influence how fat is stored and released
- Has indirect effects on appetite and reward pathways

GIP was once thought to promote weight gain, but new science shows it has complex metabolic actions—especially when combined with GLP-1.

Why GIP matters in new therapies:

- Reduces GI side effects caused by strong GLP-1 activation
- Enhances insulin sensitivity
- Boosts fat-burning mechanisms
- Works with GLP-1 to produce greater weight loss than GLP-1 alone

Example:

Tirzepatide is a dual GIP/GLP-1 agonist.

GIP = "Fine-tune insulin and fat metabolism—boost the potency of GLP-1."

3. Glucagon

Where it comes from:

Produced by alpha cells of the pancreas.

Primary role:

Glucagon typically does the opposite of insulin:

- Raises blood glucose by stimulating the liver to release stored sugar.

Metabolic functions beyond glucose:

- Increases energy expenditure → burns more calories
- Enhances fat oxidation → burns fat for fuel
- Reduces liver fat and helps improve fatty liver disease
- Helps regulate overall metabolic rate

Why controlled glucagon activation is useful in new therapies:

A small, balanced amount of glucagon activation increases calorie burning, which:

- counters metabolic slowdown during weight loss
- enhances fat loss
- improves cardiometabolic health

Example:

Retatrutide activates GLP-1 + GIP + glucagon, achieving record weight reductions (up to ~24% in trials).

Glucagon = "Burn energy, use fat stores, raise metabolic rate."

How They Work Together in Next-Gen Incretin Therapies

- **GLP-1:** reduces hunger and lowers blood glucose
- **GIP:** boosts insulin and enhances fat metabolism; improves tolerability
- **Glucagon:** increases calorie burn and fat oxidation

This synergistic combination explains why newer drugs like tirzepatide and retatrutide outperform semaglutide in clinical trials.

GIP's role is slightly different; it enhances insulin secretion under hyperglycaemic conditions and is also involved in fat metabolism regulation. Its modulation of food reward systems suggests that it could buffer against the gastrointestinal side effects seen with GLP-1 therapies, improving patient tolerability [828]. The glucagon receptor, typically associated with raising blood glucose levels, exhibits beneficial effects when partially activated, including increased energy expenditure and enhanced fat oxidation [829]. This multi-faceted approach allows for more effective targeting of metabolic pathways, potentially leading to better clinical outcomes.

Why Combine GLP-1, GIP, and Glucagon?

The limitations of existing GLP-1 selective therapies have prompted the exploration of dual and triple agonists. While GLP-1 agonists like semaglutide offer substantial glycaemic control and appetite suppression, their inability to significantly boost energy expenditure or sustain weight loss as patients acclimate to lower weights remains a challenge. Recent studies illustrate that the integration of GIP and glucagon receptors can address these limitations by providing enhanced metabolic effects, including the promotion of calorie burning and refined energy management, alongside appetite suppression [830, 831].

Thus, the hypothesis behind triple agonist therapy posits that by simultaneously activating these three pathways, one can achieve comprehensive metabolic reprogramming that facilitates greater weight loss (potentially reaching 20-25%) similar to surgical outcomes, without the invasiveness of bariatric surgery [832, 833]. Early phase trials with compounds like retatrutide indicate promising results, showcasing substantial reductions in body weight and improvement in metabolic health indicators, including HbA1c levels and liver fat content [833, 834].

Mechanism of Synergy

The mechanism underlying the synergy of these hormone interactions can be conceptualized through their distinct, overlapping actions across brain, liver, and peripheral systems. In the central nervous system, GLP-1 and GIP diminish hunger and regulate food-related behaviours, thus supporting conscious choices about food intake [835, 836]. Altogether, these hormones enact a complex control system that helps modulate hunger cues and satiety.

On a hepatic level, glucagon, in conjunction with GLP-1 and GIP, helps shift the body's metabolic processes from fat storage to fat oxidation, addressing issues of visceral fat accumulation, which is closely linked to comorbidities in obesity and diabetes [829, 837]. This is crucial as it repositions the body's fuel dynamics, promoting energy expenditure rather than storage.

Finally, the collective action of these receptors enhances whole-body metabolism, where glucagon can elevate resting energy expenditure, counteracting the metabolic slowdown that follows weight loss [829, 837]. Effectively, triple agonists manage to amplify caloric expenditure even as caloric intake is reduced, representing a significant leap in obesity pharmacotherapy.

Clinical Outcomes and Safety Considerations

Recent trials highlight the efficacy of triple agonists in achieving clinically significant weight loss and metabolic benefits. Evidence suggests that candidates such as retatrutide facilitate up to 24% weight loss in some individuals, alongside marked therapeutic improvements in lipid profiles and reductions in elevated liver fat due to NAFLD/NASH [811, 838].

However, increased potency also raises concerns about safety profiles. Gastrointestinal side effects are common and pose a risk for patient adherence. The complexities introduced by glucagon's role must also be carefully balanced, as excessive activation may counteract the glucose-lowering benefits, leading to possible hyperglycaemia [829, 832]. The long-term safety of these novel therapies remains under investigation, necessitating more data to ascertain their acceptable risk profiles over extended periods.

Future Implications

The promising efficacy of triple agonists posits them as potential first-line interventions for severe obesity and advanced metabolic syndromes [836, 839]. Should ongoing clinical trials support their safety and durability, these treatments could shift current paradigms in obesity management, potentially reducing reliance on surgical methods for weight control in selected patient populations. As with any novel class of therapies, considerations such as accessibility, cost-effectiveness, and comprehensive longitudinal safety assessments will be imperative in determining their ultimate impact on clinical practice.

The multifaceted approach inherent in GLP-1, GIP, and glucagon receptor agonists represents a significant advancement in metabolic therapy, allowing for a more comprehensive strategy to manage obesity and related metabolic disorders.

Long-Term Sustainability of Weight Loss

The long-term sustainability of weight loss achieved through pharmacological interventions such as semaglutide presents a multifaceted challenge in the landscape of obesity management. The complexities of maintaining weight loss are often compounded by biological responses and behavioural adaptations that occur post-treatment.

Significant weight loss from various interventions—such as dietary changes, bariatric surgery, or medications like semaglutide—does not guarantee lasting success. Biological mechanisms, such as increases in hunger hormones (ghrelin) and decreased satiety hormones (PPY, GLP-1) following weight loss, contribute to a rebound effect where the body becomes more efficient at conserving energy. This physiological response often results in a gradual regain of weight after stopping treatment [335, 840]. The STEP 4 trial demonstrated this phenomenon: those who continued semaglutide maintained their weight loss, while participants who discontinued treatment regained a substantial portion of their lost weight, indicating that pharmacological effects are not permanent and illustrate the challenges faced when relying solely on medications for weight management [103, 428].

While semaglutide has significant short-term impacts on reducing appetite and altering metabolic responses, these effects are inherently temporary. When patients are on semaglutide, they often experience reduced food cues and feel satisfied with smaller portions. This pharmacological support makes it easier for individuals to adhere to caloric restrictions [841]. However, when the drug is withdrawn, patients may revert back to pre-treatment metabolic states, characterized by increased appetite and energy conservation, leading to weight regain [842]. Thus, while the medication may facilitate weight loss, lasting change relies heavily on continued lifestyle modifications alongside pharmacotherapy to maintain health outcomes [843, 844].

Research indicates that long-term weight maintenance is more effectively achieved through an amalgamation of ongoing behavioural strategies. Individuals who successfully maintain weight loss often engage in consistent meal planning, regular self-monitoring (like weighing), and accountability practices [723]. High protein diets, resistance training, and sustained physical activities are associated with preserving lean muscle mass and metabolic rate, crucial components in preventing weight regain [845]. Furthermore, early intervention when experiencing weight creep—i.e., addressing small weight gains quickly—proves to be pivotal in maintaining weight loss [846].

Evidence suggests two distinct approaches for weight maintenance in the context of obesity treatment: long-term pharmacological maintenance versus stepping down medications. In the pharmacological model, continued use of medications like semaglutide, paired with structured lifestyle practices, helps maintain appetite control and proper caloric intake [847, 848]. Conversely, transitioning off medications often involves a gradual dose reduction paired with a robust focus on sustaining diet and exercise habits; however, this approach presents a higher risk of relapse, especially if structured support diminishes [849]. The blend of these strategies—initial intensive therapy followed by maintenance dosing and lifestyle support—may provide an optimal pathway for many individuals struggling with obesity [850].

Realistically, successful weight management post-treatment does not typically mean returning to one's lowest weight indefinitely. More achievable outcomes are maintaining a loss of about 10-15% of initial body weight, which can significantly lower health risks associated with obesity, such as type 2 diabetes and cardiovascular diseases [840, 846]. Weight loss sustainability focuses not on a single number but rather on achieving a health-promoting weight that reflects metabolic improvements, underscoring the essence of a broader health perspective rather than a strictly number-focused one [851, 852].

Next-generation therapies show promise in achieving even greater weight reductions; however, ongoing concerns about maintenance remain critical. Preliminary observations suggest similar biological responses to weight regain when these newer agents are paused. Continued use along with lifestyle changes consistently yields better long-term weight maintenance rates [852, 853]. The persistent nature of obesity as a chronic condition means that while treatment tools are advancing, the fundamental challenges posed by biological drives for weight regain necessitate a comprehensive, supportive, and sustainable approach to obesity management.

> While semaglutide and similar medications represent advancements in obesity treatment, the challenges of long-term weight maintenance emphasize the need for an integrated strategy that combines pharmacological options with behavioural and lifestyle adjustments to promote enduring health and weight outcomes.

How Personalised Medicine May Change Treatment Approaches

As research on obesity and metabolic diseases continues to evolve, personalized medicine is emerging as a pivotal approach in treatment strategies, moving away from traditional one-size-fits-all methods. Personalized medicine emphasizes individual characteristics such as biology, behaviour, genetics, and environmental factors, allowing for tailored treatments that target the unique needs of each patient. Evidence suggests that obesity and metabolic dysfunction stem from diverse etiological origins, including appetite regulation, insulin resistance, emotional eating, hormonal imbalances, and energy expenditure discrepancies [721, 854].

Recent advancements in pharmacotherapy, particularly with agents such as semaglutide, have demonstrated differing metabolic responses to targeted hormonal therapies. Semaglutide, a GLP-1 receptor agonist, and newer agents like tirzepatide and retatrutide showcase enhanced efficacy due to their multi-receptor targeting capabilities, providing significant therapeutic benefits for varying obesity phenotypes [721, 855]. For instance, specific genetic variants and metabolic markers can now be leveraged to predict which patients may respond favourably to GLP-1 agonists, indicating a shift towards biologically-informed prescriptions [856, 857].

The future of personalized medicine in obesity treatment also hinges on the identification and use of biomarkers. These biomarkers include genetic predispositions, gut microbiome profiles, and metabolic markers that help clinicians determine the most effective medication, dosage, and treatment duration for each patient [857, 858]. Continued research into metabolomics has shown promise in defining an "obesity signature," enhancing our understanding of metabolic health and treatment responses [857, 858]. Furthermore, integrating psychosocial factors into treatment plans is paramount, as conditions like emotional eating, ADHD, and sleep disorders necessitate distinct therapeutic strategies that include behavioural and psychological support [859, 860].

Monitoring and adjusting treatment regimens may also see significant advancements through technology. For instance, devices capable of continuous glucose monitoring and digital tracking of appetite and energy could enable clinicians to make real-time adjustments to treatment plans, ensuring optimal dosing tailored to the patient's needs [861]. This high level of precision can facilitate early identification of weight-loss plateaus and suggest personalized interventions aimed at improving outcomes [862].

Ultimately, the paradigm of personalized medicine aims to transcend mere weight loss, focusing instead on restoring comprehensive metabolic health. Emerging evidence underscores that obesity is a multifaceted, biologically complex condition rather than merely a failure of discipline, necessitating a sophisticated, integrative approach that combines genomics, behavioural science, digital health innovations, and multi-target pharmacological strategies [863, 864]. This holistic framework is poised to enhance the efficacy, safety, and sustainability of treatments aimed at combating obesity, type 2 diabetes, and related metabolic disorders.

Future Regulatory Landscapes

Personalized medicine, often referred to as precision medicine, represents a significant shift in medical treatment paradigms, particularly in managing obesity, diabetes, and related metabolic disorders. This approach emphasizes the customization of therapeutic interventions based on an individual's biological, genetic, behavioural, and environmental characteristics rather than adhering to generalized treatment protocols. As the understanding of obesity and metabolic disorders matures, personalized therapeutic strategies, such as drugs like semaglutide and next-generation incretin therapies, promise to enhance treatment efficacy and patient outcomes.

The heterogeneity of metabolic conditions such as obesity and diabetes necessitates a nuanced treatment approach. The adoption of genetic and metabolic biomarkers can provide insight into how individuals may respond to specific medications like semaglutide. Evidence from genome-wide association studies (GWAS) highlights variations in pathways related to insulin secretion and GLP-1 receptor expression, which contribute to differential responses to therapies. Specifically, certain genetic variants affecting the GLP-1 receptor locus (GLP1R) have been associated with variations in responsiveness to GLP-1 receptor agonists, thus paving the way for biomarker-driven prescription strategies similar to those used in oncology [865].

Moreover, the influence of behavioural and psychological dimensions on treatment efficacy cannot be underestimated. Research indicates that individuals exhibit different eating behaviours—ranging from emotional eating to hunger dysregulation—which can affect their weight management strategies [369]. Emerging findings suggest that various incretin-based drugs may interact differently with appetitive neural pathways, indicating a need for precision-matched medication selection. For instance, stronger agonists may be more suitable for individuals exhibiting compulsive eating behaviours, while less potent options may be more appropriate for those who are sensitive to gastrointestinal side effects [866].

In addition to pharmacological considerations, the personalization of treatment protocols also encompasses dose titration strategies. Current standard titration schedules often fail to account for individual patient variations such as gastric emptying rates and renal function. Future approaches employing continuous glucose monitoring and digital tracking may enable real-time adjustments to therapy based on individual responses, optimizing outcomes related to appetite control and metabolic improvements [867]. This shift toward individualized dosing strategies is critical for improving the tolerability of GLP-1 receptor agonists and minimizing adverse effects such as nausea or gastrointestinal discomfort, which are common following standardized titration schedules [868].

The development of combination therapies represents another significant advancement in personalized medicine. As new agents targeting diverse metabolic pathways are introduced, such as GIP and glucagon receptors, clinicians will be equipped to tailor combinations based on a patient's specific metabolic phenotype. For instance, patients with non-alcoholic fatty liver disease (NAFLD) might experience substantial benefits from combinations like GLP-1 and glucagon receptor agonists that specifically target hepatic fat accumulation [869]. This tailored approach extends to long-term maintenance strategies, where individualized care plans can help maintain weight loss or prevent metabolic disease progression, factoring in individual predispositions to weight regain.

Beyond clinical efficacy, the advent of personalized medicine in the management of metabolic disorders raises important equity and ethical questions. Enhanced diagnostic technologies and targeted therapies have the potential to improve early identification of high-risk individuals; however, disparities in access to these advancements may lead to increased health inequalities. Hence, it is essential for policymakers to develop frameworks that promote equitable access to personalized metabolic treatments across different socio-economic backgrounds [870]. Balancing the benefits of personalized medicine with considerations of health equity will be crucial as this field continues to evolve.

> Personalized medicine has the potential to transform the management of obesity, diabetes, and metabolic disorders by using a multifaceted approach that integrates genetic, behavioural, and physiological insights. Through tailored pharmacotherapy and diligent attention to individual patient characteristics, it may be possible to optimize treatment effectiveness, enhance tolerability, and ultimately improve patient outcomes in this challenging area of healthcare.

References

1. Husain, M., et al., *Semaglutide (SUSTAIN and PIONEER) Reduces Cardiovascular Events in Type 2 Diabetes Across Varying Cardiovascular Risk.* Diabetes Obesity and Metabolism, 2020. **22**(3): p. 442-451.
2. Essilfie-Quaye, K., et al., *Semaglutide-Induced Silent Aspiration: An Unrecognised Cause of Organising Pneumonia.* Respirology Case Reports, 2025. **13**(7).
3. Frías, J.P., et al., *Tirzepatide Versus Semaglutide Once Weekly in Patients With Type 2 Diabetes.* New England Journal of Medicine, 2021. **385**(6): p. 503-515.
4. Janić, M., et al., *Effect of Oral Semaglutide on Cardiovascular Parameters and Their Mechanisms in Patients With Type 2 Diabetes: Rationale and Design of the Semaglutide Anti-Atherosclerotic Mechanisms of Action Study (SAMAS).* Diabetes Therapy, 2022. **13**(4): p. 795-810.
5. Patel, S. and S.K. Niazi, *Emerging Frontiers in GLP-1 Therapeutics: A Comprehensive Evidence Base (2025).* Pharmaceutics, 2025. **17**(8): p. 1036.
6. Yanai, H., et al., *A Significant Effect of Oral Semaglutide on Cardiovascular Risk Factors in Patients With Type 2 Diabetes.* Cardiology Research, 2022. **13**(5): p. 303-308.
7. Hosseinpour, A., et al., *Glucagon-Like Peptide-1 Receptor Agonists and Major Adverse Cardiovascular Events in Patients With and Without Diabetes: A Meta-Analysis of Randomized-Controlled Trials.* Clinical Cardiology, 2024. **47**(7).
8. Pocai, A., *G Protein-Coupled Receptors and Obesity.* Frontiers in Endocrinology, 2023. **14**.
9. Saraiva, J.F.K. and D.R. Franco, *Oral GLP-1 Analogue: Perspectives and Impact on Atherosclerosis in Type 2 Diabetic Patients.* Cardiovascular Diabetology, 2021. **20**(1).
10. Prakash, S. and J.O. Coleman, *Glucagon-Like Peptide 1 Receptor Agonists and Cardiovascular Disease Risk: Findings From Real-World Data Using AI-Powered Outcomes.* 2024.
11. Ashraf, T., et al., *A Meta-Analytic Review of the Safety and Efficacy of Semaglutide in Type 2 Diabetes Mellitus and Chronic Kidney Disease Patients.* Annals of Medicine and Surgery, 2025. **87**(4): p. 2278-2285.
12. Yoshiji, S., et al., *Effects of Glucagon-like Peptide-1 Receptor Agonists on Cardiovascular and Renal Outcomes: A <scp>meta-analysis</Scp> And <scp>meta-regression</Scp> Analysis.* Diabetes Obesity and Metabolism, 2022. **24**(6): p. 1029-1037.
13. Princy, R., *Semaglutide Induced Pancreatitis.* International Journal for Multidisciplinary Research, 2024. **6**(4).
14. Buckley, S.T., et al., *Transcellular Stomach Absorption of a Derivatized Glucagon-Like Peptide-1 Receptor Agonist.* Science Translational Medicine, 2018. **10**(467).
15. Jain, A., et al., *Real-World Effectiveness Analysis of Switching From Liraglutide or Dulaglutide to Semaglutide in Patients With Type 2 Diabetes Mellitus: The Retrospective REALISE-DM Study.* Diabetes Therapy, 2020. **12**(2): p. 527-536.
16. Jensen, L., et al., *Pharmacokinetics and Tolerability of Semaglutide in People With Hepatic Impairment.* Diabetes Obesity and Metabolism, 2018. **20**(4): p. 998-1005.

17. Madsbad, S., et al., *An Overview of Once-weekly Glucagon-like Peptide-1 Receptor Agonists—available Efficacy and Safety Data and Perspectives for the Future.* Diabetes Obesity and Metabolism, 2011. **13**(5): p. 394-407.
18. Husain, M., et al., *Oral Semaglutide and Cardiovascular Outcomes in Patients With Type 2 Diabetes.* New England Journal of Medicine, 2019. **381**(9): p. 841-851.
19. Mahapatra, M.K., M. Karuppasamy, and B.M. Sahoo, *Therapeutic Potential of Semaglutide, a Newer GLP-1 Receptor Agonist, in Abating Obesity, Non-Alcoholic Steatohepatitis and Neurodegenerative Diseases: A Narrative Review.* Pharmaceutical Research, 2022. **39**(6): p. 1233-1248.
20. Rodbard, H.W., et al., *Semaglutide Added to Basal Insulin in Type 2 Diabetes (SUSTAIN 5): A Randomized, Controlled Trial.* The Journal of Clinical Endocrinology & Metabolism, 2018. **103**(6): p. 2291-2301.
21. Reed, J., S.C. Bain, and V. Kanamarlapudi, *Recent Advances in Understanding the Role of Glucagon-Like Peptide 1.* F1000research, 2020. **9**: p. 239.
22. Nauck, M.A., et al., *GLP-1 Receptor Agonists in the Treatment of Type 2 Diabetes – State-of-the-Art.* Molecular Metabolism, 2021. **46**: p. 101102.
23. Hare, K.J., et al., *The Glucagonostatic and Insulinotropic Effects of Glucagon-Like Peptide 1 Contribute Equally to Its Glucose-Lowering Action.* Diabetes, 2010. **59**(7): p. 1765-1770.
24. Ørgaard, A. and J.J. Holst, *The Role of Somatostatin in GLP-1-induced Inhibition of Glucagon Secretion in Mice.* Diabetologia, 2017. **60**(9): p. 1731-1739.
25. Müller, T.D., et al., *Glucagon-Like Peptide 1 (GLP-1).* Molecular Metabolism, 2019. **30**: p. 72-130.
26. Drucker, D.J., *The Cardiovascular Biology of Glucagon-Like Peptide-1.* Cell Metabolism, 2016. **24**(1): p. 15-30.
27. Nadkarni, P., O.G. Chepurny, and G.G. Holz, *Regulation of Glucose Homeostasis by GLP-1.* 2014: p. 23-65.
28. Pinheiro, E.G.H., et al., *The Cardioprotective Effects of Semaglutide in Obese Patients: Literature Review.* Journal of Medical Residency Review, 2024. **3**(00): p. e059.
29. Nauck, M.A., *Incretin Therapies: Highlighting Common Features and Differences in the Modes of Action of Glucagon-like Peptide-1 Receptor Agonists and Dipeptidyl Peptidase-4 Inhibitors.* Diabetes Obesity and Metabolism, 2016. **18**(3): p. 203-216.
30. Himmerich, H. and S.L. McElroy, *Glucagon-Like Peptide 1 Receptor Agonists in Psychiatry.* Journal of Clinical Psychopharmacology, 2024. **44**(3): p. 207-210.
31. Friedrichsen, M., et al., *The Effect of Semaglutide 2.4 Mg Once Weekly on Energy Intake, Appetite, Control of Eating, and Gastric Emptying in Adults With Obesity.* Diabetes Obesity and Metabolism, 2021. **23**(3): p. 754-762.
32. Wadden, T.A., et al., *Effect of Subcutaneous Semaglutide vs Placebo as an Adjunct to Intensive Behavioral Therapy on Body Weight in Adults With Overweight or Obesity.* Jama, 2021. **325**(14): p. 1403.
33. Enebo, L.B., et al., *Safety, Tolerability, Pharmacokinetics, and Pharmacodynamics of Concomitant Administration of Multiple Doses of Cagrilintide With Semaglutide 2·4 Mg for Weight Management: A Randomised, Controlled, Phase 1b Trial.* The Lancet, 2021. **397**(10286): p. 1736-1748.
34. Tóth, L.I., et al., *Semaglutide Improves Lipid Subfraction Profiles in Type 2 Diabetes: Insights From a One-Year Follow-Up Study.* International Journal of Molecular Sciences, 2025. **26**(13): p. 5951.

35. Aroda, V.R., et al., *High-Dose Semaglutide (Up to 16 Mg) in People With Type 2 Diabetes and Overweight or Obesity: A Randomized, Placebo-Controlled, Phase 2 Trial.* Diabetes Care, 2025. **48**(6): p. 905-913.
36. Martins, F.F., et al., *Semaglutide (GLP-1 Receptor Agonist) Stimulates Browning on Subcutaneous Fat Adipocytes and Mitigates Inflammation and Endoplasmic Reticulum Stress in Visceral Fat Adipocytes of Obese Mice.* Cell Biochemistry and Function, 2022. **40**(8): p. 903-913.
37. Secher, A., et al., *The Arcuate Nucleus Mediates GLP-1 Receptor Agonist Liraglutide-Dependent Weight Loss.* Journal of Clinical Investigation, 2014. **124**(10): p. 4473-4488.
38. Okamoto, A., et al., *Efficacy of Oral Semaglutide After Switching From DPP-4 Inhibitors in Japanese Type 2 Diabetes Patients With Obesity.* 2024.
39. Lau, J., et al., *Discovery of the Once-Weekly Glucagon-Like Peptide-1 (GLP-1) Analogue Semaglutide.* Journal of Medicinal Chemistry, 2015. **58**(18): p. 7370-7380.
40. Sorli, C., et al., *Efficacy and Safety of Once-Weekly Semaglutide Monotherapy Versus Placebo in Patients With Type 2 Diabetes (SUSTAIN 1): A Double-Blind, Randomised, Placebo-Controlled, Parallel-Group, Multinational, Multicentre Phase 3a Trial.* The Lancet Diabetes & Endocrinology, 2017. **5**(4): p. 251-260.
41. Hjerpsted, J., et al., *Semaglutide Improves Postprandial Glucose and Lipid Metabolism, and Delays First-hour Gastric Emptying in Subjects With Obesity.* Diabetes Obesity and Metabolism, 2017. **20**(3): p. 610-619.
42. Aroda, V.R., L. Blonde, and R.E. Pratley, *A New Era for Oral Peptides: SNAC and the Development of Oral Semaglutide for the Treatment of Type 2 Diabetes.* Reviews in Endocrine and Metabolic Disorders, 2022. **23**(5): p. 979-994.
43. Tan, H., et al., *Albumin-Binding Domain Extends Half-Life of Glucagon-Like Peptide-1.* European Journal of Pharmacology, 2021. **890**: p. 173650.
44. Xie, P., et al., *A Phase 1, Randomized, Double-blind, Placebo-controlled Trial Investigating the Pharmacokinetics, Pharmacodynamics, Safety and Tolerability of Oral Semaglutide in Healthy Chinese Subjects.* Diabetes Obesity and Metabolism, 2024. **26**(8): p. 3068-3077.
45. Overgaard, R.V., et al., *Clinical Pharmacokinetics of Oral Semaglutide: Analyses of Data From Clinical Pharmacology Trials.* Clinical Pharmacokinetics, 2021. **60**(10): p. 1335-1348.
46. Cowart, K., *Oral Semaglutide: First-in-Class Oral GLP-1 Receptor Agonist for the Treatment of Type 2 Diabetes Mellitus.* Annals of Pharmacotherapy, 2019. **54**(5): p. 478-485.
47. Mima, A., et al., *Effects of Oral Semaglutide on Renal Function in Diabetic Kidney Disease: A Short-Term Clinical Study.* In Vivo, 2023. **38**(1): p. 308-312.
48. Marbury, T., et al., *Pharmacokinetics and Tolerability of a Single Dose of Semaglutide, a Human Glucagon-Like Peptide-1 Analog, in Subjects With and Without Renal Impairment.* Clinical Pharmacokinetics, 2017. **56**(11): p. 1381-1390.
49. Kim, J.C., E.J. Park, and D.H. Na, *Gastrointestinal Permeation Enhancers for the Development of Oral Peptide Pharmaceuticals.* Pharmaceuticals, 2022. **15**(12): p. 1585.
50. Seino, Y., et al., *Safety and Efficacy of Semaglutide Once Weekly vs Sitagliptin Once Daily, Both as Monotherapy In <scp>J</Scp> Apanese People With Type 2 Diabetes.* Diabetes Obesity and Metabolism, 2017. **20**(2): p. 378-388.
51. Aroda, V.R., et al., *Efficacy and Safety of Once-Weekly Semaglutide Versus Once-Daily Insulin Glargine as Add-on to Metformin (With or Without Sulfonylureas) in Insulin-Naive*

Patients With Type 2 Diabetes (SUSTAIN 4): A Randomised, Open-Label, Parallel-Group, Multicentre, Multinational, Phase 3a Trial. The Lancet Diabetes & Endocrinology, 2017. **5**(5): p. 355-366.

52. Aroda, V.R., et al., *PIONEER 1: Randomized Clinical Trial of the Efficacy and Safety of Oral Semaglutide Monotherapy in Comparison With Placebo in Patients With Type 2 Diabetes.* Diabetes Care, 2019. **42**(9): p. 1724-1732.
53. Htike, Z.Z., et al., *Efficacy and Safety of Glucagon-like Peptide-1 Receptor Agonists in Type 2 Diabetes: <scp>A</Scp> Systematic Review and Mixed-treatment Comparison Analysis.* Diabetes Obesity and Metabolism, 2017. **19**(4): p. 524-536.
54. Isaacs, D., L. Prasad-Reddy, and S.B. Srivastava, *Role of Glucagon-Like Peptide 1 Receptor Agonists in Management of Obesity.* American Journal of Health-System Pharmacy, 2016. **73**(19): p. 1493-1507.
55. Mahapatra, M.K., M. Karuppasamy, and B.M. Sahoo, *Semaglutide, a Glucagon Like Peptide-1 Receptor Agonist With Cardiovascular Benefits for Management of Type 2 Diabetes.* Reviews in Endocrine and Metabolic Disorders, 2022. **23**(3): p. 521-539.
56. Hebsgaard, J.B., et al., *Glucagon-like Peptide-1 Receptor Expression in the Human Eye.* Diabetes Obesity and Metabolism, 2018. **20**(9): p. 2304-2308.
57. Shi, A., et al., *Pharmacokinetics, Safety and Tolerability of Once-Weekly Subcutaneous Semaglutide in Healthy Chinese Subjects: A Double-Blind, Phase 1, Randomized Controlled Trial.* Advances in Therapy, 2020. **38**(1): p. 550-561.
58. Solis-Herrera, C., M.P. Kane, and C. Triplitt, *Current Understanding of Sodium N-(8-[2-Hydroxylbenzoyl] Amino) Caprylate (SNAC) as an Absorption Enhancer: The Oral Semaglutide Experience.* Clinical Diabetes, 2023. **42**(1): p. 74-86.
59. Bækdal, T.A., et al., *Effect of Oral Semaglutide on the Pharmacokinetics of Lisinopril, Warfarin, Digoxin, and Metformin in Healthy Subjects.* Clinical Pharmacokinetics, 2019. **58**(9): p. 1193-1203.
60. Granhall, C., et al., *Pharmacokinetics, Safety and Tolerability of Oral Semaglutide in Subjects With Renal Impairment.* Clinical Pharmacokinetics, 2018. **57**(12): p. 1571-1580.
61. Helmstädter, J., et al., *Glucagon-like Peptide-1 (GLP-1) Receptor Agonists and Their Cardiovascular Benefits—The Role of the GLP-1 Receptor.* British Journal of Pharmacology, 2021. **179**(4): p. 659-676.
62. Knudsen, L.B. and J. Lau, *The Discovery and Development of Liraglutide and Semaglutide.* Frontiers in Endocrinology, 2019. **10**.
63. Nauck, M.A., et al., *Normalization of Fasting Hyperglycaemia by Exogenous Glucagon-Like Peptide 1 (7-36 Amide) in Type 2 (Non-Insulin-Dependent) Diabetic Patients.* Diabetologia, 1993. **36**(8): p. 741-744.
64. Meier, J.J., *GLP-1 Receptor Agonists for Individualized Treatment of Type 2 Diabetes Mellitus.* Nature Reviews Endocrinology, 2012. **8**(12): p. 728-742.
65. Vella, A., et al., *Effect of Glucagon-Like Peptide 1(7-36) Amide on Glucose Effectiveness and Insulin Action in People With Type 2 Diabetes.* Diabetes, 2000. **49**(4): p. 611-617.
66. Aroda, V.R., et al., *Comparative Efficacy, Safety, and Cardiovascular Outcomes With Once-Weekly Subcutaneous Semaglutide in the Treatment of Type 2 Diabetes: Insights From the SUSTAIN 1–7 Trials.* Diabetes & Metabolism, 2019. **45**(5): p. 409-418.
67. Ji, L., et al., *Efficacy and Safety of Once-weekly Semaglutide Versus Once-daily Sitagliptin as Add-on to Metformin in Patients With Type 2 Diabetes In <scp>SUSTAIN*

China</Scp> : A 30-week, Double-blind, Phase 3a, Randomized Trial. Diabetes Obesity and Metabolism, 2021. **23**(2): p. 404-414.

68. Åhrén, B., et al., *Semaglutide Induces Weight Loss in Subjects With Type 2 Diabetes Regardless of Baseline <scp>BMI</Scp> or Gastrointestinal Adverse Events in the SUSTAIN 1 to 5 Trials.* Diabetes Obesity and Metabolism, 2018. **20**(9): p. 2210-2219.
69. Liu, L., et al., *Long-Term Cost-Effectiveness of Subcutaneous Once-Weekly Semaglutide Versus Polyethylene Glycol Loxenatide for Treatment of Type 2 Diabetes Mellitus in China.* Diabetes Therapy, 2022. **14**(1): p. 93-107.
70. Menzen, M., et al., *Real-World Use of Once-Weekly Semaglutide in Type 2 Diabetes: Results From SemaglUtide Real-World Evidence (SURE) Germany.* Experimental and Clinical Endocrinology & Diabetes, 2023. **131**(04): p. 205-215.
71. Singh, G., M. Krauthamer, and M. Bjalme-Evans, *Wegovy (Semaglutide): A New Weight Loss Drug for Chronic Weight Management.* Journal of Investigative Medicine, 2022. **70**(1): p. 5-13.
72. Goldenberg, R. and O. Steen, *Semaglutide: Review and Place in Therapy for Adults With Type 2 Diabetes.* Canadian Journal of Diabetes, 2019. **43**(2): p. 136-145.
73. Aroda, V.R., et al., *Impact of Baseline Characteristics and Beta-cell Function on the Efficacy and Safety of Subcutaneous Once-weekly Semaglutide: A Patient-level, Pooled Analysis of the SUSTAIN 1-5 Trials.* Diabetes Obesity and Metabolism, 2019. **22**(3): p. 303-314.
74. Buse, J.B., et al., *Study Design and Baseline Profile for Adults With Type 2 Diabetes in the Once-Weekly Subcutaneous SEmaglutide Randomized PRAgmatic (SEPRA) Trial.* BMJ Open Diabetes Research & Care, 2023. **11**(3): p. e003206.
75. Krishnan, S., et al., *Physician Perceptions of the Safety and Efficacy of GLP-1 Receptor Agonists: Underestimation of Cardiovascular Risk Reduction and Discrepancies With Clinical Evidence.* Journal of Cardiovascular Development and Disease, 2025. **12**(1): p. 19.
76. Nanna, M.G., et al., *Population-level Impact of Semaglutide 2.4 mg in Patients With Obesity or Overweight and Cardiovascular Disease: A Modelling Study Based on The <scp>SELECT</Scp> Trial.* Diabetes Obesity and Metabolism, 2025. **27**(6): p. 3442-3452.
77. Lǐ, Y., et al., *Semaglutide and Major Adverse Cardiovascular Events in Patients With and Without DM: A Systematic Review and Meta-Analysis.* 2024.
78. Fisher, M., *Series: Cardiovascular Outcome Trials for Diabetes Drugs Semaglutide and SUSTAIN-6.* British Journal of Diabetes, 2021. **21**(1): p. 110-112.
79. Marso, S.P., et al., *Semaglutide and Cardiovascular Outcomes in Patients With Type 2 Diabetes.* New England Journal of Medicine, 2016. **375**(19): p. 1834-1844.
80. Katz, G., *Efficacy, Safety, and Future of GLP-1 Receptor Agonists: A Systematic Literature Review and Meta-Analysis.* Hormone and Metabolic Research, 2025. **57**(05): p. 326-337.
81. Uzoigwe, C., et al., *Semaglutide Once-Weekly Persistence and Adherence Versus Other GLP-1 RAs in Patients With Type 2 Diabetes in a US Real-World Setting.* Diabetes Therapy, 2021. **12**(5): p. 1475-1489.
82. Alkhezi, O.S., et al., *Comparative Effectiveness of Glucagon-like Peptide-1 Receptor Agonists for the Management of Obesity in Adults Without Diabetes: A Network Meta-analysis of Randomized Clinical Trials.* Obesity Reviews, 2022. **24**(3).

83. Fang, Z., et al., *Glucagon-Like Peptide-1 Mimetics, Optimal for Asian Type 2 Diabetes Patients With and Without Overweight/Obesity: Meta-Analysis of Randomized Controlled Trials*. Scientific Reports, 2017. **7**(1).
84. Kushner, R.F., et al., *Semaglutide 2.4 Mg for the Treatment of Obesity: Key Elements of the STEP Trials 1 to 5*. Obesity, 2020. **28**(6): p. 1050-1061.
85. Viljoen, A., et al., *Evaluation of the Long-term Cost-effectiveness of Once-weekly Semaglutide Versus Dulaglutide for Treatment of Type 2 Diabetes Mellitus in the UK*. Diabetes Obesity and Metabolism, 2018. **21**(3): p. 611-621.
86. Mody, R., et al., *Adherence and Persistence Among Patients With Type 2 Diabetes Initiating Dulaglutide Compared With Semaglutide and Exenatide <scp>BCise</Scp>: 6-month Follow-up From <scp>US Real-world</Scp> Data*. Diabetes Obesity and Metabolism, 2020. **23**(1): p. 106-115.
87. Witkowski, M., et al., *A Systematic Literature Review and Network Meta-Analysis Comparing Once-Weekly Semaglutide With Other GLP-1 Receptor Agonists in Patients With Type 2 Diabetes Previously Receiving 1–2 Oral Anti-Diabetic Drugs*. Diabetes Therapy, 2018. **9**(3): p. 1149-1167.
88. Rubino, D., et al., *Effect of Weekly Subcutaneous Semaglutide vs Daily Liraglutide on Body Weight in Adults With Overweight or Obesity Without Diabetes*. Jama, 2022. **327**(2): p. 138.
89. Liu, L., et al., *Comparative Efficacy and Safety of Glucagon-Like Peptide-1 Receptor Agonists in Children and Adolescents With Obesity or Overweight: A Systematic Review and Network Meta-Analysis*. Pharmaceuticals, 2024. **17**(7): p. 828.
90. Kahn, S.E., et al., *Effect of Semaglutide on Regression and Progression of Glycemia in People With Overweight or Obesity but Without Diabetes in the SELECT Trial*. Diabetes Care, 2024. **47**(8): p. 1350-1359.
91. Colhoun, H.M., et al., *Long-Term Kidney Outcomes of Semaglutide in Obesity and Cardiovascular Disease in the SELECT Trial*. Nature Medicine, 2024. **30**(7): p. 2058-2066.
92. Johansen, P., A. Sandberg, and M. Capehorn, *A Relative Cost of Control Analysis of Once-Weekly Semaglutide Versus Exenatide Extended-Release, Dulaglutide and Liraglutide in the UK*. Advances in Therapy, 2020. **37**(3): p. 1248-1259.
93. Lingvay, I., et al., *An Indirect Treatment Comparison of Semaglutide 2.0 Mg vs Dulaglutide 3.0 Mg and 4.5 Mg Using Multilevel Network Meta-Regression*. The Journal of Clinical Endocrinology & Metabolism, 2021. **107**(5): p. 1461-1469.
94. Guo, X., et al., *The Antiobesity Effect and Safety of GLP-1 Receptor Agonist In Overweight/Obese Patients Without Diabetes: A Systematic Review And Meta-Analysis*. Hormone and Metabolic Research, 2022. **54**(07): p. 458-471.
95. Granhall, C., et al., *Safety and Pharmacokinetics of Single and Multiple Ascending Doses of the Novel Oral Human GLP-1 Analogue, Oral Semaglutide, in Healthy Subjects and Subjects With Type 2 Diabetes*. Clinical Pharmacokinetics, 2018. **58**(6): p. 781-791.
96. Sofogianni, A. and K. Τζιόμαλος, *Oral Semaglutide, a New Option in the Management of Type 2 Diabetes Mellitus: A Narrative Review*. Advances in Therapy, 2020. **37**(10): p. 4165-4174.
97. Evans, M., et al., *Meeting the Challenge of Virtual Diabetes Care: A Consensus Viewpoint on the Positioning and Value of Oral Semaglutide in Routine Clinical Practice*. Diabetes Therapy, 2022. **13**(2): p. 225-240.

98. Jordy, A.B., et al., *Effect of Oral Semaglutide on the Pharmacokinetics of Levonorgestrel and Ethinylestradiol in Healthy Postmenopausal Women and Furosemide and Rosuvastatin in Healthy Subjects.* Clinical Pharmacokinetics, 2021. **60**(9): p. 1171-1185.
99. Majanović, S.K., et al., *Effectiveness of Oral Versus Injectable Semaglutide in Adults With Type 2 Diabetes: Results From a Retrospective Observational Study in Croatia.* Diabetology, 2024. **5**(1): p. 60-68.
100. Tilinca, M.C., et al., *Untitled.* Farmacia, 2023. **71**(1).
101. Davies, M.J., et al., *Effect of Oral Semaglutide Compared With Placebo and Subcutaneous Semaglutide on Glycemic Control in Patients With Type 2 Diabetes.* Jama, 2017. **318**(15): p. 1460.
102. Mikhail, N., *Oral Semaglutide for the Treatment of Type 2 Diabetes: A Mini Review.* Series of Endocrinology Diabetes and Metabolism, 2019. **1**(3): p. 62-66.
103. Rubino, D., et al., *Effect of Continued Weekly Subcutaneous Semaglutide vs Placebo on Weight Loss Maintenance in Adults With Overweight or Obesity.* Jama, 2021. **325**(14): p. 1414.
104. Alabduljabbar, K., W. Al-Najim, and C.W.l. Roux, *The Impact Once-Weekly Semaglutide 2.4 Mg Will Have on Clinical Practice: A Focus on the STEP Trials.* Nutrients, 2022. **14**(11): p. 2217.
105. Garvey, W.T., et al., *Two-Year Effects of Semaglutide in Adults With Overweight or Obesity: The STEP 5 Trial.* Nature Medicine, 2022. **28**(10): p. 2083-2091.
106. Chakhtoura, M., et al., *Pharmacotherapy of Obesity: An Update on the Available Medications and Drugs Under Investigation.* Eclinicalmedicine, 2023. **58**: p. 101882.
107. Salvatore, M., et al., *Real-World Comparative Outcomes of GLP-1 RA and Semaglutide Prescription Among Individuals With Type 2 Diabetes.* 2025.
108. Mital, S. and H.V. Nguyen, *Cost-Effectiveness of Antiobesity Drugs for Adolescents With Severe Obesity.* Jama Network Open, 2023. **6**(10): p. e2336400.
109. Wilding, J., et al., *Weight Regain and Cardiometabolic Effects After Withdrawal of Semaglutide: The <scp>STEP</Scp> 1 Trial Extension.* Diabetes Obesity and Metabolism, 2022. **24**(8): p. 1553-1564.
110. Arillotta, D., et al., *GLP-1 Receptor Agonists and Related Mental Health Issues; Insights From a Range of Social Media Platforms Using a Mixed-Methods Approach.* Brain Sciences, 2023. **13**(11): p. 1503.
111. Daneshgaran, G., O. Shauly, and D.J. Gould, *"Ozempic Face" in Plastic Surgery: A Systematic Review of the Literature on GLP-1 Receptor Agonist Mediated Weight Loss and Analysis of Public Perceptions.* Aesthetic Surgery Journal Open Forum, 2025. **7**.
112. Bloom, B.E., et al., *How Glucagon-Like Peptide-1 Medications Are Depicted in Instagram Posts Regarding Women's Health, Nontraditional Access, and Barriers to Access: Content Analysis.* Journal of Medical Internet Research, 2025. **27**: p. e66400.
113. Alibilli, A.S., et al., *Harnessing Facebook to Investigate Real-World Mentions of Adverse Events of Glucagon-Like Peptide-1 Receptor Agonist (GLP-1 RA) Medications: Observational Study of Facebook Posts From 2022 to 2024.* Jmir Infodemiology, 2025. **5**: p. e73619-e73619.
114. Gribble, F.M., et al., *A Novel Glucose-Sensing Mechanism Contributing to Glucagon-Like Peptide-1 Secretion From the GLUTag Cell Line.* Diabetes, 2003. **52**(5): p. 1147-1154.
115. Sodum, N., et al., *Nutrient Combinations Sensed by L-Cell Receptors Potentiate GLP-1 Secretion.* International Journal of Molecular Sciences, 2024. **25**(2): p. 1087.

116. Nauck, M.A. and J.J. Meier, *Incretin Hormones: Their Role in Health and Disease.* Diabetes Obesity and Metabolism, 2018. **20**(S1): p. 5-21.
117. Degn, K.B., et al., *One Week's Treatment With the Long-Acting Glucagon-Like Peptide 1 Derivative Liraglutide (NN2211) Markedly Improves 24-H Glycemia and A- And B-Cell Function and Reduces Endogenous Glucose Release in Patients With Type 2 Diabetes.* Diabetes, 2004. **53**(5): p. 1187-1194.
118. Shu, Y., et al., *Gastrointestinal Adverse Events Associated With Semaglutide: A Pharmacovigilance Study Based on FDA Adverse Event Reporting System.* Frontiers in Public Health, 2022. **10**.
119. Moellmann, J., et al., *Glucagon-Like Peptide 1 and Its Cleavage Products Are Renoprotective in Murine Diabetic Nephropathy.* Diabetes, 2018. **67**(11): p. 2410-2419.
120. Anini, Y. and P.L. Brubaker, *Role of Leptin in the Regulation of Glucagon-Like Peptide-1 Secretion.* Diabetes, 2003. **52**(2): p. 252-259.
121. Zhang, F., et al., *Impaired Secretion of Total Glucagon-Like Peptide-1 in People With Impaired Fasting Glucose Combined Impaired Glucose Tolerance.* International Journal of Medical Sciences, 2012. **9**(7): p. 574-581.
122. Yang, W., et al., *Liraglutide Provides Similar Glycaemic Control as Glimepiride (Both in Combination With Metformin) and Reduces Body Weight and Systolic Blood Pressure in Asian Population With Type 2 Diabetes From China, South Korea and India: A 16-week, Randomized, Double-blind, Active Control Trial [*].* Diabetes Obesity and Metabolism, 2010. **13**(1): p. 81-88.
123. Laverdure, R., et al., *A Role for Methanogens and Methane in the Regulation of <scp>GLP</Scp>-1.* Endocrinology Diabetes & Metabolism, 2017. **1**(1).
124. Holst, J.J., *The Physiology of Glucagon-Like Peptide 1.* Physiological Reviews, 2007. **87**(4): p. 1409-1439.
125. Rakipovski, G., et al., *The GLP-1 Analogs Liraglutide and Semaglutide Reduce Atherosclerosis In ApoE−/− and LDLr−/− Mice By a Mechanism That Includes Inflammatory Pathways.* Jacc Basic to Translational Science, 2018. **3**(6): p. 844-857.
126. Malavazos, A.E., et al., *Semaglutide Therapy Decreases Epicardial Fat Inflammation and Improves Psoriasis Severity in Patients Affected by Abdominal Obesity and Type-2 Diabetes.* Endocrinology Diabetes and Metabolism Case Reports, 2023. **2023**(3).
127. Shaman, A.M., et al., *Effect of the Glucagon-Like Peptide-1 Receptor Agonists Semaglutide and Liraglutide on Kidney Outcomes in Patients With Type 2 Diabetes: Pooled Analysis of SUSTAIN 6 and LEADER.* Circulation, 2022. **145**(8): p. 575-585.
128. Flint, A., et al., *Randomised Clinical Trial: Semaglutide Versus Placebo Reduced Liver Steatosis but Not Liver Stiffness in Subjects With Non-alcoholic Fatty Liver Disease Assessed by Magnetic Resonance Imaging.* Alimentary Pharmacology & Therapeutics, 2021. **54**(9): p. 1150-1161.
129. Yang, H.M., *GLP-1 Agonists in Cardiovascular Diseases: Mechanisms, Clinical Evidence, and Emerging Therapies.* Journal of Clinical Medicine, 2025. **14**(19): p. 6758.
130. Vilsbøll, T., et al., *Semaglutide, Reduction in Glycated Haemoglobin and the Risk of Diabetic Retinopathy.* Diabetes Obesity and Metabolism, 2018. **20**(4): p. 889-897.
131. Wilding, J., et al., *Impact of Semaglutide on Body Composition in Adults With Overweight or Obesity: Exploratory Analysis of the STEP 1 Study.* Journal of the Endocrine Society, 2021. **5**(Supplement_1): p. A16-A17.

132. Sheahan, K.H., E.A. Wahlberg, and M.P. Gilbert, *An Overview of GLP-1 Agonists and Recent Cardiovascular Outcomes Trials*. Postgraduate Medical Journal, 2019. **96**(1133): p. 156-161.
133. Nuhoho, S., et al., *Orally Administered Semaglutide Versus GLP-1 RAs in Patients With Type 2 Diabetes Previously Receiving 1–2 Oral Antidiabetics: Systematic Review and Network Meta-Analysis*. Diabetes Therapy, 2019. **10**(6): p. 2183-2199.
134. Evans, M., et al., *Evaluating the Long-Term Cost-Effectiveness of Once-Weekly Semaglutide 1 mg Versus Liraglutide 1.8 Mg: A Health Economic Analysis in the UK*. Diabetes Therapy, 2023. **14**(6): p. 1005-1021.
135. Toraih, E.A., et al., *The Risk of Vestibular Disorders With Semaglutide and Tirzepatide: Findings From a Large Real-World Cohort*. Biomedicines, 2025. **13**(5): p. 1049.
136. Andréadis, P., et al., *Semaglutide for Type 2 Diabetes Mellitus: A Systematic Review and Meta-analysis*. Diabetes Obesity and Metabolism, 2018. **20**(9): p. 2255-2263.
137. Malkin, S.J.P., et al., *The Management of Type 2 Diabetes With Once-Weekly Semaglutide Versus Dulaglutide: A Long-Term Cost-Effectiveness Analysis in Slovakia*. Advances in Therapy, 2019. **36**(8): p. 2034-2051.
138. Samanta, A., et al., *Glucagon-Like Peptide-1 Receptor Agonists in the Management of Diabetic Retinopathy*. International Ophthalmology Clinics, 2024. **65**(1): p. 23-26.
139. Johansen, P., et al., *Evaluating the Long-Term Cost-Effectiveness of Once-Weekly Semaglutide Versus Once-Daily Liraglutide for the Treatment of Type 2 Diabetes in the UK*. Advances in Therapy, 2020. **37**(5): p. 2427-2441.
140. Stenberg, E. and E. Näslund, *Major Adverse Cardiovascular Events Among Patients With Type-2 Diabetes, a Nationwide Cohort Study Comparing Primary Metabolic and Bariatric Surgery to GLP-1 Receptor Agonist Treatment*. International Journal of Obesity, 2023. **47**(4): p. 251-256.
141. García-Vega, D., et al., *Semaglutide Modulates Prothrombotic and Atherosclerotic Mechanisms, Associated With Epicardial Fat, Neutrophils and Endothelial Cells Network*. Cardiovascular Diabetology, 2024. **23**(1).
142. Torimoto, K., Y. Okada, and Y. Tanaka, *Hypoglycemia Abrogates the Vascular Endothelial Protective Effect of Exenatide in Type 2 Diabetes Mellitus*. Diabetes Therapy, 2019. **10**(3): p. 1127-1132.
143. Grieve, D., R. Cassidy, and B.D. Green, *Emerging Cardiovascular Actions of the Incretin Hormone Glucagon-like Peptide-1: Potential Therapeutic Benefits Beyond Glycaemic Control?* British Journal of Pharmacology, 2009. **157**(8): p. 1340-1351.
144. Yin, Y., et al., *Efficacy of <scp>GLP</Scp>-1 Receptor Agonist-Based Therapies on Cardiovascular Events and Cardiometabolic Parameters in Obese Individuals Without Diabetes: A Meta-Analysis of Randomized Controlled Trials*. Journal of Diabetes, 2025. **17**(4).
145. Кониг, M., et al., *Exploring Potential Mediators of the Cardiovascular Benefit of Dulaglutide in Type 2 Diabetes Patients in REWIND*. Cardiovascular Diabetology, 2021. **20**(1).
146. McLean, B.A., et al., *Differential Importance of Endothelial and Hematopoietic Cell GLP-1Rs for Cardiometabolic Versus Hepatic Actions of Semaglutide*. Jci Insight, 2021. **6**(22).
147. Cheng, X., et al., *Semaglutide Attenuates Diabetic Retinopathy Progression via Ameliorating Retinal Vasculopathy and Oxidative Stress in Vivo and in Vitro*. Diabetes Obesity and Metabolism, 2025.

148. Røder, M., *Clinical Potential of Treatment With Semaglutide in Type 2 Diabetes Patients.* Drugs in Context, 2019. **8**: p. 1-11.
149. Chen, Y., et al., *Real-World Effectiveness of GLP-1 Receptor Agonist-Based Treatment Strategies on "Time in Range" in Patients With Type 2 Diabetes.* Frontiers in Pharmacology, 2024. **15**.
150. Shi, C., et al., *Effectiveness and Safety of Once-weekly Subcutaneous Semaglutide Versus Other Glucose-lowering Agents in Real-world Patients With Type 2 Diabetes: A Retrospective, Observational Post-marketing Study.* Diabetes Obesity and Metabolism, 2024. **26**(6): p. 2513-2516.
151. Bucheit, J.D., et al., *Oral Semaglutide: A Review of the First Oral Glucagon-Like Peptide 1 Receptor Agonist.* Diabetes Technology & Therapeutics, 2020. **22**(1): p. 10-18.
152. Qin, J. and L. Song, *Glucagon-Like Peptide-1 (GLP-1) Receptor Agonists and Cardiovascular Events in Patients With Type 2 Diabetes Mellitus: A Meta-Analysis of Double-Blind, Randomized, Placebo-Controlled Clinical Trials.* 2020.
153. Kang, Y.M., et al., *Glucagon-like Peptide-1 Receptor Agonists Lower Risk of Cardiovascular and Non-cardiovascular Mortality: A Meta-analysis of Eleven Cardiovascular Outcome Trials.* Diabetes Obesity and Metabolism, 2025. **27**(7): p. 4017-4021.
154. Ghusn, W., et al., *Weight Loss Outcomes Associated With Semaglutide Treatment for Patients With Overweight or Obesity.* Jama Network Open, 2022. **5**(9): p. e2231982.
155. Catalfamo, L., F.S.D. Ponte, and D.D. Rinaldis, *"Ozempic Face": An Emerging Drug-Related Aesthetic Concern and Its Treatment With Endotissutal Bipolar Radiofrequency (RF)—Our Experience.* Journal of Clinical Medicine, 2025. **14**(15): p. 5269.
156. Infante, M., et al., *Unveiling the Therapeutic Potential of the Second-Generation Incretin Analogs Semaglutide and Tirzepatide in Type 1 Diabetes and Latent Autoimmune Diabetes in Adults.* Journal of Clinical Medicine, 2025. **14**(4): p. 1303.
157. McGowan, B., et al., *Impact of <scp>BMI</Scp> and Comorbidities on Efficacy of Once-weekly Semaglutide: Post Hoc Analyses of the <scp>STEP</Scp> 1 Randomized Trial.* Obesity, 2023. **31**(4): p. 990-999.
158. Bensignor, M.O., A.S. Kelly, and S. Arslanian, *Anti-Obesity Pharmacotherapy for Treatment of Pediatric Type 2 Diabetes: Review of the Literature and Lessons Learned From Adults.* Frontiers in Endocrinology, 2022. **13**.
159. Rubino, D., et al., *Effect of Continued Weekly Subcutaneous Semaglutide vs Placebo on Weight Loss Maintenance in Adults With Overweight or Obesity.* Jama, 2021. **325**(14): p. 1414.
160. Gasoyan, H., et al., *One-Year Weight Reduction With Semaglutide or Liraglutide in Clinical Practice.* Jama Network Open, 2024. **7**(9): p. e2433326.
161. Fornes, A., et al., *Once-Weekly Semaglutide for Weight Management: A Clinical Review.* Journal of Pharmacy Technology, 2022. **38**(4): p. 239-246.
162. Aroda, V.R., et al., *Safety and Tolerability of Semaglutide Across The <scp>SUSTAIN</Scp> And <scp>PIONEER</Scp> Phase <scp>IIIa</Scp> Clinical Trial Programmes.* Diabetes Obesity and Metabolism, 2023. **25**(5): p. 1385-1397.
163. Lingvay, I., et al., *Semaglutide for Cardiovascular Event Reduction in People With Overweight or Obesity: <scp>SELECT</Scp> Study Baseline Characteristics.* Obesity, 2022. **31**(1): p. 111-122.

164. Husain, M., et al., *Effects of Semaglutide on Risk of Cardiovascular Events Across a Continuum of Cardiovascular Risk: Combined Post Hoc Analysis of the SUSTAIN and PIONEER Trials*. Cardiovascular Diabetology, 2020. **19**(1).
165. Verma, S., et al., *Effects of Glucagon -like Peptide -1 Receptor Agonists Liraglutide and Semaglutide on Cardiovascular and Renal Outcomes Across Body Mass Index Categories in Type 2 Diabetes: Results of The <scp>LEADER</Scp> And <scp>SUSTAIN</Scp> 6 Trials*. Diabetes Obesity and Metabolism, 2020. **22**(12): p. 2487-2492.
166. Rossing, P., et al., *Effect of Semaglutide on Major Adverse Cardiovascular Events by Baseline Kidney Parameters in Participants With Type 2 Diabetes and at High Risk of Cardiovascular Disease: SUSTAIN 6 and PIONEER 6 Post Hoc Pooled Analysis*. Cardiovascular Diabetology, 2023. **22**(1).
167. Verma, S., et al., *Duration of Diabetes and Cardiorenal Efficacy of Liraglutide and Semaglutide: A Post Hoc Analysis of the LEADER and SUSTAIN 6 Clinical Trials*. Diabetes Obesity and Metabolism, 2019. **21**(7): p. 1745-1751.
168. Strain, W.D., et al., *Effects of Semaglutide on Stroke Subtypes in Type 2 Diabetes: Post Hoc Analysis of the Randomized SUSTAIN 6 and PIONEER 6*. Stroke, 2022. **53**(9): p. 2749-2757.
169. Rosenstock, J., et al., *Oral Semaglutide Versus Empagliflozin in Patients With Type 2 Diabetes Uncontrolled on Metformin: The PIONEER 2 Trial*. Diabetes Care, 2019. **42**(12): p. 2272-2281.
170. Fisher, M., *Series: Cardiovascular Outcome Trials for Diabetes Drugs*. British Journal of Diabetes, 2022. **22**(2): p. 105-111.
171. Devasia, A.G., A. Ramasamy, and C.H. Leo, *Current Therapeutic Landscape for Metabolic Dysfunction-Associated Steatohepatitis*. International Journal of Molecular Sciences, 2025. **26**(4): p. 1778.
172. Salazar, M.A., et al., *Natural History of Metabolic Dysfunction-Associated Steatotic Liver Disease: From Metabolic Syndrome to Hepatocellular Carcinoma*. Medicina, 2025. **61**(1): p. 88.
173. Kanwal, F., et al., *Metabolic Dysfunction–associated Steatotic Liver Disease: Update and Impact of New Nomenclature on the American Association for the Study of Liver Diseases Practice Guidance on Nonalcoholic Fatty Liver Disease*. Hepatology, 2023. **79**(5): p. 1212-1219.
174. Theel, W., et al., *Evaluation of the Prevalence of MASLD, MASH and Liver Fibrosis in a Dutch Bariatric Cohort*. Plos One, 2025. **20**(6): p. e0324813.
175. Radosavljević, T., et al., *Altered Mitochondrial Function in MASLD: Key Features and Promising Therapeutic Approaches*. Antioxidants, 2024. **13**(8): p. 906.
176. Rinella, M.E., et al., *A Multisociety Delphi Consensus Statement on New Fatty Liver Disease Nomenclature*. Hepatology, 2023. **78**(6): p. 1966-1986.
177. Hwang, J., et al., *Bariatric Intervention Improves Metabolic Dysfunction-Associated Steatohepatitis in Patients With Obesity: A Systematic Review and Meta-Analysis*. Clinical and Molecular Hepatology, 2024. **30**(3): p. 561-576.
178. Aldroubi, B., et al., *Cell-Specific Regulation of Insulin Action and Hepatic Fibrosis by CEACAM1*. Metabolism and Target Organ Damage, 2024. **4**(4).
179. Norlin, J., et al., *The Combination of Zalfermin and Semaglutide Has Additive Therapeutic Effects in a Diet-Induced Obese and Biopsy-Confirmed Mouse Model of MASH*. Plos One, 2025. **20**(10): p. e0331665.

180. Nasr, P., et al., *The Amount of Liver Fat Predicts Mortality and Development of Type 2 Diabetes in Non-alcoholic Fatty Liver Disease*. Liver International, 2020. **40**(5): p. 1069-1078.
181. Habermaass, V., et al., *Lipid Dysmetabolism in Canine Chronic Liver Disease: Relationship Between Clinical, Histological and Immunohistochemical Features*. Veterinary Sciences, 2025. **12**(3): p. 220.
182. Sergi, C., *NAFLD (MASLD)/NASH (MASH): Does It Bother to Label at All? A Comprehensive Narrative Review*. International Journal of Molecular Sciences, 2024. **25**(15): p. 8462.
183. Zhang, Y., et al., *Glucagon-Like Peptide-1 Receptor Agonists Decrease Hyperinsulinemia and Hyperandrogenemia in Dehydroepiandrosterone-Induced Polycystic Ovary Syndrome Mice and Are Associated With Mitigating Inflammation and Inducing Browning of White Adipose Tissue*. Biology of Reproduction, 2023. **108**(6): p. 945-959.
184. Alshenqiti, A. and G. Almohammadi, *Overview of the Role of Glucagon Like Peptide-1 Receptor Agonists in the Management of Polycystic Ovary Syndrome*. Journal of Pharmaceutical Research International, 2021: p. 312-318.
185. Çelik, Ö., et al., *GLP-1 Receptor Analogs: Evidence Linking to Effect on Metabolic and Reproductive Functions in Patients With PCOS and Obesity*. Obesity Facts, 2025: p. 1-15.
186. Babar, A., R. Ali, and V. Zuhair, *Glucagon-Like Peptide 1 Agonists: A Ray of Hope for the Treatment of Polycystic Ovarian Syndrome*. Journal of the Pakistan Medical Association, 2023. **73**(12): p. 2521-2522.
187. Ma, R., et al., *Short-Term Combined Treatment With Exenatide and Metformin for Overweight/Obese Women With Polycystic Ovary Syndrome*. Chinese Medical Journal, 2021. **134**(23): p. 2882-2889.
188. Bednarz, K., et al., *The Role of GLP-1 Receptor Agonists in Insulin Resistance With Concomitant Obesity Treatment in Polycystic Ovary Syndrome*. International Journal of Molecular Sciences, 2022. **23**(8): p. 4334.
189. He, K., et al., *Once-weekly semaglutide for Obesity or Overweight: A Systematic Review and Meta-analysis*. Diabetes Obesity and Metabolism, 2021. **24**(4): p. 722-726.
190. Bader, S., et al., *A Systematic Review of GLP-1 on Anthropometrics, Metabolic and Endocrine Parameters in Patients With PCOS*. Women S Health, 2024. **20**.
191. Akel, M., et al., *Exploring the Therapeutic Potential of Glucagon-Like Peptide 1 (GLP-1) Receptor Agonists in Polycystic Ovary Syndrome*. Cureus, 2024.
192. Liao, M., et al., *Effects and Plasma Proteomic Analysis of GLP-1RA Versus CPA/EE, in Combination With Metformin, on Overweight PCOS Women: A Randomized Controlled Trial*. Endocrine, 2023. **83**(1): p. 227-241.
193. Jensterle, M., S. Ferjan, and A. Janež, *The Maintenance of Long-Term Weight Loss After Semaglutide Withdrawal in Obese Women With PCOS Treated With Metformin: A 2-Year Observational Study*. Frontiers in Endocrinology, 2024. **15**.
194. Cena, H., L. Chiovato, and R.E. Nappi, *Obesity, Polycystic Ovary Syndrome, and Infertility: A New Avenue for GLP-1 Receptor Agonists*. The Journal of Clinical Endocrinology & Metabolism, 2020. **105**(8): p. e2695-e2709.
195. Hudanich, M., et al., *The Effects of Glucagon-Like Peptide-1 (GLP-1) Receptor Agonists on Polycystic Ovarian Syndrome: A Scoping Review*. Cureus, 2025.

196. Szczęsnowicz, A., et al., *Do GLP-1 Analogs Have a Place in the Treatment of PCOS? New Insights and Promising Therapies*. Journal of Clinical Medicine, 2023. **12**(18): p. 5915.
197. Lin, A.-C., et al., *Elevated Hedgehog-Interacting Protein Levels in Subjects With Prediabetes and Type 2 Diabetes*. Journal of Clinical Medicine, 2019. **8**(10): p. 1635.
198. Stull, A.J., *Lifestyle Approaches and Glucose Intolerance*. American Journal of Lifestyle Medicine, 2016. **10**(6): p. 406-416.
199. Pascot, A., et al., *Contribution of Visceral Obesity to the Deterioration of the Metabolic Risk Profile in Men With Impaired Glucose Tolerance*. Diabetologia, 2000. **43**(9): p. 1126-1135.
200. Perreault, L., et al., *Changes in Glucose Metabolism and Glycemic Status With Once-Weekly Subcutaneous Semaglutide 2.4 Mg Among Participants With Prediabetes in the STEP Program*. Diabetes Care, 2022. **45**(10): p. 2396-2405.
201. Qin, W., et al., *Efficacy and Safety of Semaglutide 2.4 mg for Weight Loss in Overweight or Obese Adults Without Diabetes: An Updated Systematic Review and Meta-analysis Including the 2-year <scp>STEP</Scp> 5 Trial*. Diabetes Obesity and Metabolism, 2023. **26**(3): p. 911-923.
202. Nabila, S., et al., *Associations Between Modifiable Risk Factors and Changes in Glycemic Status Among Individuals With Prediabetes*. Diabetes Care, 2023. **46**(3): p. 535-543.
203. Kumari, N., D.K. Verma, and B.K. Binawara, *A Study to Assess the Future 10-Year Cardiovascular And8-Year Diabetic Risk by Using Framingham Heartscale in Prediabetic Subjects*. International Journal of Endocrinology (Ukraine), 2022. **18**(5): p. 245-250.
204. Kushner, R.F., et al., *Safety Profile of Semaglutide Versus Placebo in the <scp>SELECT</Scp> Study: A Randomized Controlled Trial*. Obesity, 2025. **33**(3): p. 452-462.
205. Lincoff, A.M., et al., *Semaglutide and Cardiovascular Outcomes in Obesity Without Diabetes*. New England Journal of Medicine, 2023. **389**(24): p. 2221-2232.
206. Kahal, H. and C. Walton, *Critique of Semaglutide (Wegovy®) for Obesity Management NICE Technology Appraisal TA875*. British Journal of Diabetes, 2024. **24**(1): p. 13-15.
207. Sandhu, H., et al., *Once-Weekly Subcutaneous Semaglutide 2.4 Mg Injection Is Cost-Effective for Weight Management in the United Kingdom*. Advances in Therapy, 2023. **40**(3): p. 1282-1291.
208. Miguel, L.S., et al., *Cost-Effectiveness of Semaglutide 2.4 mg in Chronic Weight Management in Portugal*. Diabetology & Metabolic Syndrome, 2024. **16**(1).
209. Liotta, M., *Examining the pros and cons of semaglutide* in *NewsGP*. 2025, The Royal Australian College of General Practitioners (RACGP).
210. Yang, Z., et al., *GLP-1 Receptor Agonist-Associated Tumor Adverse Events: A Real-World Study From 2004 to 2021 Based on FAERS*. Frontiers in Pharmacology, 2022. **13**.
211. Bing, S., et al., *Efficacy and Safety of cAMP Signalling-Biased GLP-1 Analogue Ecnoglutide Monotherapy Versus Placebo in Patients With Type 2 Diabetes (EECOH-1): A Randomised, Double-Blind, Placebo-Controlled, Phase 3 Trial*. 2025.
212. Sarwal, A., et al., *Glycemic Therapies and the Risk of Gastrointestinal Adverse Events In Veterans With Type 2 Diabetes*. Diabetes Obesity and Metabolism, 2025. **27**(10): p. 5865-5877.
213. Eleftheriadou, A., et al., *Risk of Diabetic Retinopathy and Diabetic Macular Oedema With Sodium–glucose Cotransporter 2 Inhibitors and Glucagon-Like Peptide 1 Receptor*

Agonists in Type 2 Diabetes: A Real-World Data Study From a Global Federated Database. Diabetologia, 2024. **67**(7): p. 1271-1282.

214. Zhong, P., et al., *Efficacy and Safety of Subcutaneous and Oral Semaglutide Administration in Patients With Type 2 Diabetes: A Meta-Analysis*. Frontiers in Pharmacology, 2021. **12**.

215. Petri, K.C.C., et al., *Semaglutide s.c. Once-Weekly in Type 2 Diabetes: A Population Pharmacokinetic Analysis*. Diabetes Therapy, 2018. **9**(4): p. 1533-1547.

216. Ikushima, I., et al., *A Randomized Trial Investigating the Pharmacokinetics, Pharmacodynamics, and Safety of Subcutaneous Semaglutide Once-Weekly in Healthy Male Japanese and Caucasian Subjects*. Advances in Therapy, 2018. **35**(4): p. 531-544.

217. Kapitza, C., et al., *Effects of Semaglutide on Beta Cell Function and Glycaemic Control in Participants With Type 2 Diabetes: A Randomised, Double-Blind, Placebo-Controlled Trial*. Diabetologia, 2017. **60**(8): p. 1390-1399.

218. Shapira-Furman, T., et al., *The Synthesis of SNAC Phenolate Salts and the Effect on Oral Bioavailability of Semaglutide*. Molecules, 2024. **29**(16): p. 3909.

219. Avgerinos, I., et al., *Oral Semaglutide for Type 2 Diabetes: A Systematic Review and Meta-analysis*. Diabetes Obesity and Metabolism, 2019. **22**(3): p. 335-345.

220. Choe, H.J. and Y.M. Cho, *Peptidyl and Non-Peptidyl Oral Glucagon-Like Peptide-1 Receptor Agonists*. Endocrinology and Metabolism, 2021. **36**(1): p. 22-29.

221. Wharton, S., et al., *Gastrointestinal Tolerability of Once-weekly Semaglutide 2.4 mg in Adults With Overweight or Obesity, and the Relationship Between Gastrointestinal Adverse Events and Weight Loss*. Diabetes Obesity and Metabolism, 2021. **24**(1): p. 94-105.

222. Petri, K.C.C., et al., *Exposure-response Analysis for Evaluation of Semaglutide Dose Levels in Type 2 Diabetes*. Diabetes Obesity and Metabolism, 2018. **20**(9): p. 2238-2245.

223. Tzoulis, P., M. Batavanis, and S. Baldeweg, *A Real-World Study of the Effectiveness and Safety of Semaglutide for Weight Loss*. Cureus, 2024.

224. Roux, C.W.l., et al., *Tirzepatide for the Treatment of Obesity: Rationale and Design of the <scp>SURMOUNT</Scp> Clinical Development Program*. Obesity, 2022. **31**(1): p. 96-110.

225. Singhal, R., et al., *Unmasking Semaglutide-Induced Gastroparesis: The Dangers of Rapid Dose Escalation in a Diabetic Patient*. Cureus, 2025.

226. Xu, Y., et al., *Titration and Discontinuation of Semaglutide for Weight Management in Commercially Insured US Adults*. Obesity, 2025. **33**(7): p. 1243-1248.

227. Samuels, J.M., et al., *Real-world Titration, Persistence &Amp; Weight Loss of Semaglutide and Tirzepatide in an Academic Obesity Clinic*. Diabetes Obesity and Metabolism, 2025. **27**(11): p. 6200-6209.

228. Gao, X., et al., *Efficacy and Safety of Semaglutide on Weight Loss in Obese or Overweight Patients Without Diabetes: A Systematic Review and Meta-Analysis of Randomized Controlled Trials*. Frontiers in Pharmacology, 2022. **13**.

229. Alkhalifah, M., et al., *Semaglutide for the Management of Diabesity: The Real-World Experience*. World Journal of Methodology, 2024. **14**(3).

230. Newsome, P.N., et al., *Effect of Semaglutide on Liver Enzymes and Markers of Inflammation in Subjects With Type 2 Diabetes and/or Obesity*. Alimentary Pharmacology & Therapeutics, 2019. **50**(2): p. 193-203.

231. Frías, J.P., et al., *Efficacy and Safety of Once-Weekly Semaglutide 2·0 Mg Versus 1·0 Mg in Patients With Type 2 Diabetes (SUSTAIN FORTE): A Double-Blind, Randomised, Phase 3B Trial.* The Lancet Diabetes & Endocrinology, 2021. **9**(9): p. 563-574.
232. Strathe, A., et al., *A Model-based Approach to Predict Individual Weight Loss With Semaglutide in People With Overweight or Obesity.* Diabetes Obesity and Metabolism, 2023. **25**(11): p. 3171-3180.
233. Bergmann, N.C., et al., *Semaglutide for the Treatment of Overweight and Obesity: A Review.* Diabetes Obesity and Metabolism, 2022. **25**(1): p. 18-35.
234. Bhopale, K.K. and M.P. Srinivasan, *Therapeutics for Metabolic Dysfunction-Associated Fatty Liver Disease (MAFLD).* Livers, 2023. **3**(4): p. 597-617.
235. Мисникова, И.В., et al., *A Randomized Controlled Trial to Assess the Impact of Proper Insulin Injection Technique Training on Glycemic Control.* Diabetes Therapy, 2017. **8**(6): p. 1309-1318.
236. Campinos, C., et al., *An Effective Intervention for Diabetic Lipohypertrophy: Results of a Randomized, Controlled, Prospective Multicenter Study in France.* Diabetes Technology & Therapeutics, 2017. **19**(11): p. 623-632.
237. Gibney, M.A., et al., *Skin and Subcutaneous Adipose Layer Thickness in Adults With Diabetes at Sites Used for Insulin Injections: Implications for Needle Length Recommendations.* Current Medical Research and Opinion, 2010. **26**(6): p. 1519-1530.
238. Presti, D.L., C. Ingegnosi, and K. Strauss, *Skin and Subcutaneous Thickness at Injecting Sites in Children With Diabetes: Ultrasound Findings and Recommendations for Giving Injection.* Pediatric Diabetes, 2012. **13**(7): p. 525-533.
239. Rini, C.J., et al., *Evaluating the Impact of Human Factors and Pen Needle Design on Insulin Pen Injection.* Journal of Diabetes Science and Technology, 2019. **13**(3): p. 533-545.
240. Snitker, S., et al., *Comparison of the Injection-site Experience of Semaglutide in a Single-dose and a Multidose Pen-injector.* Diabetes Obesity and Metabolism, 2022. **24**(8): p. 1643-1646.
241. Attia, N., Y. Marzouk, and N.I. Marzouk, *First Case Report: Breakage of an Insulin Pen Needle in Subcutaneous Tissue.* Diabetes Case Reports, 2017. **02**(01).
242. Frid, A., et al., *Effects of Accidental Intramuscular Injection on Insulin Absorption in IDDM.* Diabetes Care, 1988. **11**(1): p. 41-45.
243. Seddio, A.E., et al., *Lower Risk of Postoperative Complications and Rotator Cuff Retear Associated With Semaglutide Use in Patients With Type II Diabetes Mellitus Undergoing Arthroscopic Rotator Cuff Repair.* Arthroscopy the Journal of Arthroscopic and Related Surgery, 2025. **41**(2): p. 199-206.
244. Christou, G.A., et al., *Semaglutide as a Promising Antiobesity Drug.* Obesity Reviews, 2019. **20**(6): p. 805-815.
245. Gallwitz, B. and F. Giorgino, *Clinical Perspectives on the Use of Subcutaneous and Oral Formulations of Semaglutide.* Frontiers in Endocrinology, 2021. **12**.
246. Haggag, A.Z., et al., *Non-clinical and First-in-human Characterization Of <scp>ECC5004</Scp> / <scp>AZD5004</Scp> , a Novel Once-daily, Oral Small-molecule <scp>GLP</Scp> -1 Receptor Agonist.* Diabetes Obesity and Metabolism, 2024. **27**(2): p. 551-562.
247. Bækdal, T.A., et al., *Relationship Between Oral Semaglutide Tablet Erosion and Pharmacokinetics: A Pharmacoscintigraphic Study.* Clinical Pharmacology in Drug Development, 2021. **10**(5): p. 453-462.

248. R.Hassanein, M.R., et al., *808-P: Impact of Fasting on Adherence to Dosing Instructions and Efficacy of Oral Semaglutide During Ramadan in People With Type 2 Diabetes in Real-World Setting—O-Sema-Fast Subanalysis*. Diabetes, 2024. **73**(Supplement_1).
249. Overgaard, R.V., et al., *Population Pharmacokinetics of Semaglutide for Type 2 Diabetes*. Diabetes Therapy, 2019. **10**(2): p. 649-662.
250. Zinman, B., et al., *Efficacy, Safety, and Tolerability of Oral Semaglutide Versus Placebo Added to Insulin With or Without Metformin in Patients With Type 2 Diabetes: The PIONEER 8 Trial*. Diabetes Care, 2019. **42**(12): p. 2262-2271.
251. Bækdal, T.A., et al., *Effect of Various Dosing Conditions on the Pharmacokinetics of Oral Semaglutide, a Human Glucagon-Like Peptide-1 Analogue in a Tablet Formulation*. Diabetes Therapy, 2021. **12**(7): p. 1915-1927.
252. Bain, S.C., et al., *Oral Semaglutide Versus Empagliflozin, Sitagliptin and Liraglutide in the UK: Long-Term Cost-Effectiveness Analyses Based on the PIONEER Clinical Trial Programme*. Diabetes Therapy, 2019. **11**(1): p. 259-277.
253. O'Neill, E.S., et al., *Injectable Weight Loss Medications in Plastic Surgery: What We Know, Perioperative Considerations, and Recommendations for the Future*. Plastic & Reconstructive Surgery Global Open, 2024. **12**(1): p. e5516.
254. Wojtara, M., et al., *Glucagon-Like Peptide-1 Receptor Agonists for Chronic Weight Management*. Advances in Medicine, 2023. **2023**: p. 1-7.
255. Abasheva, D., A. Ortíz, and B. Fernández-Fernández, *GLP-1 Receptor Agonists in Patients With Chronic Kidney Disease and Either Overweight or Obesity*. Clinical Kidney Journal, 2024. **17**(Supplement_2): p. ii19-ii35.
256. Lee, C.Y., *Glucagon-Like Peptide-1 Formulation – The Present and Future Development in Diabetes Treatment*. Basic & Clinical Pharmacology & Toxicology, 2015. **118**(3): p. 173-180.
257. Gad, A.I., et al., *Therapeutic Effects of Semaglutide on Nonalcoholic Fatty Liver Disease With Type 2 Diabetes Mellitus and Obesity: An Open-Label Controlled Trial*. Diseases, 2024. **12**(8): p. 186.
258. Haider, S., et al., *8752 the Ethical Concerns of Improper Semaglutide Administration After Acquisition From a Compounded Pharmacy*. Journal of the Endocrine Society, 2024. **8**(Supplement_1).
259. Drucker, D.J., *Mechanisms of Action and Therapeutic Application of Glucagon-Like Peptide-1*. Cell Metabolism, 2018. **27**(4): p. 740-756.
260. Candido, R., et al., *Real-World Retrospective Study Into the Effects of Oral Semaglutide (As a Switchover or Add-on Therapy) in Type 2 Diabetes*. Journal of Clinical Medicine, 2023. **12**(18): p. 6052.
261. Jain, A., et al., *Use of Once-daily Oral Semaglutide and Associated Clinical Outcomes Among Adults With Type 2 Diabetes in Routine Clinical Practice in Canada: A Multicentre, Prospective Real-world Study (<scp>PIONEER REAL</scp> Canada)*. Diabetes Obesity and Metabolism, 2024. **26**(5): p. 1799-1807.
262. Wang, M. and T. Hng, *HbA1c: More than just a number*. Australian Journal of General Practice, 2021. **50**: p. 628-632.
263. Morieri, M.L., et al., *Clinical Features, Cardiovascular Risk Profile, and Therapeutic Trajectories of Patients With Type 2 Diabetes Candidate for Oral Semaglutide Therapy in the Italian Specialist Care*. Diabetes Therapy, 2023. **14**(12): p. 2159-2172.

264. Frazer, M., et al., *Real-World Hemoglobin A1c Changes, Prescribing Provider Types, and Medication Dose Among Patients With Type 2 Diabetes Mellitus Initiating Treatment With Oral Semaglutide.* Advances in Therapy, 2023. **40**(11): p. 5102-5114.
265. Maiorino, M.I., et al., *Improvement of Glycemic Control and Reduction of Major Cardiovascular Events in 18 Cardiovascular Outcome Trials: An Updated Meta-Regression.* Cardiovascular Diabetology, 2021. **20**(1).
266. Barer, Y., O. Cohen, and T. Cukierman-Yaffe, *Effect of Glycaemic Control on Cardiovascular Disease in Individuals With Type 2 Diabetes With Pre-existing Cardiovascular Disease: A Systematic Review and Meta-analysis.* Diabetes Obesity and Metabolism, 2018. **21**(3): p. 732-735.
267. Chen, H., et al., *Comparative Efficacy and Safety of Glucagon-Like Peptide 1 Receptor Agonists for the Treatment of Type 2 Diabetes: A Network Meta-Analysis.* Medicine, 2023. **102**(27): p. e34122.
268. Gu, Y., et al., *Comparative Efficacy of 5 Sodium-Glucose Cotransporter Protein-2 (SGLT-2) Inhibitor and 4 Glucagon-Like Peptide-1 (GLP-1) Receptor Agonist Drugs in Non-Alcoholic Fatty Liver Disease: A GRADE-assessed Systematic Review and Network Meta-Analysis of Randomized Controlled Trials.* Frontiers in Pharmacology, 2023. **14**.
269. Evans, M.L., et al., *The Impact of Flash Glucose Monitoring on Glycaemic Control as Measured by HbA1c: A Meta-Analysis of Clinical Trials and Real-World Observational Studies.* Diabetes Therapy, 2019. **11**(1): p. 83-95.
270. Ding, L., et al., *Comparing the Efficacy and Safety of Glucagon-Like Peptide 1 Receptor Agonists With Sodium-Glucose Cotransporter 2 Inhibitors for Obese Type 2 Diabetes Patients Uncontrolled on Metformin: A Systematic Review and Meta-Analysis of Randomized Clinical Trials.* International Journal of Endocrinology, 2020. **2020**: p. 1-7.
271. Qarni, A.A., et al., *The Impact of Diabetes Type 2 Treatment Interventions on Cardiovascular Outcomes – A Comprehensive Review.* Series of Endocrinology Diabetes and Metabolism, 2023. **5**(2): p. 68-91.
272. Bethel, M.A., et al., *HbA1c Change and Diabetic Retinopathy During GLP-1 Receptor Agonist Cardiovascular Outcome Trials: A Meta-Analysis and Meta-Regression.* Diabetes Care, 2020. **44**(1): p. 290-296.
273. Stefanou, M.I., et al., *Risk of Major Adverse Cardiovascular Events and All-Cause Mortality Under Treatment With GLP-1 RAs or the Dual GIP/GLP-1 Receptor Agonist Tirzepatide in Overweight or Obese Adults Without Diabetes: A Systematic Review and Meta-Analysis.* Therapeutic Advances in Neurological Disorders, 2024. **17**.
274. Palazzi, S., et al., *Real-World Analysis of Short-Term Effectiveness of Oral Semaglutide: Impact on Glycometabolic Control and Cardiovascular Risk.* Pharmaceuticals, 2025. **18**(6): p. 856.
275. Nekidy, W.S.E., et al., *Comparing the Efficacy of Liraglutide and Semaglutide on Weight Loss: Experience From the Middle East Gulf Region and Literature Review.* Hospital Pharmacy, 2025. **60**(5): p. 432-440.
276. Colin, I.M. and A. Gérard, *Once-Weekly 2.4 Mg Semaglutide for Weight Management in Obesity: A Game Changer?* Touchreviews in Endocrinology, 2022. **18**(1): p. 35.
277. Gu, W., et al., *Efficacy and Safety of Once-weekly Semaglutide 2.4 mg for Weight Management in Participants From China: A Prespecified Analysis of the <scp>STEP</Scp> 7 Randomized Clinical Trial.* Diabetes Obesity and Metabolism, 2025. **27**(5): p. 2540-2551.

278. Kosiborod, M., et al., *Semaglutide Improves Cardiometabolic Risk Factors in Adults With Overweight or Obesity: <scp>STEP</Scp> 1 and 4 Exploratory Analyses*. Diabetes Obesity and Metabolism, 2022. **25**(2): p. 468-478.
279. Tchang, B.G., et al., *Effect of Semaglutide 2.4 mg on Use of Antihypertensive and Lipid-lowering Treatment in Five Randomized Controlled <scp>STEP</Scp> Trials*. Obesity, 2025. **33**(2): p. 267-277.
280. Kaku, K., et al., *Safety and Efficacy of Once-weekly Semaglutide vs Additional Oral Antidiabetic Drugs in Japanese People With Inadequately Controlled Type 2 Diabetes: A Randomized Trial*. Diabetes Obesity and Metabolism, 2018. **20**(5): p. 1202-1212.
281. Mamas, M., et al., *Tirzepatide Compared With Semaglutide and 10-Year Cardiovascular Disease Risk Reduction in Obesity: <i>post-Hoc</I> Analysis of the SURMOUNT-5 Trial*. European Heart Journal Open, 2025. **5**(5).
282. Ryan, D.H., et al., *Long-Term Weight Loss Effects of Semaglutide in Obesity Without Diabetes in the SELECT Trial*. Nature Medicine, 2024. **30**(7): p. 2049-2057.
283. Mikhail, N. and S. Wali, *Semaglutide: The First Anti-Obesity Agent Shown to Decrease Cardiovascular Events*. Annals of Cardiovascular Diseases, 2024. **8**(1): p. 1-4.
284. Bjørnholm, K.D., et al., *Liraglutide Treatment Improves Endothelial Function in the <i>Ldlr−/−</I> Mouse Model of Atherosclerosis and Affects Genes Involved in Vascular Remodelling and Inflammation*. Basic & Clinical Pharmacology & Toxicology, 2020. **128**(1): p. 103-114.
285. Temporelli, P.L., *Role of Glucagon-Like Peptide-1 Agonists in Obesity and Heart Failure With Preserved Ejection Fraction*. European Heart Journal Supplements, 2024. **26**(Supplement_1): p. i127-i130.
286. Porter, S.A., et al., *Abdominal Subcutaneous Adipose Tissue: A Protective Fat Depot?* Diabetes Care, 2009. **32**(6): p. 1068-1075.
287. Powell-Wiley, T.M., et al., *Obesity and Cardiovascular Disease: A Scientific Statement From the American Heart Association*. Circulation, 2021. **143**(21).
288. Erhabor, J., M. Khorsandi, and M.J. Blaha, *National and State Estimates of SELECT Trial Eligibility and Its Public Health Impact in the US*. Jama Network Open, 2024. **7**(7): p. e2420105.
289. Hargovan, S., et al., *Is Semaglutide Cost-effective at Closing the Gap for Aboriginal and Torres Strait Islander Australians With Cardiovascular Disease and Obesity Without Type 2 Diabetes?* Internal Medicine Journal, 2025. **55**(10): p. 1725-1732.
290. Kotit, S. and M. Sous, *SELECT: Glucagon-Like Peptide-1 Receptor Agonist in Obese Patients With Cardiovascular Disease in the Absence of Diabetes*. Global Cardiology Science and Practice, 2024. **2024**(4).
291. Bain, S.C., et al., *Cardiovascular Safety of Oral Semaglutide in Patients With Type 2 Diabetes: Rationale, Design and Patient Baseline Characteristics for the PIONEER 6 Trial*. Diabetes Obesity and Metabolism, 2018. **21**(3): p. 499-508.
292. Hu, E.-H., et al., *A Review and Meta-Analysis of the Safety and Efficacy of Using Glucagon-Like Peptide-1 Receptor Agonists*. Medicina, 2024. **60**(3): p. 357.
293. Phizackerley, D., *Semaglutide Reduces the Absolute Risk of Major Cardiovascular Events by 1.5%*. BMJ, 2024: p. q53.
294. Khoo, J., et al., *Comparative Effects of Liraglutide 3 Mg vs Structured Lifestyle Modification on Body Weight, Liver Fat and Liver Function in Obese Patients With Non-alcoholic Fatty Liver Disease: A Pilot Randomized Trial*. Diabetes Obesity and Metabolism, 2017. **19**(12): p. 1814-1817.

295. Hudert, C., et al., *Genetic Determinants of Steatosis and Fibrosis Progression in Paediatric Non-alcoholic Fatty Liver Disease.* Liver International, 2018. **39**(3): p. 540-556.
296. Xia, M., et al., *NAFLD-related Gene Polymorphisms and All-cause and Cause-specific Mortality in an Asian Population: The Shanghai Changfeng Study.* Alimentary Pharmacology & Therapeutics, 2022. **55**(6): p. 705-721.
297. Donati, B., et al., *MBOAT7 Rs641738 Variant and Hepatocellular Carcinoma in Non-Cirrhotic Individuals.* Scientific Reports, 2017. **7**(1).
298. Kleinstein, S.E., et al., *Whole-Exome Sequencing Study of Extreme Phenotypes of NAFLD.* Hepatology Communications, 2018. **2**(9): p. 1021-1029.
299. Sookoian, S., et al., *Genetic Variation in Transmembrane 6 Superfamily Member 2 and the Risk of Nonalcoholic Fatty Liver Disease and Histological Disease Severity.* Hepatology, 2015. **61**(2): p. 515-525.
300. Wu, J., et al., *Independent and Joint Correlation of PNPLA3 I148M and TM6SF2 E167K Variants With the Risk of Coronary Heart Disease in Patients With Non-Alcoholic Fatty Liver Disease.* Lipids in Health and Disease, 2020. **19**(1).
301. Wang, X., et al., *Additive Effects of the Risk Alleles of PNPLA3 and TM6SF2 on Non-Alcoholic Fatty Liver Disease (NAFLD) in a Chinese Population.* Frontiers in Genetics, 2016. **7**.
302. Luo, Q., et al., *Efficacy of Off-Label Therapy for Non-Alcoholic Fatty Liver Disease in Improving Non-Invasive and Invasive Biomarkers: A Systematic Review and Network Meta-Analysis of Randomized Controlled Trials.* Frontiers in Medicine, 2022. **9**.
303. Mantovani, A., et al., *Glucagon-Like Peptide-1 Receptor Agonists for Treatment of Nonalcoholic Fatty Liver Disease and Nonalcoholic Steatohepatitis: An Updated Meta-Analysis of Randomized Controlled Trials.* Metabolites, 2021. **11**(2): p. 73.
304. Qin, J. and L. Song, *Glucagon-Like Peptide-1 (GLP-1) Receptor Agonists and Cardiovascular Events in Patients With Type 2 Diabetes Mellitus: A Meta-Analysis of Double-Blind, Randomized, Placebo-Controlled Clinical Trials.* BMC Endocrine Disorders, 2022. **22**(1).
305. Husain, M., et al., *Oral Semaglutide and Cardiovascular Outcomes in Patients With Type 2 Diabetes.* Boston Medical and Surgical Journal, 2019. **381**(9): p. 841-851.
306. Pojskic, L., D. Mršić, and A. Macić-Džanković, *The Benefits of GLP1 Receptors in Cardiovascular Diseases.* Frontiers in Clinical Diabetes and Healthcare, 2023. **4**.
307. Kang, Y.M. and C.H. Jung, *Cardiovascular Effects of Glucagon-Like Peptide-1 Receptor Agonists.* Endocrinology and Metabolism, 2016. **31**(2): p. 258.
308. Dahl, K., et al., *Oral Semaglutide Improves Postprandial Glucose and Lipid Metabolism, and Delays Gastric Emptying, in Subjects With Type <scp>2</Scp> Diabetes.* Diabetes Obesity and Metabolism, 2021. **23**(7): p. 1594-1603.
309. Volpe, S., et al., *Once-Weekly Subcutaneous Semaglutide Improves Fatty Liver Disease in Patients With Type 2 Diabetes: A 52-Week Prospective Real-Life Study.* Nutrients, 2022. **14**(21): p. 4673.
310. Newsome, P.N., et al., *A Placebo-Controlled Trial of Subcutaneous Semaglutide in Nonalcoholic Steatohepatitis.* Boston Medical and Surgical Journal, 2021. **384**(12): p. 1113-1124.
311. Edholm, T., et al., *Differential Incretin Effects of GIP and GLP-1 on Gastric Emptying, Appetite, and Insulin-Glucose Homeostasis.* Neurogastroenterology & Motility, 2010. **22**(11): p. 1191-e315.

312. João, A.L., F. Reis, and R. Fernandes, *The Incretin System ABCs in Obesity and Diabetes – Novel Therapeutic Strategies for Weight Loss and Beyond.* Obesity Reviews, 2016. **17**(7): p. 553-572.
313. Ghazi, T., et al., *Acute Metabolic Effects of Exenatide in Patients With Type 1 Diabetes With and Without Residual Insulin to Oral and Intravenous Glucose Challenges.* Diabetes Care, 2013. **37**(1): p. 210-216.
314. Dubé, M.C., M. D'Amours, and S.J. Weisnagel, *Beyond Glycaemic Control: A Cross-over, Double-blinded, 24-week Intervention With Liraglutide in Type 1 Diabetes.* Diabetes Obesity and Metabolism, 2017. **20**(1): p. 178-184.
315. Falkén, Y., et al., *Actions of Prolonged Ghrelin Infusion on Gastrointestinal Transit and Glucose Homeostasis in Humans.* Neurogastroenterology & Motility, 2010. **22**(6): p. e192-e200.
316. Hadzhibozheva, P., et al., *Appetite–regulating Hormones in Rats With Fructose-Induced Metabolic Changes.* Pharmacia, 2023. **70**(1): p. 1-7.
317. Xie, F., et al., *Therapeutic Potential of Molecular Hydrogen in Metabolic Diseases From Bench to Bedside.* Pharmaceuticals, 2023. **16**(4): p. 541.
318. Chen, S.M., et al., *Interleukin-4 Inhibits the Hypothalamic Appetite Control by Modulating the Insulin<scp>-AKT</Scp> and <scp>JAK-STAT</Scp> Signaling in Leptin Mutant Mice.* Environmental Toxicology, 2024. **39**(7): p. 3980-3990.
319. Anastasiou, I.A., et al., *Hormonal Alterations in Individuals With Obesity After Metabolic Bariatric Surgery: A Narrative Review.* Medicina, 2025. **61**(10): p. 1724.
320. Alzahrani, M.A., et al., *Effect of Once Weekly Semaglutide in Patients With Type 2 Diabetes in National Guard Primary Health Care, Jeddah, Saudi Arabia: A Retrospective Cohort Study.* 2023.
321. Paiva, I.H.R.d., et al., *Semaglutide Attenuates Anxious and Depressive-Like Behaviors and Reverses the Cognitive Impairment in a Type 2 Diabetes Mellitus Mouse Model via the Microbiota-Gut-Brain Axis.* Journal of Neuroimmune Pharmacology, 2024. **19**(1).
322. Phillips, A.C. and J.N. Clements, *Clinical Review of Subcutaneous Semaglutide for Obesity.* Journal of Clinical Pharmacy and Therapeutics, 2021. **47**(2): p. 184-193.
323. Rosenstock, J., et al., *Effect of Additional Oral Semaglutide vs Sitagliptin on Glycated Hemoglobin in Adults With Type 2 Diabetes Uncontrolled With Metformin Alone or With Sulfonylurea.* Jama, 2019. **321**(15): p. 1466.
324. Lean, M.E.J., et al., *Tolerability of Nausea and Vomiting and Associations With Weight Loss in a Randomized Trial of Liraglutide in Obese, Non-Diabetic Adults.* International Journal of Obesity, 2013. **38**(5): p. 689-697.
325. Jensterle, M., et al., *Semaglutide Delays 4-hour Gastric Emptying in Women With Polycystic Ovary Syndrome and Obesity.* Diabetes Obesity and Metabolism, 2023. **25**(4): p. 975-984.
326. Gruzmark, F., et al., *Exploring the Role Of <scp>GLP</Scp> -1 Agents in Managing Diabetic Foot Ulcers: A Narrative and Systematic Review.* Wound Repair and Regeneration, 2025. **33**(5).
327. Farr, O.M., et al., *GLP-1 Receptors Exist in the Parietal Cortex, Hypothalamus and Medulla of Human Brains and the GLP-1 Analogue Liraglutide Alters Brain Activity Related to Highly Desirable Food Cues in Individuals With Diabetes: A Crossover, Randomised, Placebo-Controlled Trial.* Diabetologia, 2016. **59**(5): p. 954-965.

328. Feinglos, M.N., et al., *Effects of Liraglutide (NN2211), a Long-acting GLP-1 Analogue, on Glycaemic Control and Bodyweight in Subjects With Type 2 Diabetes.* Diabetic Medicine, 2005. **22**(8): p. 1016-1023.
329. Davies, M.L., D.Q. Pham, and S.R. Drab, *<scp>GLP</Scp>1-<scp>RA</Scp> Add-on Therapy in Patients With Type 2 Diabetes Currently on a Bolus Containing Insulin Regimen.* Pharmacotherapy the Journal of Human Pharmacology and Drug Therapy, 2016. **36**(8): p. 893-905.
330. Witkowski, M., et al., *A Systematic Literature Review and Network Meta-Analysis Comparing Once-Weekly Semaglutide With Other GLP-1 Receptor Agonists in Patients With Type 2 Diabetes Previously Receiving Basal Insulin.* Diabetes Therapy, 2018. **9**(3): p. 1233-1251.
331. Liu, L., et al., *Association Between Different GLP-1 Receptor Agonists and Gastrointestinal Adverse Reactions: A Real-World Disproportionality Study Based on FDA Adverse Event Reporting System Database.* Frontiers in Endocrinology, 2022. **13**.
332. Krajnc, N., et al., *Treatment With GLP-1 Receptor Agonists Is Associated With Significant Weight Loss and Favorable Headache Outcomes in Idiopathic Intracranial Hypertension.* 2023.
333. Iqbal, J., et al., *Effect of Glucagon-like Peptide-1 Receptor Agonists on Body Weight in Adults With Obesity Without Diabetes Mellitus—a Systematic Review and Meta-analysis of Randomized Control Trials.* Obesity Reviews, 2022. **23**(6).
334. Bando, H., et al., *Clinical Response to Xultophy Possibly Varies From Each Different Metabolic Function.* Edelweiss Applied Science and Technology, 2021: p. 21-24.
335. Qin, W., et al., *Efficacy and Safety of Once-Weekly Tirzepatide for Weight Management Compared to Placebo: An Updated Systematic Review and Meta-Analysis Including the Latest SURMOUNT-2 Trial.* Endocrine, 2024. **86**(1): p. 70-84.
336. Urva, S., et al., *The Novel Dual Glucose-dependent Insulinotropic Polypeptide and Glucagon-like Peptide-1 (<scp>GLP</Scp> -1) Receptor Agonist Tirzepatide Transiently Delays Gastric Emptying Similarly to Selective <scp>long-acting GLP</scp> -1 Receptor Agonists.* Diabetes Obesity and Metabolism, 2020. **22**(10): p. 1886-1891.
337. Johanson, J.F. and J. Kralstein, *Chronic Constipation: A Survey of the Patient Perspective.* Alimentary Pharmacology & Therapeutics, 2007. **25**(5): p. 599-608.
338. Jangid, V., et al., *Water Intake, Dietary Fibre, Defecatory Habits and Its Association With Chronic Functional Constipation.* Current Research in Nutrition and Food Science Journal, 2016. **4**(2): p. 90-95.
339. Markland, A.D., et al., *Association of Low Dietary Intake of Fiber and Liquids With Constipation: Evidence From the National Health and Nutrition Examination Survey.* The American Journal of Gastroenterology, 2013. **108**(5): p. 796-803.
340. Arnaud, M.J., *Mild Dehydration: A Risk Factor of Constipation?* European Journal of Clinical Nutrition, 2003. **57**(S2): p. S88-S95.
341. Attaluri, A., et al., *Randomised Clinical Trial: Dried Plums (Prunes) vs. Psyllium for Constipation.* Alimentary Pharmacology & Therapeutics, 2011. **33**(7): p. 822-828.
342. Rijnaarts, I., et al., *A High-Fibre Personalised Dietary Advice Given via a Web Tool Reduces Constipation Complaints in Adults.* Journal of Nutritional Science, 2022. **11**.
343. Towers, A.L., et al., *Constipation in the Elderly: Influence of Dietary, Psychological, and Physiological Factors.* Journal of the American Geriatrics Society, 1994. **42**(7): p. 701-706.

344. Yusop, N.B.M. and N.Q.A.M. Yasin, *Association Between Dietary Intake, Physical Activity and Stress Level With Constipation Among Undergraduate Students.* Malaysian Journal of Nutrition, 2021. **27**(2).
345. Bryant, A.P., et al., *Linaclotide Is a Potent and Selective Guanylate Cyclase C Agonist That Elicits Pharmacological Effects Locally in the Gastrointestinal Tract.* Life Sciences, 2010. **86**(19-20): p. 760-765.
346. Lee, W.T.K., et al., *Increased Prevalence of Constipation in Pre-school Children Is Attributable to Under-consumption of Plant Foods: A Community-based Study.* Journal of Paediatrics and Child Health, 2007. **44**(4): p. 170-175.
347. Guimarães, E.V., E. Goulart, and F.J. Penna, *Dietary Fiber Intake, Stool Frequency and Colonic Transit Time in Chronic Functional Constipation in Children.* Brazilian Journal of Medical and Biological Research, 2001. **34**(9): p. 1147-1153.
348. Loening-Baucke, V., E. Miele, and A. Staiano, *Fiber (Glucomannan) Is Beneficial in the Treatment of Childhood Constipation.* Pediatrics, 2004. **113**(3): p. e259-e264.
349. Hongisto, S.M., et al., *A Combination of Fibre-Rich Rye Bread and Yoghurt Containing Lactobacillus GG Improves Bowel Function in Women With Self-Reported Constipation.* European Journal of Clinical Nutrition, 2005. **60**(3): p. 319-324.
350. Mandarino, F.V., et al., *Gastroparesis: The Complex Interplay With Microbiota and the Role of Exogenous Infections in the Pathogenesis of the Disease.* Microorganisms, 2023. **11**(5): p. 1122.
351. Camilleri, M., *Functional Dyspepsia and Gastroparesis.* Digestive Diseases, 2016. **34**(5): p. 491-499.
352. Anaparthy, R., et al., *Gastroparesis and Gastroparesis-Like Syndrome: Response to Therapy and Its Predictors.* Digestive Diseases and Sciences, 2009. **54**(5): p. 1003-1010.
353. Lei, Y., et al., *Rectal Distension Modulates Canine Gastric Tone and Accommodation.* Digestive Diseases and Sciences, 2005. **50**(11): p. 2134-2140.
354. Agrawal, A.K., et al., *Bloating and Distension in Irritable Bowel Syndrome: The Role of Gastrointestinal Transit.* The American Journal of Gastroenterology, 2009. **104**(8): p. 1998-2004.
355. Bouin, M., et al., *Intolerance to Visceral Distension in Functional Dyspepsia or Irritable Bowel Syndrome: An Organ Specific Defect or a Pan Intestinal Dysregulation?* Neurogastroenterology & Motility, 2004. **16**(3): p. 311-314.
356. Hasler, W.L., *Gastroparesis: Pathogenesis, Diagnosis and Management.* Nature Reviews Gastroenterology & Hepatology, 2011. **8**(8): p. 438-453.
357. Gourcerol, G., et al., *Impaired Fasting Pyloric Compliance in Gastroparesis and the Therapeutic Response to Pyloric Dilatation.* Alimentary Pharmacology & Therapeutics, 2014. **41**(4): p. 360-367.
358. Salet, G., et al., *Responses to Gastric Distension in Functional Dyspepsia.* Gut, 1998. **42**(6): p. 823-829.
359. Leeuwen, N.M.v., et al., *Gastrointestinal Symptom Severity and Progression in Systemic Sclerosis.* Rheumatology, 2022. **61**(10): p. 4024-4034.
360. Sands, G., *Adverse Events in Patients With Blood Loss: A Pooled Analysis of 51 Clinical Studies From the Celecoxib Clinical Trial Database.* The Open Rheumatology Journal, 2012. **6**(1): p. 44-49.
361. Lim, Y.J. and C.H. Yang, *Non-Steroidal Anti-Inflammatory Drug-Induced Enteropathy.* Clinical Endoscopy, 2012. **45**(2): p. 138.

362. Martínez, J.J.G., et al., *Clinical Recommendations to Manage Gastrointestinal Adverse Events in Patients Treated With GLP-1 Receptor Agonists: A Multidisciplinary Expert Consensus*. Journal of Clinical Medicine, 2022. **12**(1): p. 145.

363. Little, T.J., M. Horowitz, and C. Feinle-Bisset, *Modulation by High-Fat Diets of Gastrointestinal Function and Hormones Associated With the Regulation of Energy Intake: Implications for the Pathophysiology of Obesity*. American Journal of Clinical Nutrition, 2007. **86**(3): p. 531-541.

364. Camilleri, M., et al., *Performance Characteristics of Scintigraphic Measurement of Gastric Emptying of Solids in Healthy Participants*. Neurogastroenterology & Motility, 2012. **24**(12): p. 1076.

365. Varni, J.W., et al., *Gastrointestinal Symptoms Profile in Gastroparesis Compared to Other Functional and Organic Gastrointestinal Diseases*. Journal of Pediatric Gastroenterology and Nutrition, 2023. **77**(1).

366. Lee, K.J., et al., *A Pilot Study on Duodenal Acid Exposure and Its Relationship to Symptoms in Functional Dyspepsia With Prominent Nausea*. The American Journal of Gastroenterology, 2004. **99**(9): p. 1765-1773.

367. Farré, R., et al., *In Functional Dyspepsia, Hypersensitivity to Postprandial Distention Correlates With Meal-Related Symptom Severity*. Gastroenterology, 2013. **145**(3): p. 566-573.

368. Kang, Y.M., et al., *Comparative Efficacy and Tolerability of Currently Approved Incretin Mimetics: A Systematic Analysis of Placebo‐controlled Clinical Trials*. Diabetes Obesity and Metabolism, 2025. **27**(7): p. 3736-3746.

369. Newsome, P.N., et al., *A Placebo-Controlled Trial of Subcutaneous Semaglutide in Nonalcoholic Steatohepatitis*. New England Journal of Medicine, 2021. **384**(12): p. 1113-1124.

370. Mayer, C.S. and P. Fontelo, *Semaglutide Use in People With Obesity and Type 2 Diabetes From Real‐world Utilization Data: An Analysis of the All of US Program*. Diabetes Obesity and Metabolism, 2024. **26**(11): p. 4989-4995.

371. Melo, C.A.d., et al., *Exocrine Pancreatic Insufficiency During the Use of Semaglutide: A Case Report*. Cureus, 2024.

372. Li, L., et al., *Incretin Treatment and Risk of Pancreatitis in Patients With Type 2 Diabetes Mellitus: Systematic Review and Meta-Analysis of Randomised and Non-Randomised Studies*. BMJ, 2014. **348**(apr15 2): p. g2366-g2366.

373. Elashoff, M., et al., *Pancreatitis, Pancreatic, and Thyroid Cancer With Glucagon-Like Peptide-1–Based Therapies*. Gastroenterology, 2011. **141**(1): p. 150-156.

374. Alenzi, K.A., et al., *Pancreatitis With Use of New Diabetic Medications: A Real-World Data Study Using the Post-Marketing FDA Adverse Event Reporting System (FAERS) Database*. Frontiers in Pharmacology, 2024. **15**.

375. Patel, F., et al., *Acute Pancreatitis in a Patient Taking Semaglutide*. Cureus, 2023.

376. Nohomovich, B., A. Shah, and N. Hughes, *Severe, Complicated Pancreatitis With an Unclear Etiology*. Cureus, 2023.

377. Ayoub, M., et al., *Pancreatitis Risk Associated With GLP-1 Receptor Agonists, Considered as a Single Class, in a Comorbidity-Free Subgroup of Type 2 Diabetes Patients in the United States: A Propensity Score-Matched Analysis*. Journal of Clinical Medicine, 2025. **14**(3): p. 944.

378. Talha, A., A. Farouk, and I. Hasouna, *Cholelithiasis After Weight Loss Surgery: Challenge and Prophylaxis*. Ain Shams Journal of Surgery, 2016. **15**(2): p. 267-274.

379. Bennion, L.J. and S.M. Grundy, *Effects of Obesity and Caloric Intake on Biliary Lipid Metabolism in Man.* Journal of Clinical Investigation, 1975. **56**(4): p. 996-1011.
380. Stender, S., B.G. Nordestgaard, and A. Tybjærg-Hansen, *Elevated Body Mass Index as a Causal Risk Factor for Symptomatic Gallstone Disease: A Mendelian Randomization Study.* Hepatology, 2013. **58**(6): p. 2133-2141.
381. Pizzimenti, V., et al., *Incretin-Based Therapy and Acute Cholecystitis: A Review of Case Reports and EudraVigilance Spontaneous Adverse Drug Reaction Reporting Database.* Journal of Clinical Pharmacy and Therapeutics, 2016. **41**(2): p. 116-118.
382. Anjum, R., et al., *Gallbladder Stones – Pathogenesis and Treatment.* 2023.
383. Sassenrath, K., B.B. Phillips, and R.H. Stone, *Evaluation of GLP-1 Receptor Agonists in Combination With Multiple Daily Insulin Injections for Type 2 Diabetes.* Journal of Pharmacy Practice, 2021. **35**(6): p. 979-990.
384. Bajaj, H.S., et al., *Lowest Glucose Variability and Hypoglycemia Are Observed With the Combination of a GLP-1 Receptor Agonist and Basal Insulin (VARIATION Study).* Diabetes Care, 2016. **40**(2): p. 194-200.
385. Seino, Y., et al., *Combination Therapy With Liraglutide and Insulin in Japanese Patients With Type 2 Diabetes: A 36-week, Randomized, Double-blind, Parallel-group Trial.* Journal of Diabetes Investigation, 2016. **7**(4): p. 565-573.
386. Rana, K.B., et al., *Comparison of the Effectiveness of Liraglutide vs Semaglutide in a Veteran Population.* Journal of Pharmacy Practice, 2022. **36**(5): p. 1095-1101.
387. Wilkinson, L., et al., *Cost of Achieving HbA1c Treatment Targets and Weight Loss Responses With Once-Weekly Semaglutide Versus Dulaglutide in the United States.* Diabetes Therapy, 2018. **9**(3): p. 951-961.
388. Jones, M. and J.J. Cappola, *GLP-1 Receptor Agonists in Diabetes and Obesity: A Case Report and Review of Bowel Obstruction Risks and Management.* Cureus, 2025.
389. Chaudhry, A., et al., *Tendency of Semaglutide to Induce Gastroparesis: A Case Report.* Cureus, 2024.
390. Brito, J.P., et al., *GLP-1RA Use and Thyroid Cancer Risk.* Jama Otolaryngology–head & Neck Surgery, 2025. **151**(3): p. 243.
391. Παππά, Θ., *GLP-1 Receptor Agonists and the Risk of Thyroid Cancer.* Clinical Thyroidology, 2023. **35**(1): p. 18-20.
392. Ycaza, A.E.E.D., et al., *Glucagon-Like Peptide-1 Receptor Agonists and Thyroid Cancer: A Narrative Review.* Thyroid, 2024.
393. Hegedüs, L., et al., *No Evidence of Increase in Calcitonin Concentrations or Development of C-Cell Malignancy in Response to Liraglutide for Up to 5 Years in the LEADER Trial.* Diabetes Care, 2017. **41**(3): p. 620-622.
394. Pollack, R. and J. Stokar, *Long-Term Glucagon-Like Peptide 1 Receptor Agonist Use Is Not Associated With Increased Risk of Thyroid Cancer in Adults With Type 2 Diabetes.* Diabetes/Metabolism Research and Reviews, 2025. **41**(8).
395. Marso, S.P., et al., *Liraglutide and Cardiovascular Outcomes in Type 2 Diabetes.* New England Journal of Medicine, 2016. **375**(4): p. 311-322.
396. Sherman, S.I., et al., *No Calcitonin Change in a Person Taking Dulaglutide Diagnosed With Pre-existing Medullary Thyroid Cancer.* Diabetic Medicine, 2018. **35**(3): p. 381-385.
397. Haymart, M.R., et al., *Thyroid Ultrasound and the Increase in Diagnosis of Low-Risk Thyroid Cancer.* The Journal of Clinical Endocrinology & Metabolism, 2018. **104**(3): p. 785-792.

398. Hu, W., et al., *Use of GLP-1 Receptor Agonists and Occurrence of Thyroid Disorders: A Meta-Analysis of Randomized Controlled Trials.* Frontiers in Endocrinology, 2022. **13**.
399. Zou, S.Z., et al., *Multifocal C-Cell Hyperplasia and Marked Hypercalcitoninemia in a Diabetic Patient Treated With Glucagon-Like Peptide-1 Agonist With Concurrent Multinodular Goiter and Hyperparathyroidism.* Cureus, 2023.
400. Dong, S. and C. Sun, *Can Glucagon-Like Peptide-1 Receptor Agonists Cause Acute Kidney Injury? An Analytical Study Based on Post-Marketing Approval Pharmacovigilance Data.* Frontiers in Endocrinology, 2022. **13**.
401. Safwan, M., et al., *Gastrointestinal Safety of Semaglutide and Tirzepatide vs. Placebo in Obese Individuals Without Diabetes: A Systematic Review and Meta Analysis.* Annals of Saudi Medicine, 2025. **45**(2): p. 129-143.
402. Morehouse, Z.P. and J.D. Ledford, *Problematic Pharmacokinetics: A Case of Recurrent Pancreatitis Post Discontinuation of a Glucagon-Like Peptide 1 Receptor Agonists.* Journal of Pharmacy Practice, 2024. **38**(1): p. 187-192.
403. Begum, F., et al., *Semaglutide-Associated Kidney Injury.* Clinical Kidney Journal, 2024. **17**(9).
404. Rossing, P., et al., *Effects of Semaglutide With or Without Concomitant Mineralocorticoid Receptor Antagonist Use in Participants With Type 2 Diabetes and Chronic Kidney Disease: A FLOW Trial Prespecified Secondary Analysis.* Diabetes Care, 2025. **48**(11): p. 1878-1887.
405. Dayel, F.F.B., et al., *Evaluation of Pre-Treatment Assessment of Semaglutide Users: Balancing the Benefits of Weight Loss vs. Potential Health Consequences.* Healthcare, 2025. **13**(15): p. 1827.
406. Dalbøge, L.S., et al., *Nephroprotective Effects of Semaglutide as Mono- And Combination Treatment With Lisinopril in a Mouse Model of Hypertension-Accelerated Diabetic Kidney Disease.* Biomedicines, 2022. **10**(7): p. 1661.
407. Borkum, M., et al., *Semaglutide-Associated Acute Interstitial Nephritis: A Case Report.* Kidney Medicine, 2022. **4**(12): p. 100561.
408. Holmes, P., et al., *Real-World Use of Once-Weekly Semaglutide in Type 2 Diabetes: Results From the SURE UK Multicentre, Prospective, Observational Study.* Diabetes Therapy, 2021. **12**(11): p. 2891-2905.
409. Mikhail, N., *Once Weekly Semaglutide for Treatment of Obesity.* Journal of Clinical and Laboratory Research, 2021. **2**(3): p. 01-04.
410. Muller, D.R.P., et al., *Effects of GLP-1 Agonists and SGLT2 Inhibitors During Pregnancy and Lactation on Offspring Outcomes: A Systematic Review of the Evidence.* Frontiers in Endocrinology, 2023. **14**.
411. Mikhail, N. and S. Wali, *Semaglutide as Treatment for Obesity in Adolescents.* International Journal of Diabetes Management, 2023.
412. Cousminer, D.L., et al., *Genetically Determined Later Puberty Impacts Lowered Bone Mineral Density in Childhood and Adulthood.* Journal of Bone and Mineral Research, 2017. **33**(3): p. 430-436.
413. Zaitoon, H., et al., *Beyond Weight Loss: Optimizing GLP-1 Receptor Agonist Use in Children.* Children, 2025. **12**(11): p. 1427.
414. Kanaoka, Y., et al., *Long-Term Effects of Hormone Replacement Therapy on Bone Mineral Density in Girls Oophorectomized in Adolescence.* Gynecologic and Obstetric Investigation, 2003. **55**(3): p. 168-172.

415. Yadav, S., R.K. Marwaha, and P. Sharma, *Bone Metabolism in Relation to Puberty Among North Indian Boys.* Journal of Pediatric Biochemistry, 2016. **03**(02): p. 107-112.
416. Soyka, L.A., et al., *The Effects of Anorexia Nervosa on Bone Metabolism in Female Adolescents.* Obstetrical & Gynecological Survey, 2000. **55**(5): p. 295-297.
417. Tan, H.C., O.A. Dampil, and M.M. Marquez, *Efficacy and Safety of Semaglutide for Weight Loss in Obesity Without Diabetes: A Systematic Review and Meta-Analysis.* Journal of the Asean Federation of Endocrine Societies, 2022. **37**(2): p. 65-72.
418. Warren, M., et al., *Semaglutide as a Therapeutic Option for Elderly Patients With Type 2 Diabetes: Pooled Analysis of the SUSTAIN 1-5 Trials.* Diabetes Obesity and Metabolism, 2018. **20**(9): p. 2291-2297.
419. Mohamad, A.A., *A Case Report of Semaglutide Induced Sarcopenia: Causes of Fatigue in Older Adults.* Korean Journal of Family Medicine, 2025. **46**(4): p. 288-291.
420. Cortes, T., et al., *Effect of Semaglutide on Physical Function, Body Composition, and Biomarkers of Aging in Older Adults With Overweight and Insulin Resistance: Protocol for an Open-Labeled Randomized Controlled Trial.* Jmir Research Protocols, 2024. **13**: p. e62667.
421. Cork, S., *Wegovy and Mounjaro might affect how well your contraceptives work – here's why* 2025, The Converstation.
422. Lin, L.-Y., et al., *Interactive Effects of Sleep Duration and Dietary Patterns on Obesity Moderated by Age.* Scientific Reports, 2025. **15**(1).
423. Młynarska, E., et al., *Obesity as a Multifactorial Chronic Disease: Molecular Mechanisms, Systemic Impact, and Emerging Digital Interventions.* Current Issues in Molecular Biology, 2025. **47**(10): p. 787.
424. Xian, J., et al., *Recent Advances in the Anti-Obesity Benefits of Phytoconstituents: From Phytochemistry to Targeting Novel-Systems.* Phytotherapy Research, 2024. **39**(2): p. 630-660.
425. Stathori, G., et al., *Obesity- And High-Fat-Diet-Induced Neuroinflammation: Implications for Autonomic Nervous System Dysfunction and Endothelial Disorders.* International Journal of Molecular Sciences, 2025. **26**(9): p. 4047.
426. Tolvanen, L., et al., *Weight Loss History and Its Association With Self-Esteem and Eating Behaviors in Adolescents and Young Adults With Obesity.* Obesity Facts, 2023. **16**(3): p. 293-300.
427. Hawkins, M.A.W., et al., *Cognitive and Self-Regulatory Mechanisms of Obesity Study (COSMOS): Study Protocol for a Randomized Controlled Weight Loss Trial Examining Change in Biomarkers, Cognition, and Self-Regulation Across Two Behavioral Treatments.* Contemporary Clinical Trials, 2018. **66**: p. 20-27.
428. Paddu, N.U., et al., *Weight Maintenance on Cost-effective Antiobesity Medications After 1 year of <scp>GLP-1</Scp> Receptor Agonist Therapy: A Real-world Study.* Obesity, 2024. **32**(12): p. 2255-2263.
429. Wharton, S., et al., *Two-year Effect of Semaglutide 2.4 mg on Control of Eating in Adults With Overweight/Obesity: <scp>STEP</Scp> 5.* Obesity, 2023. **31**(3): p. 703-715.
430. Zapata, R.C., et al., *Adipocytes Control Food Intake and Weight Regain via Vacuolar-Type H+ ATPase.* Nature Communications, 2022. **13**(1).
431. Chen, X., et al., *Key Genes Involved in Nonalcoholic Steatohepatitis Improvement After Bariatric Surgery.* Frontiers in Endocrinology, 2024. **15**.
432. Magwire, M., et al., *Addressing Obesity in Diabetes.* Adces in Practice, 2024. **12**(6): p. 24-38.

433. Doyle, J., et al., *How Adolescents Decide on Bariatric Surgery: An Interpretative Phenomenological Analysis*. Clinical Obesity, 2018. **8**(2): p. 114-121.
434. Lin, X. and H. Li, *Obesity: Epidemiology, Pathophysiology, and Therapeutics*. Frontiers in Endocrinology, 2021. **12**.
435. Kataria, I., et al., *Development and Evaluation of a Digital, Community-Based Intervention to Reduce Noncommunicable Disease Risk in a Low-Resource Urban Setting in Malaysia: A Research Protocol*. Implementation Science Communications, 2020. **1**(1).
436. Baur, L.A., *Child and Adolescent Obesity in the 21st Century: An Australian Perspective*. Asia Pacific Journal of Clinical Nutrition, 2002. **11**(s3).
437. Krishan, J. and A.K. Poonia, *Evaluation the Pervasiveness of Obesity Among Children's at National Institute of Medical Science and Research Jaipur Rajasthan*. International Journal of Paediatrics and Geriatrics, 2018. **1**(2): p. 22-25.
438. Paniagua, J.A., *Nutrition, Insulin Resistance and Dysfunctional Adipose Tissue Determine the Different Components of Metabolic Syndrome*. World Journal of Diabetes, 2016. **7**(19): p. 483.
439. Lappalainen, T., et al., *Association of the Fat Mass and Obesity-Associated (<i>FTO</I>) Gene Variant (Rs9939609) With Dietary Intake in the Finnish Diabetes Prevention Study*. British Journal of Nutrition, 2012. **108**(10): p. 1859-1865.
440. Berk-Clark, C.v.d., et al., *Association Between Posttraumatic Stress Disorder and Lack of Exercise, Poor Diet, Obesity, and Co-Occuring Smoking: A Systematic Review and Meta-Analysis*. Health Psychology, 2018. **37**(5): p. 407-416.
441. Abdella, H.M., et al., *Influence of Gender on the Relationship Between Eating Behaviors, Age and BMI in People in Benghazi, Benghazi, Libya*. European Journal of Theoretical and Applied Sciences, 2023. **1**(2): p. 57-65.
442. Aphramor, L., *Validity of Claims Made in Weight Management Research: A Narrative Review of Dietetic Articles*. Nutrition Journal, 2010. **9**(1).
443. McCormick, S. and C. Clarke, *Prevention and Management of Overweight/Obesity in the Community*. Nutrition Bulletin, 2004. **29**(3): p. 274-279.
444. Jung, J., et al., *Salacia Reticulata Extract Suppresses Fat Accumulation by Regulating Lipid Metabolism*. Foods, 2023. **12**(17): p. 3149.
445. Bray, G.A., K.K. Kim, and J. Wilding, *Obesity: A Chronic Relapsing Progressive Disease Process. A Position Statement of the World Obesity Federation*. Obesity Reviews, 2017. **18**(7): p. 715-723.
446. Glazer, S., *The Management of Obesity in 2023: An Update*. Canadian Primary Care Today, 2023.
447. Doll, H., S. Petersen, and S. Stewart-Brown, *Obesity and Physical and Emotional Well-Being: Associations Between Body Mass Index, Chronic Illness, and the Physical and Mental Components of the SF-36 Questionnaire*. Obesity Research, 2000. **8**(2): p. 160-170.
448. Tsai, A.G., et al., *Evidence of a Gap in Understanding Obesity Among Physicians*. Obesity Science & Practice, 2018. **4**(1): p. 46-51.
449. Schumacher, L.M., J.D. Ard, and D.B. Sarwer, *Promise and Unrealized Potential: 10 years of the American Medical Association Classifying Obesity as a Disease*. Frontiers in Public Health, 2023. **11**.
450. Shabatian, H., *The Set Point Theory Explained*. 2025, West Medical.

451. Sumithran, P., et al., *Ketosis and Appetite-Mediating Nutrients and Hormones After Weight Loss*. European Journal of Clinical Nutrition, 2013. **67**(7): p. 759-764.
452. Calcaterra, V., et al., *Long-Term Outcome After Robotic-Assisted Gastroplication in Adolescents: Hunger Hormone and Food Preference Changes Two Case Reports*. Journal of Clinical Research in Pediatric Endocrinology, 2016. **8**(2): p. 250-256.
453. MacLean, P.S., et al., *Regular Exercise Attenuates the Metabolic Drive to Regain Weight After Long-Term Weight Loss*. Ajp Regulatory Integrative and Comparative Physiology, 2009. **297**(3): p. R793-R802.
454. MacLean, P.S., et al., *Biology's Response to Dieting: The Impetus for Weight Regain*. Ajp Regulatory Integrative and Comparative Physiology, 2011. **301**(3): p. R581-R600.
455. Jung, C., et al., *Energy Expenditure During Sleep, Sleep Deprivation and Sleep Following Sleep Deprivation in Adult Humans*. The Journal of Physiology, 2010. **589**(1): p. 235-244.
456. Hebert, M., et al., *Single Rapamycin Administration Induces Prolonged Downward Shift in Defended Body Weight in Rats*. Plos One, 2014. **9**(5): p. e93691.
457. Larraufie, P., et al., *Important Role of the GLP-1 Axis for Glucose Homeostasis After Bariatric Surgery*. Cell Reports, 2019. **26**(6): p. 1399-1408.e6.
458. Speakman, J.R., et al., *Set Points, Settling Points and Some Alternative Models: Theoretical Options to Understand How Genes and Environments Combine to Regulate Body Adiposity*. Disease Models & Mechanisms, 2011. **4**(6): p. 733-745.
459. Mekjavić, I.B., et al., *Energy Intake of Men With Excess Weight During Normobaric Hypoxic Confinement*. Frontiers in Physiology, 2022. **12**.
460. Hamby, M., et al., *The Impact of Asic2 Deletion on Metabolic Homeostasis in Mice*. Physiological Reports, 2025. **13**(17).
461. Ravussin, Y., et al., *Effects of Chronic Leptin Infusion on Subsequent Body Weight and Composition in Mice: Can Body Weight Set Point Be Reset?A*. Molecular Metabolism, 2014. **3**(4): p. 432-440.
462. Considine, R.V., et al., *Serum Immunoreactive-Leptin Concentrations in Normal-Weight and Obese Humans*. New England Journal of Medicine, 1996. **334**(5): p. 292-295.
463. Salehi, M. and J.Q. Purnell, *The Role of Glucagon-Like Peptide-1 in Energy Homeostasis*. Metabolic Syndrome and Related Disorders, 2019. **17**(4): p. 183-191.
464. Zanchi, D., et al., *The Impact of Gut Hormones on the Neural Circuit of Appetite and Satiety: A Systematic Review*. Neuroscience & Biobehavioral Reviews, 2017. **80**: p. 457-475.
465. Richards, P., N.A. Thornberry, and S. Pinto, *The Gut–brain Axis: Identifying New Therapeutic Approaches for Type 2 Diabetes, Obesity, and Related Disorders*. Molecular Metabolism, 2021. **46**: p. 101175.
466. Wachsmuth, H.R., S.N. Weninger, and F.A. Duca, *Role of the Gut–brain Axis in Energy and Glucose Metabolism*. Experimental & Molecular Medicine, 2022. **54**(4): p. 377-392.
467. Cork, S.C., *The Role of the Vagus Nerve in Appetite Control: Implications for the Pathogenesis of Obesity*. Journal of Neuroendocrinology, 2018. **30**(11).
468. Burcelin, R. and P. Gourdy, *Harnessing Glucagon-like Peptide-1 Receptor Agonists for the Pharmacological Treatment of Overweight and Obesity*. Obesity Reviews, 2016. **18**(1): p. 86-98.
469. Pizarroso, N., et al., *A Review on the Role of Food-Derived Bioactive Molecules and the Microbiota–Gut–Brain Axis in Satiety Regulation*. Nutrients, 2021. **13**(2): p. 632.

470. Charpentier, J., et al., *Lixisenatide Requires a Functional Gut-Vagus Nerve-Brain Axis to Trigger Insulin Secretion in Controls and Type 2 Diabetic Mice.* Ajp Gastrointestinal and Liver Physiology, 2018. **315**(5): p. G671-G684.
471. Yan, M., et al., *Gut Liver Brain Axis in Diseases: The Implications for Therapeutic Interventions.* Signal Transduction and Targeted Therapy, 2023. **8**(1).
472. Dragano, N.R.V., et al., *Polyunsaturated Fatty Acid Receptors, GPR40 and GPR120, Are Expressed in the Hypothalamus and Control Energy Homeostasis and Inflammation.* Journal of Neuroinflammation, 2017. **14**(1).
473. Hamamah, S., A. Hajnal, and M. Covașă, *Influence of Bariatric Surgery on Gut Microbiota Composition and Its Implication on Brain and Peripheral Targets.* Nutrients, 2024. **16**(7): p. 1071.
474. Longo, S., S. Rizza, and M. Federici, *Microbiota-Gut-Brain Axis: Relationships Among the Vagus Nerve, Gut Microbiota, Obesity, and Diabetes.* Acta Diabetologica, 2023. **60**(8): p. 1007-1017.
475. Chuong, V., et al., *The Glucagon-Like Peptide-1 (GLP-1) Analogue Semaglutide Reduces Alcohol Drinking and Modulates Central GABA Neurotransmission.* Jci Insight, 2023. **8**(12).
476. Rastelli, M., et al., *Intestinal NAPE-PLD Contributes to Short-Term Regulation of Food Intake via Gut-to-Brain Axis.* Ajp Endocrinology and Metabolism, 2020. **319**(3): p. E647-E657.
477. Cabou, C. and R. Burcelin, *GLP-1, the Gut-Brain, and Brain-Periphery Axes.* The Review of Diabetic Studies, 2011. **8**(3): p. 418-431.
478. Gabery, S., et al., *Semaglutide Lowers Body Weight in Rodents via Distributed Neural Pathways.* Jci Insight, 2020. **5**(6).
479. Figueredo, Y., et al., *Weight Loss Effects of Glucagon-Like Peptide-One Receptor Analog Treatment in a Severely Obese Patient During Hospital Admission.* Cureus, 2023.
480. Alyar, G., F.Z. Umudum, and N. Akbaş, *Changes in Ghrelin, GLP-1, and PYY Levels After Diet and Exercise in Obese Individuals.* Revista Da Associação Médica Brasileira, 2024. **70**(1).
481. Ma, T., et al., *Distinct Effects of Semaglutide and Tirzepatide on Metabolic and Inflammatory Gene Expression in Brown Adipose Tissue of Mice Fed a High-Fat, High-Fructose Diet.* Frontiers in Nutrition, 2025. **12**.
482. Beauregard, N., et al., *Energy Balance and Obesity: The Emerging Role of Glucagon Like Peptide-1 Receptor Agonists.* Current Opinion in Clinical Nutrition & Metabolic Care, 2024. **27**(6): p. 472-478.
483. Henderson, S., et al., *Robust Anti-obesity and Metabolic Effects of a Dual <scp>GLP</Scp> -1/Glucagon Receptor Peptide Agonist in Rodents and Non-human Primates.* Diabetes Obesity and Metabolism, 2016. **18**(12): p. 1176-1190.
484. Dhar, R., A. Kumar, and S. Karmakar, *The Craze With Semaglutide.* Asian Journal of Medical Sciences, 2024. **15**(6): p. 1-2.
485. Akhtar, S.J., et al., *The Effect of Insurance Status on Bariatric Surgery Outcomes: A Retrospective Chart Review Study.* The American Surgeon, 2022. **89**(5): p. 1887-1892.
486. Sankar, A., et al., *Actual Weight Loss Trajectories After Bariatric Surgery Compared With the SOPHIA Prediction Tool: An Observational Comparison Study.* Diabetes Obesity and Metabolism, 2025. **27**(4): p. 2206-2213.

487. Touzot, M., P. Ureña-Torres, and O. Dupuy, *Semaglutide for Treatment of Obesity in Hemodialysis Patients Waiting for a Kidney Transplant: New Hope?* Clinical Kidney Journal, 2022. **15**(9): p. 1782-1784.
488. Giorelli, G., et al., *Body Composition Changes With Semaglutide: A Systematic Review and Meta-Analysis*. 2025.
489. Alsugair, H.A., et al., *Weekly Semaglutide vs. Liraglutide Efficacy Profile: A Network Meta-Analysis*. Healthcare, 2021. **9**(9): p. 1125.
490. Leahey, T.M., et al., *A Randomized Controlled Trial Testing an Internet Delivered Cost–benefit Approach to Weight Loss Maintenance*. Preventive Medicine, 2016. **92**: p. 51-57.
491. Alsaad, N., et al., *Outcomes of Semaglutide Use in Achieving Target Body Mass Index Before Renal Transplant in Five End-Stage Renal Disease Patients: A Case Series*. Cureus, 2024.
492. Petrova, L., et al., *Systematic Review of the Efficacy and Safety of GLP-1 Receptor Agonists in the Treatment of Patients With Type 2 Diabetes Mellitus*. Pharmacia, 2024. **71**: p. 1-17.
493. Arterburn, D., et al., *Comparative Effectiveness of Bariatric Surgery vs. Nonsurgical Treatment of Type 2 Diabetes Among Severely Obese Adults*. Obesity Research & Clinical Practice, 2013. **7**(4): p. e258-e268.
494. Purnell, J.Q., et al., *Type 2 Diabetes Remission Rates After Laparoscopic Gastric Bypass and Gastric Banding: Results of the Longitudinal Assessment of Bariatric Surgery Study*. Diabetes Care, 2016. **39**(7): p. 1101-1107.
495. Coleman, K.J., et al., *Long-Term Microvascular Disease Outcomes in Patients With Type 2 Diabetes After Bariatric Surgery: Evidence for the Legacy Effect of Surgery*. Diabetes Care, 2016. **39**(8): p. 1400-1407.
496. Ribeiro, G.d.M., et al., *The Effectiveness of Bariatric Surgery in the Control of Type 2 Diabetes Mellitus: An Integrative Review*. International Journal of Health Science, 2023. **3**(47): p. 2-9.
497. Wilding, J., et al., *Once-Weekly Semaglutide in Adults With Overweight or Obesity*. New England Journal of Medicine, 2021. **384**(11): p. 989-1002.
498. He, L., et al., *Association of Glucagon-Like Peptide-1 Receptor Agonist Use With Risk of Gallbladder and Biliary Diseases*. Jama Internal Medicine, 2022. **182**(5): p. 513.
499. Faillie, J.L., et al., *Pancreatitis Associated With the Use of GLP-1 Analogs and DPP-4 Inhibitors: A Case/Non-Case Study From the French Pharmacovigilance Database*. Acta Diabetologica, 2013.
500. Meng, Z., *Long-Term Safety Profile of Semaglutide in the Management of Type 2 Diabetes and Obesity*. Medscien, 2025. **1**(3).
501. Diec, C.B., E.A. Cook, and N.T. Nguyen, *Asymptomatic Subcutaneous Semaglutide Overdose: A Case Report and Literature Review*. Journal of Pharmacy Practice, 2025.
502. Chen, A.S., et al., *Efficacy of Antiobesity Medications for Weight Reduction in Older Adults: A Systematic Review*. Obesity, 2024.
503. Kruse, T., et al., *Development of Cagrilintide, a Long-Acting Amylin Analogue*. Journal of Medicinal Chemistry, 2021. **64**(15): p. 11183-11194.
504. Camilleri, M. and A. Acosta, *Newer Pharmacological Interventions Directed at Gut Hormones for Obesity*. British Journal of Pharmacology, 2023. **181**(8): p. 1153-1164.
505. D'Ascanio, A.M., J. Mullally, and W.H. Frishman, *Cagrilintide: A Long-Acting Amylin Analog for the Treatment of Obesity*. Cardiology in Review, 2023. **32**(1): p. 83-90.

506. Wang, Y., Z. Feng, and L. Yu, *The Next Frontier in Metabolic Health: Cagrilintide-Semaglutide and the Evolving Landscape of Therapies*. The Innovation Medicine, 2025. **3**(3): p. 100150.
507. Jin, T., et al., *Comparative Efficacy and Safety of Semaglutide, Cagrilintide, and CagriSema for the Treatment of Type 2 Diabetes Mellitus: A Bayesian Network Meta-Analysis*. Journal of Clinical Question, 2025. **2**(5): p. e90.
508. Mikhail, N., *Cagrilintide Combined With Semaglutide: A New Approach for Treatment of Obesity and Type 2 Diabetes*. Clinical Research and Clinical Trials, 2023. **8**(3): p. 01-04.
509. Podolsky, M.I., et al., *Factors Associated With Semaglutide Initiation Among Adults With Obesity*. Jama Network Open, 2025. **8**(1): p. e2455222.
510. Lautenbach, A., et al., *The Potential of Semaglutide Once-Weekly in Patients Without Type 2 Diabetes With Weight Regain or Insufficient Weight Loss After Bariatric Surgery—a Retrospective Analysis*. Obesity Surgery, 2022. **32**(10): p. 3280-3288.
511. Blüher, M., et al., *New Insights Into the Treatment of Obesity*. Diabetes Obesity and Metabolism, 2023. **25**(8): p. 2058-2072.
512. Rivero-Moreno, Y., et al., *Semaglutide vs Revisional Bariatric Surgery: What Is the Best Option for Suboptimal Clinical Response or Recurrent Weight Gain After MBS?* . 2025.
513. Schauer, P.R., et al., *Bariatric Surgery Versus Intensive Medical Therapy in Obese Patients With Diabetes*. New England Journal of Medicine, 2012. **366**(17): p. 1567-1576.
514. Schauer, P.R., et al., *Bariatric Surgery Versus Intensive Medical Therapy for Diabetes — 3-Year Outcomes*. New England Journal of Medicine, 2014. **370**(21): p. 2002-2013.
515. Arterburn, D., et al., *Benefits and Risks of Bariatric Surgery in Adults*. Jama, 2020. **324**(9): p. 879.
516. Courcoulas, A.P., *Weight Change and Health Outcomes at 3 Years After Bariatric Surgery Among Individuals With Severe Obesity*. Jama, 2013.
517. Courcoulas, A.P., et al., *Three-Year Outcomes of Bariatric Surgery vs Lifestyle Intervention for Type 2 Diabetes Mellitus Treatment*. Jama Surgery, 2015. **150**(10): p. 931.
518. Brethauer, S.A., et al., *Can Diabetes Be Surgically Cured? Long-Term Metabolic Effects of Bariatric Surgery in Obese Patients With Type 2 Diabetes Mellitus*. Annals of Surgery Open, 2013. **258**(4): p. 628-637.
519. Lautenbach, A., et al., *Sustained Weight Loss With Semaglutide Once Weekly in Patients Without Type 2 Diabetes and Post-bariatric Treatment Failure*. Clinical Obesity, 2023. **13**(5).
520. Louis, M. and E.J. Velazquez, *The Impact of New Weight-Loss Medications on Bariatric Surgery and Surgeon Employment*. Cureus, 2025.
521. Doyle, W.N., et al., *Anti-Obesity Medication Use for Adolescent Metabolic and Bariatric Surgery Patients: A Systematic Literature Review*. Cureus, 2023.
522. Admani, B., M. Fahim, and H. Ahmed, *Semaglutide and Weight Loss – A Concern for Diabetics and Pharmaceuticals*. Journal of the Pakistan Medical Association, 2024. **74**(6): p. 1204-1204.
523. Heimann, N., I. Handzlik, and B. Myszkowska, *The Ozempic Pregnancy Phenomenon: What Medical Research Reveals*. Clinical Medicine and Health Research Journal, 2025. **5**(05): p. 1455-1459.
524. Kolli, R., et al., *Rebound or Retention: A Meta-Analysis of Weight Regain After the Discontinuation of Glucagon-Like Peptide-1 (GLP-1) Receptor Agonists and Other Anti-Obesity Drugs*. Cureus, 2025.

525. Nathan, B.M., et al., *Predictors of Weight-loss Response With Glucagon-like Peptide-1 Receptor Agonist Treatment Among Adolescents With Severe Obesity.* Clinical Obesity, 2015. **6**(1): p. 73-78.
526. Schirra, J., et al., *GLP-1 Regulates Gastroduodenal Motility Involving Cholinergic Pathways.* Neurogastroenterology & Motility, 2009. **21**(6): p. 609.
527. Witaszek, T., et al., *Gastrointestinal Symptoms in Obesity Therapy: Mechanisms, Epidemiology, and Management Strategies.* Biomedicines, 2025. **13**(10): p. 2362.
528. Camilleri, M., et al., *Clinical Guideline: Management of Gastroparesis.* The American Journal of Gastroenterology, 2013. **108**(1): p. 18-37.
529. Kenz, Z., C. Vallejo, and S. Siler, *Weight Loss and Nausea From Subcutaneous and Oral Semaglutide Accurately Simulated With a QSP Model.* 2024.
530. Mori, H., et al., *Gastrointestinal Hormones and Regulation of Gastric Emptying.* Current Opinion in Endocrinology Diabetes and Obesity, 2022. **29**(2): p. 191-199.
531. Huo, R.R., et al., *Effects of Mediterranean-Style Diet on Glycemic Control, Weight Loss and Cardiovascular Risk Factors Among Type 2 Diabetes Individuals: A Meta-Analysis.* European Journal of Clinical Nutrition, 2014. **69**(11): p. 1200-1208.
532. Barrea, L., et al., *A Multidisciplinary Perspective on Semaglutide Treatment and Medical Nutrition Therapy in Obesity Management.* Current Obesity Reports, 2025. **14**(1).
533. Carbonneau, É., et al., *Effects of the Mediterranean Diet Before and After Weight Loss on Eating Behavioral Traits in Men With Metabolic Syndrome.* Nutrients, 2017. **9**(3): p. 305.
534. Pedrollo, E.F., et al., *Effect of an Intensive Nutrition Intervention of a High Protein and Low Glycemic-Index Diet on Weight of Kidney Transplant Recipients: Study Protocol for a Randomized Clinical Trial.* Trials, 2017. **18**(1).
535. Larsen, T.M., et al., *Diets With High or Low Protein Content and Glycemic Index for Weight-Loss Maintenance.* New England Journal of Medicine, 2010. **363**(22): p. 2102-2113.
536. Li, S.S., et al., *Dietary Pulses, Satiety and Food Intake: A Systematic Review and Meta-analysis of Acute Feeding Trials.* Obesity, 2014. **22**(8): p. 1773-1780.
537. Ponzo, V., et al., *Exploring Dietary Intake in Adults With Type 2 Diabetes Using GLP-1 Receptor Agonists: A Cross-Sectional Analysis.* Nutrients, 2025. **17**(21): p. 3318.
538. He, L., et al., *Pharmacovigilance Study of GLP-1 Receptor Agonists for Metabolic and Nutritional Adverse Events.* Frontiers in Pharmacology, 2024. **15**.
539. García-Gorrita, C., et al., *Beyond GLP-1 Agonists: An Adaptive Ketogenic–Mediterranean Protocol to Counter Metabolic Adaptation in Obesity Management.* Nutrients, 2025. **17**(16): p. 2699.
540. Wilson, P.R., K.H. Bridges, and S.H. Wilson, *Particulate Gastric Contents in Patients Prescribed Glucagon-Like Peptide 1 Receptor Agonists After Appropriate Perioperative Fasting: A Report of 2 Cases.* A&a Practice, 2023. **17**(8): p. e01712.
541. Acosta, A., et al., *Exenatide in Obesity With Accelerated Gastric Emptying: A Randomized, Pharmacodynamics Study.* Physiological Reports, 2015. **3**(11): p. e12610.
542. Blundell, J.E., et al., *Effects of Once-weekly Semaglutide on Appetite, Energy Intake, Control of Eating, Food Preference and Body Weight in Subjects With Obesity.* Diabetes Obesity and Metabolism, 2017. **19**(9): p. 1242-1251.
543. Ahajumobi, N.E., et al., *Effect of Water Intake on Constipation and Bowel Movement.* Asian Journal of Medicine and Health, 2022: p. 1-10.

544. Frąckiewicz, J. and K. Szewczyk, *Is There an Association Between Hydration Status, Beverage Consumption Frequency, Blood Pressure, Anthropometric Characteristics, and Urinary Biomarkers in Adults?* Nutrients, 2025. **17**(6): p. 952.
545. Kushner, R.F., J.P. Almandoz, and D. Rubino, *Managing Adverse Effects of Incretin-Based Medications for Obesity.* Jama, 2025. **334**(9): p. 822.
546. Horswill, C.A. and L.M. Janas, *Hydration and Health.* American Journal of Lifestyle Medicine, 2011. **5**(4): p. 304-315.
547. Costilla, V. and A.E. Foxx–Orenstein, *Constipation in Adults: Diagnosis and Management.* Current Treatment Options in Gastroenterology, 2014. **12**(3): p. 310-321.
548. Hayat, U., M. Dugum, and S. Garg, *Chronic Constipation: Update on Management.* Cleveland Clinic Journal of Medicine, 2017. **84**(5): p. 397-408.
549. Maddi, V.I., *Regulation of Bowel Function by a Laxative/Stool Softener Preparation in Aged Nursing Home Patients.* Journal of the American Geriatrics Society, 1979. **27**(10): p. 464-468.
550. Bril, S., Y. Shoham, and J.S. Marcus, *The 'Mystery' of Opioid-Induced Diarrhea.* Pain Research and Management, 2011. **16**(3): p. 197-199.
551. Thosani, S., et al., *Constipation: An Overlooked, Unmanaged Symptom of Patients With Pheochromocytoma and Sympathetic Paraganglioma.* European Journal of Endocrinology, 2015. **173**(3): p. 377-387.
552. Tomasiewicz, A., et al., *Semaglutide and Body Composition: A Narrative Review of Its Effects on Lean Mass and Strategies for Preservation.* International Journal of Innovative Technologies in Social Science, 2025. **4**(3(47)).
553. Delmonico, M.J. and I.E. Lofgren, *Resistance Training During Weight Loss in Overweight and Obese Older Adults: What Are the Benefits?* American Journal of Lifestyle Medicine, 2010. **4**(4): p. 309-313.
554. Murphy, C.H., S.N. McCarthy, and H.M. Roche, *Nutrition Strategies to Counteract Sarcopenia: A Focus on Protein, LC <i>n</I>-3 PUFA and Precision Nutrition.* Proceedings of the Nutrition Society, 2023. **82**(3): p. 419-431.
555. Cava, E., N.C. Yeat, and B. Mittendorfer, *Preserving Healthy Muscle During Weight Loss.* Advances in Nutrition, 2017. **8**(3): p. 511-519.
556. Jiang, B. and D.T. Villareal, *The Benefits of Exercise Training in Combination With Weight Loss Therapies.* Diabetes, 2025.
557. Lenz, T.L., *Leucine With Resistance Training for the Treatment of Sarcopenia.* American Journal of Lifestyle Medicine, 2010. **4**(4): p. 317-319.
558. Lee, S., et al., *Aerobic Exercise but Not Resistance Exercise Reduces Intrahepatic Lipid Content and Visceral Fat and Improves Insulin Sensitivity in Obese Adolescent Girls: A Randomized Controlled Trial.* Ajp Endocrinology and Metabolism, 2013. **305**(10): p. E1222-E1229.
559. Κανελλοπούλου, K., *The Effect of Exercise on Cardiovascular Function of Patients With Chronic Kidney Disease.* Journal of Research and Practice on the Musculoskeletal System, 2022. **06**(03): p. 88-92.
560. Swift, D.L., et al., *The Role of Exercise and Physical Activity in Weight Loss and Maintenance.* Progress in Cardiovascular Diseases, 2014. **56**(4): p. 441-447.
561. González, A., et al., *Impact of Exercise Training on Sarcopenia Associated With Non-Alcoholic Fatty Liver Disease (NAFLD) in Humans: A Systematic Review and Meta-Analysis.* 2020.

562. Ceviz, E., *Relationship Between Visceral Fat Tissue and Exercise.* Türk Spor Bilimleri Dergisi, 2024. **7**(1): p. 10-20.
563. Lee, S., Y. Kim, and J.L. Kuk, *What Is the Role of Resistance Exercise in Improving the Cardiometabolic Health of Adolescents With Obesity?* Journal of Obesity & Metabolic Syndrome, 2019. **28**(2): p. 76-91.
564. Forbes, S.C., J.P. Little, and D.G. Candow, *Exercise and Nutritional Interventions for Improving Aging Muscle Health.* Endocrine, 2012. **42**(1): p. 29-38.
565. Galiassi, G.E.R., et al., *The Use of Semaglutide (Analog of GLP-1) in the Treatment of Obesity.* International Journal of Health Science, 2022. **2**(43): p. 2-6.
566. Fujishima, Y., et al., *Efficacy of Liraglutide, a Glucagon-Like Peptide-1 (GLP-1) Analogue, on Body Weight, Eating Behavior, and Glycemic Control, in Japanese Obese Type 2 Diabetes.* Cardiovascular Diabetology, 2012. **11**(1).
567. Okamoto, A., et al., *Efficacy and Safety of Semaglutide in Glycemic Control, Body Weight Management, Lipid Profiles and Other Biomarkers Among Obese Type 2 Diabetes Patients Initiated or Switched to Semaglutide From Other GLP-1 Receptor Agonists.* Journal of Diabetes & Metabolic Disorders, 2021. **20**(2): p. 2121-2128.
568. Gibbons, C., et al., *Effects of Oral Semaglutide on Energy Intake, Food Preference, Appetite, Control of Eating and Body Weight in Subjects With Type 2 Diabetes.* Diabetes Obesity and Metabolism, 2020. **23**(2): p. 581-588.
569. Heise, T., et al., *Tirzepatide Reduces Appetite, Energy Intake, and Fat Mass in People With Type 2 Diabetes.* Diabetes Care, 2023. **46**(5): p. 998-1004.
570. Bloemendaal, L.v., et al., *GLP-1 Receptor Activation Modulates Appetite- And Reward-Related Brain Areas in Humans.* Diabetes, 2014. **63**(12): p. 4186-4196.
571. Kapitza, C., et al., *Semaglutide, a Once-weekly Human GLP-1 Analog, Does Not Reduce the Bioavailability of the Combined Oral Contraceptive, Ethinylestradiol/Levonorgestrel.* The Journal of Clinical Pharmacology, 2015. **55**(5): p. 497-504.
572. Hartman, R.L., et al., *Cannabis Effects on Driving Lateral Control With and Without Alcohol.* Drug and Alcohol Dependence, 2015. **154**: p. 25-37.
573. Thomas, T., et al., *Case Report: Medical Cannabis—warfarin Drug-Drug Interaction.* Journal of Cannabis Research, 2022. **4**(1).
574. Kruger, D.J. and J.S. Kruger, *Consumer Experiences With Delta-8-Thc: Medical Use, Pharmaceutical Substitution, and Comparisons With Delta-9-THC.* Cannabis and Cannabinoid Research, 2023. **8**(1): p. 166-173.
575. Hutten, N.R.P.W., et al., *Cannabis Containing Equivalent Concentrations of Delta-9-Tetrahydrocannabinol (THC) and Cannabidiol (CBD) Induces Less State Anxiety Than THC-dominant Cannabis.* Psychopharmacology, 2022. **239**(11): p. 3731-3741.
576. Pertwee, R.G., *The Ring Test: A Quantitative Method for Assessing the 'Cataleptic' Effect of Cannabis in Mice.* British Journal of Pharmacology, 1972. **46**(4): p. 753-763.
577. Lineham, J., E. Wadsworth, and D. Hammond, *Self-reported <scp>THC</Scp> Content and Associations With Perceptions of Feeling High Among Cannabis Consumers.* Drug and Alcohol Review, 2023. **42**(5): p. 1142-1152.
578. Arkell, T.R., et al., *Cannabidiol (CBD) Content in Vaporized Cannabis Does Not Prevent Tetrahydrocannabinol (THC)-induced Impairment of Driving and Cognition.* Psychopharmacology, 2019. **236**(9): p. 2713-2724.
579. Ahmad, E., et al., *Where Does Metformin Stand in Modern Day Management of Type 2 Diabetes?* Pharmaceuticals, 2020. **13**(12): p. 427.

580. Žunić, T. and M. Ponjavić, *The Role of Novel Antihyperglycaemic Agents in the Treatment of Type 2 Diabetes: From Glycaemic Control to Cardiovascular Protection.* Arhiv Za Farmaciju, 2020. **70**(4): p. 198-223.
581. Jia, W., et al., *Standards of Medical Care for Type 2 Diabetes in China 2019.* Diabetes/Metabolism Research and Reviews, 2019. **35**(6).
582. Gašparini, D., et al., *Oral Semaglutide Improves Glycemic Control and Lowers Blood Lipids: Evidence From a Real-World Study.* Cardiovascular Endocrinology & Metabolism, 2024. **13**(4).
583. Coke, L.A., et al., *GLP-1 Receptor Agonists and Cardiovascular Outcomes in Patients With Type 2 Diabetes: Clinical Evidence and Best Practice.* Journal of the American Association of Nurse Practitioners, 2022. **34**(2): p. 418-440.
584. Tian, L., et al., *Cardiovascular and Renal Outcomes With Sodium Glucose Co-Transporter 2 Inhibitors in Patients With Type 2 Diabetes Mellitus: A System Review and Network Meta-Analysis.* Frontiers in Pharmacology, 2022. **13**.
585. Voors, A.A., et al., *The SGLT2 Inhibitor Empagliflozin in Patients Hospitalized for Acute Heart Failure: A Multinational Randomized Trial.* Nature Medicine, 2022. **28**(3): p. 568-574.
586. Tesař, V.r., *SGLT2 Inhibitors in Non-Diabetic Kidney Disease.* Advances in Clinical and Experimental Medicine, 2022. **31**(2): p. 105-107.
587. Herrington, W.G., et al., *Empagliflozin in Patients With Chronic Kidney Disease.* New England Journal of Medicine, 2023. **388**(2): p. 117-127.
588. Sonesson, C., et al., *Cardiovascular Effects of Dapagliflozin in Patients With Type 2 Diabetes and Different Risk Categories: A Meta-Analysis.* Cardiovascular Diabetology, 2016. **15**(1).
589. Mil, D.v., et al., *Baseline, Early Changes, and Residual Albuminuria.* Clinical Journal of the American Society of Nephrology, 2024. **19**(12): p. 1574-1584.
590. Jongs, N., et al., *Effect of Dapagliflozin on Urinary Albumin Excretion in Patients With Chronic Kidney Disease With and Without Type 2 Diabetes: A Prespecified Analysis From the DAPA-CKD Trial.* The Lancet Diabetes & Endocrinology, 2021. **9**(11): p. 755-766.
591. Xu, B., et al., *The Current Role of Sodium-Glucose Cotransporter 2 Inhibitors in Type 2 Diabetes Mellitus Management.* Cardiovascular Diabetology, 2022. **21**(1).
592. Qiu, M., et al., *Safety of Four SGLT2 Inhibitors in Three Chronic Diseases: A Meta-Analysis of Large Randomized Trials of SGLT2 Inhibitors.* Diabetes and Vascular Disease Research, 2021. **18**(2).
593. Wan, N., et al., *The Effects of Sodium-Glucose Cotransporter 2 Inhibitors on Sympathetic Nervous Activity.* Frontiers in Endocrinology, 2018. **9**.
594. Saisho, Y., *SGLT2 Inhibitors: The Star in the Treatment of Type 2 Diabetes?* Diseases, 2020. **8**(2): p. 14.
595. Wheeler, D.C., et al., *The Dapagliflozin and Prevention of Adverse Outcomes in Chronic Kidney Disease (DAPA-CKD) Trial: Baseline Characteristics.* Nephrology Dialysis Transplantation, 2020. **35**(10): p. 1700-1711.
596. Cherney, D.Z.I., et al., *The Effect of Sodium Glucose Cotransporter 2 Inhibition With Empagliflozin on Microalbuminuria and Macroalbuminuria in Patients With Type 2 Diabetes.* Diabetologia, 2016. **59**(9): p. 1860-1870.
597. Wainstein, J., et al., *Insulin Pump Therapy vs. Multiple Daily Injections in Obese Type 2 Diabetic Patients.* Diabetic Medicine, 2005. **22**(8): p. 1037-1046.

598. Rosenstock, J., et al., *Alogliptin Added to Insulin Therapy in Patients With Type 2 Diabetes Reduces HbA _{1c} Without Causing Weight Gain or Increased Hypoglycaemia*. Diabetes Obesity and Metabolism, 2009. **11**(12): p. 1145-1152.
599. Meyer, J., et al., *The Effects of Adding Semaglutide to High Daily Dose Insulin Regimens in Patients With Type 2 Diabetes*. Annals of Pharmacotherapy, 2022. **57**(3): p. 241-250.
600. Vilsbøll, T., et al., *Real-world Impact of Once-weekly Subcutaneous Semaglutide After 2 years of Follow-up: Results From a Nationwide Observational Study in People With Type 2 Diabetes*. Diabetes Obesity and Metabolism, 2023. **25**(6): p. 1740-1749.
601. Rosenstock, J., et al., *Impact of a Weekly Glucagon-Like Peptide 1 Receptor Agonist, Albiglutide, on Glycemic Control and on Reducing Prandial Insulin Use in Type 2 Diabetes Inadequately Controlled on Multiple Insulin Therapy: A Randomized Trial*. Diabetes Care, 2020. **43**(10): p. 2509-2518.
602. Rosenstock, J., et al., *Advancing Basal Insulin Replacement in Type 2 Diabetes Inadequately Controlled With Insulin Glargine Plus Oral Agents: A Comparison of Adding Albiglutide, a Weekly GLP-1 Receptor Agonist, Versus Thrice-Daily Prandial Insulin Lispro*. Diabetes Care, 2014. **37**(8): p. 2317-2325.
603. Whitley, H.P. and W.D. Smith, *Adjusting Background Insulin Therapy in Type 2 Diabetes When Initiating a Glucagon-Like Peptide 1 Receptor Agonist: A Case Series*. Journal of Case Reports and Images in Medicine, 2023. **9**(1): p. 4-10.
604. Bonora, B.M., et al., *Long-Term Effectiveness of Once-Weekly Semaglutide in Patients With Type 2 Diabetes Previously Treated With Insulin. A Multicentre Real-World Study*. Diabetes/Metabolism Research and Reviews, 2025. **41**(4).
605. Rodriguez, P., et al., *De-intensification of Basal-bolus Therapy by Replacing Prandial Insulin With Once-weekly Subcutaneous Semaglutide in Individuals With Well-controlled Type 2 Diabetes: A Single-centre, Open-label Randomised Trial (<scp>TRANSITION</Scp> - <scp>T2D</Scp>)*. Diabetes Obesity and Metabolism, 2024. **27**(2): p. 642-651.
606. Giugliano, D., et al., *Feasibility of Simplification From a Basal-Bolus Insulin Regimen to a Fixed-Ratio Formulation of Basal Insulin Plus a GLP-1RA or to Basal Insulin Plus an SGLT2 Inhibitor: BEYOND, a Randomized, Pragmatic Trial*. Diabetes Care, 2021. **44**(6): p. 1353-1360.
607. Kim, H.S., et al., *Dulaglutide as an Effective Replacement for Prandial Insulin in Kidney Transplant Recipients With Type 2 Diabetes Mellitus: A Retrospective Review*. Diabetes & Metabolism Journal, 2021. **45**(6): p. 948-953.
608. Shi, F.H., et al., *Efficacy and Safety of Once-Weekly Semaglutide for the Treatment of Type 2 Diabetes*. Medicine, 2018. **97**(16): p. e0420.
609. Costa, S., et al., *Effectiveness and Safety of Daily Oral Semaglutide in People With Type 2 Diabetes Mellitus Switching From Sulfonylureas: A Real-world Retrospective Study*. Diabetes Obesity and Metabolism, 2025. **27**(6): p. 3084-3093.
610. Ahern, S.P., *Allodynia and Dysesthesia Associated With Semaglutide and Tirzepatide*. Cureus, 2025.
611. Karagiannis, T., et al., *Management of Type 2 Diabetes With the Dual GIP/GLP-1 Receptor Agonist Tirzepatide: A Systematic Review and Meta-Analysis*. Diabetologia, 2022. **65**(8): p. 1251-1261.
612. Bhagavathula, A.S., K. Vidyasagar, and W. Tesfaye, *Efficacy and Safety of Tirzepatide in Patients With Type 2 Diabetes Mellitus: A Systematic Review and Meta-Analysis of Randomized Phase II/III Trials*. Pharmaceuticals, 2021. **14**(10): p. 991.

613. Samms, R.J., et al., *GIPR Agonism Mediates Weight-Independent Insulin Sensitization by Tirzepatide in Obese Mice.* Journal of Clinical Investigation, 2021. **131**(12).
614. Mody, R., et al., *Cost Per Patient Achieving Treatment Targets and Number Needed to Treat With Tirzepatide Versus Semaglutide 1 mg in Patients With Type 2 Diabetes in the United States.* Diabetes Therapy, 2023. **14**(12): p. 2045-2055.
615. Kayed, A., et al., *OXM-104, a Potential Candidate for the Treatment of Obesity, NASH and Type 2 Diabetes.* 2021.
616. Buckley, A., et al., *Real World Use of Tirzepatide in the Treatment of Type 2 Diabetes in an Arab Population.* Diabetes Obesity and Metabolism, 2024. **26**(8): p. 3381-3391.
617. Block, C.D., et al., *Tirzepatide for the Treatment of Adults With Type 2 Diabetes: An Endocrine Perspective.* Diabetes Obesity and Metabolism, 2022. **25**(1): p. 3-17.
618. Al-Sabah, S., et al., *Effect of Dual Glucagon-Like Peptide 1/Glucose-Dependent Insulinotropic Polypeptide Receptor Agonist (Tirzepatide) Versus Bariatric Surgery on Weight Loss and Nonalcoholic Fatty Liver Disease.* Medical Principles and Practice, 2024. **33**(5): p. 478-490.
619. Iwamoto, Y., et al., *Tirzepatide, a Dual Glucose-dependent Insulinotropic Polypeptide/Glucagon-like Peptide 1 Receptor Agonist, Exhibits Favourable Effects on Pancreatic Β-cells and Hepatic Steatosis in Obese Type 2 Diabetic Db/Db Mice.* Diabetes Obesity and Metabolism, 2024. **26**(12): p. 5982-5994.
620. Thomas, M.K., et al., *Dual GIP and GLP-1 Receptor Agonist Tirzepatide Improves Beta-Cell Function and Insulin Sensitivity in Type 2 Diabetes.* The Journal of Clinical Endocrinology & Metabolism, 2020. **106**(2): p. 388-396.
621. Mikhail, N., *Tirzepatide: A Useful Addition for Treatment of Type 2 Diabetes and Obesity.* Gastroenterology Pancreatology and Hepatobilary Disorders, 2021. **5**(5): p. 01-04.
622. Frías, J.P., et al., *Tirzepatide in Hispanic/Latino Patients With Type 2 Diabetes: A Subgroup Analysis of the SURPASS Program.* The Journal of Clinical Endocrinology & Metabolism, 2023. **109**(2): p. 557-568.
623. Katsi, V., et al., *Retatrutide—A Game Changer in Obesity Pharmacotherapy.* Biomolecules, 2025. **15**(6): p. 796.
624. Vilsbøll, T., et al., *<scp>HbA1c</Scp> Reduction With Tirzepatide in People With Type 2 Diabetes: The Contribution of Weight Loss Assessed by a Mediation Analysis.* Diabetes Obesity and Metabolism, 2025. **27**(10): p. 5498-5505.
625. Zakir, M., et al., *Cardiovascular Complications of Diabetes: From Microvascular to Macrovascular Pathways.* Cureus, 2023.
626. Bzowyckyj, A.S., *Managing the Multifaceted Nature of Type 2 Diabetes Using Once-weekly Injectable GLP-1 Receptor Agonist Therapy.* Journal of Clinical Pharmacy and Therapeutics, 2020. **45**(S1): p. 7-16.
627. Boyle, J.G., R. Livingstone, and J.R. Petrie, *Cardiovascular Benefits of GLP-1 Agonists in Type 2 Diabetes: A Comparative Review.* Clinical Science, 2018. **132**(15): p. 1699-1709.
628. Halimi, J.M., et al., *Expert Perspectives on Incorporating Glucagon-Like Peptide-1 Receptor Agonist in Diabetes and Chronic Kidney Disease: Challenges and Opportunities.* European Journal of Preventive Cardiology, 2025.
629. Bazargaliyev, S.Y., et al., *Non-Alcoholic Fatty Liver Disease and Its Relationship With Metabolic Syndrome: Modern Approaches to Treatment and Prevention.* Farmaciâ Kazahstana, 2025(6): p. 69-80.

630. Bzoma, M., et al., *GLP-1 Receptor Agonists in Metabolic Dysfunction-Associated Steatotic Liver Disease: Therapeutic Potential and Clinical Challenges.* International Journal of Innovative Technologies in Social Science, 2025(3(47)).
631. Lewis, J.E., et al., *The Impact of Semaglutide on Wound Healing in Diabetes Related Foot Ulcer Patients: A TriNetX Database Study.* Diabetes and Vascular Disease Research, 2025. **22**(2).
632. Demmel, V., et al., *No QTc Prolongation With Semaglutide: A Thorough QT Study in Healthy Subjects.* Diabetes Therapy, 2018. **9**(4): p. 1441-1456.
633. Soubry, E., et al., *Orale Semaglutide: Een Nieuwe en Eerste Orale GLP1-receptoragonist.* Tijdschrift Voor Geneeskunde, 2022.
634. Dahl, K., et al., *Oral semaglutide improves postprandial glucose and lipid metabolism, and delays gastric emptying, in subjects with type 2 diabetes.* Diabetes, Obesity and Metabolism, 2021. **23**(7): p. 1594-1603.
635. Urva, S., et al., *The novel dual glucose-dependent insulinotropic polypeptide and glucagon-like peptide-1 (GLP-1) receptor agonist tirzepatide transiently delays gastric emptying similarly to selective long-acting GLP-1 receptor agonists.* Diabetes, Obesity and Metabolism, 2020. **22**(10): p. 1886-1891.
636. Calvarysky, B., et al., *Drug-drug interactions between glucagon-like peptide 1 receptor agonists and oral medications: a systematic review.* Drug Safety, 2024. **47**(5): p. 439-451.
637. Reardon, D.P. and P.S. Yoo, *Levothyroxine tablet malabsorption associated with gastroparesis corrected with gelatin capsule formulation.* Case reports in endocrinology, 2016. **2016**(1): p. 1316724.
638. Mazokopakis, E.E., *Semaglutide-induced subclinical hypothyroidism: a case report.* European Journal of Medical and Health Sciences, 2023. **5**(3): p. 8-9.
639. Korytkowski, M.T., *Sulfonylurea treatment of type 2 diabetes mellitus: focus on glimepiride.* Pharmacotherapy: The Journal of Human Pharmacology and Drug Therapy, 2004. **24**(5): p. 606-620.
640. Leonard, C.E., et al., *Comparative risk of serious hypoglycemia with oral antidiabetic monotherapy: a retrospective cohort study.* Pharmacoepidemiology and drug safety, 2018. **27**(1): p. 9-18.
641. Douros, A., et al., *Pharmacologic differences of sulfonylureas and the risk of adverse cardiovascular and hypoglycemic events.* Diabetes care, 2017. **40**(11): p. 1506-1513.
642. Leonard, C.E., et al., *Severe hypoglycemia in users of sulfonylurea antidiabetic agents and antihyperlipidemics.* Clinical Pharmacology & Therapeutics, 2016. **99**(5): p. 538-547.
643. Xu, H., M. Murray, and A.J. McLachlan, *Influence of genetic polymorphisms on the pharmacokinetics and pharmacodynamics of sulfonylurea drugs.* Current drug metabolism, 2009. **10**(6): p. 643-658.
644. Pakkir Maideen, N.M., G. Manavalan, and K. Balasubramanian, *Drug interactions of meglitinide antidiabetics involving CYP enzymes and OATP1B1 transporter.* Therapeutic advances in endocrinology and metabolism, 2018. **9**(8): p. 259-268.
645. Philip, J. and C.J. Fernandez, *Efficacy and cardiovascular safety of meglitinides.* Current Drug Safety, 2021. **16**(2): p. 207-216.
646. Guardado-Mendoza, R., et al., *State of the art paper The role of nateglinide and repaglinide, derivatives of meglitinide, in the treatment of type 2 diabetes mellitus.* Archives of medical science, 2013. **9**(5): p. 936-943.

647. Calvarysky, B., et al., *Drug-Drug Interactions Between Glucagon-Like Peptide 1 Receptor Agonists and Oral Medications: A Systematic Review.* Medical Toxicology and Adverse Drug Experience, 2024. **47**(5): p. 439-451.
648. Sproule, B., et al., *Selective Serotonin Reuptake Inhibitors and CNS Drug Interactions.* Clinical Pharmacokinetics, 1997. **33**(6): p. 454-471.
649. Nazarova, V.A., et al., *Treatment of ADHD: Drugs, Psychological Therapies, Devices, Complementary and Alternative Methods as Well as the Trends in Clinical Trials.* Frontiers in Pharmacology, 2022. **13**.
650. Hejdak, D., et al., *Interaction of Semaglutide and Ziprasidone in a Patient With Schizophrenia: A Case Report.* Cureus, 2024.
651. Hausner, H., et al., *Effect of Semaglutide on the Pharmacokinetics of Metformin, Warfarin, Atorvastatin and Digoxin in Healthy Subjects.* Clinical Pharmacokinetics, 2017. **56**(11): p. 1391-1401.
652. Pontikes, T., Z. Bloomberg, and A. Halaris, *Utility of Pharmacogenomics in Management of Attention-Deficit/Hyperactivity Disorder in Children and Adolescents: A Case Series.* Journal of Medical Case Reports and Case Series, 2021.
653. Bækdal, T.A., et al., *Pharmacokinetics, Safety, and Tolerability of Oral Semaglutide in Subjects With Hepatic Impairment.* The Journal of Clinical Pharmacology, 2018. **58**(10): p. 1314-1323.
654. Petta, S., et al., *Focus on Semaglutide 2.4 mg/week for the Treatment of Metabolic Dysfunction-Associated Steatohepatitis.* Liver International, 2025. **45**(11).
655. Ghazanfar, H., et al., *Role of Glucagon-Like Peptide-1 Receptor Agonists in the Management of Non-Alcoholic Steatohepatitis: A Clinical Review Article.* Cureus, 2021.
656. Ki, S., et al., *Development of Guidelines on the Primary Prevention of Frailty in Community-Dwelling Older Adults.* Annals of Geriatric Medicine and Research, 2021. **25**(4): p. 237-244.
657. Mate, K.S., et al., *Evidence for the 4Ms: Interactions and Outcomes Across the Care Continuum.* Journal of Aging and Health, 2021. **33**(7-8): p. 469-481.
658. Hsu, H.F., et al., *Polypharmacy and Pattern of Medication Use in Community-dwelling Older Adults: A Systematic Review.* Journal of Clinical Nursing, 2020. **30**(7-8): p. 918-928.
659. Poelgeest, E.P.v., et al., *Optimizing Pharmacotherapy and Deprescribing Strategies in Older Adults Living With Multimorbidity and Polypharmacy: EuGMS SIG on Pharmacology Position Paper.* European Geriatric Medicine, 2023. **14**(6): p. 1195-1209.
660. Elmotia, K., et al., *Geriatric Syndromes in Older Adults With and Without Diabetes: A Systematic Review and Meta-Analysis.* Research in Gerontological Nursing, 2025. **18**(2): p. 99-108.
661. Bhagavathula, A.S., E.A. Gebreyohannes, and D. Fialová, *Prevalence of Polypharmacy and Risks of Potentially Inappropriate Medication Use in the Older Population in a Developing Country: A Systematic Review and Meta-Analysis.* Gerontology, 2021. **68**(2): p. 136-145.
662. Sabbagh, M.N., et al., *Safety Considerations of Semaglutide in the Potential Treatment of Alzheimer's Disease: A Pooled Analysis of Semaglutide in Adults Aged ≥ 65 Years.* Alzheimer S & Dementia Translational Research & Clinical Interventions, 2025. **11**(2).
663. Onoviran, O.F., et al., *Effects of Glucagon-Like Peptide 1 Receptor Agonists on Comorbidities in Older Patients With Diabetes Mellitus.* Therapeutic Advances in Chronic Disease, 2019. **10**.

664. Davis, T.M.E., *Severe Hypomagnesemia and Hypocalcemia Linked to Semaglutide in Type 2 Diabetes: A Case Report*. American Journal of Case Reports, 2024. **26**.
665. Goddard, G., S. Rajagopal, and M.A. Raji, *Metabolic Syndrome in Older Adults: Through the Lens of Institute for Healthcare Improvement's (IHI) 4Ms Framework and Social Determinants of Health*. Life, 2025. **15**(9): p. 1370.
666. Engels, L., et al., *Medication Management in Patients With Polypharmacy in Primary Care: A Scoping Review of Clinical Practice Guidelines*. Journal of Evidence-Based Medicine, 2025. **18**(1).
667. Sattar, N., et al., *Cardiovascular, Mortality, and Kidney Outcomes With GLP-1 Receptor Agonists in Patients With Type 2 Diabetes: A Systematic Review and Meta-Analysis of Randomised Trials*. The Lancet Diabetes & Endocrinology, 2021. **9**(10): p. 653-662.
668. Rosenberg, A.E., et al., *Albiglutide and Cardiovascular Outcomes in Patients With Type 2 Diabetes and Cardiovascular Disease (Harmony Outcomes): A Double-Blind, Randomised Placebo-Controlled Trial*. The Lancet, 2018. **392**(10157): p. 1519-1529.
669. Li, P., et al., *Prescribing Trends of Glucagon-Like Peptide 1 Receptor Agonists for Type 2 Diabetes or Obesity*. Jama Network Open, 2025. **8**(10): p. e2540890.
670. Verma, S., et al., *Impact of Microvascular Disease on Cardiovascular Outcomes in Type 2 Diabetes: Results From The <scp>LEADER</Scp> And <scp>SUSTAIN</Scp> 6 Clinical Trials*. Diabetes Obesity and Metabolism, 2020. **22**(11): p. 2193-2198.
671. Webb, J., et al., *Cardiovascular Risk Profiles: A Cross-sectional Study Evaluating the Generalizability of the Glucagon-like Peptide-1 Receptor Agonist Cardiovascular Outcome Trials <scp>REWIND</Scp>, <scp>LEADER</Scp> And <scp>SUSTAIN</Scp>-6 to the Real-world Type 2 Diabetes Population in The <scp>United Kingdom</Scp>*. Diabetes Obesity and Metabolism, 2021. **24**(2): p. 289-295.
672. Yin, W., S. Baín, and T. Min, *The Effect of Glucagon-Like Peptide-1 Receptor Agonists on Renal Outcomes in Type 2 Diabetes*. Diabetes Therapy, 2020. **11**(4): p. 835-844.
673. Baden, C.S., et al., *Safety of Glucagon-Like Peptide-1 Receptor Agonists for Weight Management in Adults, Adolescents, and Children With Obesity: A Scoping Review*. Adverse Drug Reaction Bulletin, 2023. **339**(1): p. 1315-1318.
674. Pantalone, K.M., et al., *Cardiovascular Outcomes Trials With Glucagon-like Peptide-1 Receptor Agonists: A Comparison of Study Designs, Populations and Results*. Diabetes Obesity and Metabolism, 2020. **22**(12): p. 2209-2226.
675. Iqbal, P.M.R., O. Maadarani, and Z. Bitar, *Tirzepatide-Induced Ketoacidosis in Non-Diabetic Patients*. European Journal of Case Reports in Internal Medicine, 2024. **11**(4).
676. Moreno, Ó., et al., *Real-world Effectiveness and Safety of Oral Semaglutide in People Living With Type 2 Diabetes: A Nationwide Multicentre Retrospective Observational Study (<scp> Endo ² S-rwd </Scp>)*. Diabetes Obesity and Metabolism, 2023. **26**(4): p. 1519-1523.
677. Xie, Z., et al., *Comparison of the Efficacy and Safety of 10 Glucagon-Like Peptide-1 Receptor Agonists as Add-on to Metformin in Patients With Type 2 Diabetes: A Systematic Review*. Frontiers in Endocrinology, 2023. **14**.
678. Sinha, R., et al., *Efficacy and Safety of Tirzepatide in Type 2 Diabetes and Obesity Management*. Journal of Obesity & Metabolic Syndrome, 2023. **32**(1): p. 25-45.
679. Buse, J.B., et al., *DURATION-1: Exenatide Once Weekly Produces Sustained Glycemic Control and Weight Loss Over 52 Weeks*. Diabetes Care, 2010. **33**(6): p. 1255-1261.

680. Gentilella, R., et al., *Glucagon-like Peptide-1 Receptor Agonists in Type 2 Diabetes Treatment: Are They All the Same?* Diabetes/Metabolism Research and Reviews, 2018. **35**(1).
681. Matza, L.S., et al., *Assessing Patient PREFERence Between the Dulaglutide Pen and the Semaglutide Pen: A Crossover Study (PREFER).* Diabetes Obesity and Metabolism, 2019. **22**(3): p. 355-364.
682. Mather, K.J., et al., *Greater Improvement in Insulin Sensitivity Per Unit Weight Loss Associated With Tirzepatide Versus Semaglutide: An Exploratory Analysis.* Diabetes Obesity and Metabolism, 2025. **27**(3): p. 1507-1514.
683. Rodriguez, P.J., et al., *Semaglutide vs Tirzepatide for Weight Loss in Adults With Overweight or Obesity.* Jama Internal Medicine, 2024. **184**(9): p. 1056.
684. Roux, C.W.l., et al., *Tirzepatide 10 and 15 mg Compared With Semaglutide 2.4 mg for the Treatment of Obesity: An Indirect Treatment Comparison.* Diabetes Obesity and Metabolism, 2023. **25**(9): p. 2626-2633.
685. Frías, J.P., et al., *Tirzepatide Improved Markers of Islet Cell Function and Insulin Sensitivity in People With T2D (SURPASS-2).* The Journal of Clinical Endocrinology & Metabolism, 2024. **109**(7): p. 1745-1753.
686. Vadher, K., et al., *Efficacy of Tirzepatide 5, 10 and 15 mg Versus Semaglutide 2 mg in Patients With Type 2 Diabetes: An Adjusted Indirect Treatment Comparison.* Diabetes Obesity and Metabolism, 2022. **24**(9): p. 1861-1868.
687. Pearson, E.R., et al., *Predictors of Initial and Sustained Glycemic and Weight Response to Tirzepatide: A Post Hoc Analysis of SURPASS-4.* Diabetes, 2025. **74**(10): p. 1850-1862.
688. Feng, Z., et al., *Cost-Effectiveness Analysis of Once-Daily Oral Semaglutide Versus Placebo and Subcutaneous Glucagon-Like Peptide-1 Receptor Agonists Added to Insulin in Patients With Type 2 Diabetes in China.* Frontiers in Pharmacology, 2023. **14**.
689. Chubb, B., et al., *Once-Daily Oral Semaglutide Versus Injectable GLP-1 RAs in People With Type 2 Diabetes Inadequately Controlled on Basal Insulin: Systematic Review and Network Meta-Analysis.* Diabetes Therapy, 2021. **12**(5): p. 1325-1339.
690. Khawaji, A., et al., *Weight Loss Efficacy of Tirzepatide Compared to Placebo or GLP-1 Receptor Agonists in Adults With Obesity or Overweight: A Meta-Analysis of Randomized Controlled Trials With ≥ 20 Weeks Treatment Duration.* Journal of Obesity, 2025. **2025**(1).
691. Samms, R.J., et al., *Tirzepatide Induces a Thermogenic-Like Amino Acid Signature in Brown Adipose Tissue.* Molecular Metabolism, 2022. **64**: p. 101550.
692. Åhrén, B., *GLP-1 Receptor Agonists in the Treatment of Type 2 Diabetes.* Diabetes Management, 2013. **3**(5): p. 401-413.
693. Prasad-Reddy, L. and D. Isaacs, *A Clinical Review of GLP-1 Receptor Agonists: Efficacy and Safety in Diabetes and Beyond.* Drugs in Context, 2015. **4**: p. 1-19.
694. Dutta, D., et al., *Efficacy and Safety of Novel Twincretin Tirzepatide, a Dual GIP/GLP-1 Receptor Agonist, as an Anti-Obesity Medicine in Individuals Without Diabetes: A Systematic Review and Meta-Analysis.* Touchreviews in Endocrinology, 2024. **20**(2).
695. Dahl, D., et al., *Effect of Subcutaneous Tirzepatide vs Placebo Added to Titrated Insulin Glargine on Glycemic Control in Patients With Type 2 Diabetes.* Jama, 2022. **327**(6): p. 534.
696. Khatri, T., T. Siddiqui, and P.R. Doultani, *Tirzepatide (Mounjaro) - A Novel Pharmacotherapeutic Agent for Obesity.* Journal of the Pakistan Medical Association, 2023. **73**(05): p. 1171-1171.

697. Hathaway, J.T., et al., *Risk of Nonarteritic Anterior Ischemic Optic Neuropathy in Patients Prescribed Semaglutide.* Jama Ophthalmology, 2024. **142**(8): p. 732.
698. Trujillo, J., W. Nuffer, and B.A. Smith, *GLP-1 Receptor Agonists: An Updated Review of Head-to-Head Clinical Studies.* Therapeutic Advances in Endocrinology and Metabolism, 2021. **12**.
699. Schafheutle, E., K. Hassell, and P. Noyce, *Access to Medicines: Cost as an Influence on the Views and Behaviour of Patients.* Health & Social Care in the Community, 2002. **10**(3): p. 187-195.
700. Liu, X., et al., *Coverage and Prior Authorization Policies for Semaglutide and Tirzepatide in Medicare Part D Plans.* Jama Network Open, 2025. **8**(8): p. e2529842.
701. Shi, I., et al., *Semaglutide Eligibility Across All Current Indications for US Adults.* Jama Cardiology, 2025. **10**(1): p. 96.
702. Sarpatwari, A., et al., *Glucagon-Like Peptide-1 Receptor Agonist Order Fills and Out-of-Pocket Costs by Race, Ethnicity, and Indication.* Jama Health Forum, 2025. **6**(10): p. e254258.
703. Rada, A.G., *Spanish Officials Investigate Novo Nordisk's Obesity Awareness Campaign.* BMJ, 2025. **389**: p. r1319.
704. Lewis, K.H., et al., *Effectiveness and Safety of Drugs for Obesity.* BMJ, 2024: p. e072686.
705. Lau, D.C.W., et al., *Once-Weekly Cagrilintide for Weight Management in People With Overweight and Obesity: A Multicentre, Randomised, Double-Blind, Placebo-Controlled and Active-Controlled, Dose-Finding Phase 2 Trial.* The Lancet, 2021. **398**(10317): p. 2160-2172.
706. Larsen, A.T., et al., *The Calcitonin Receptor Plays a Major Role in Glucose Regulation as a Function of Dual Amylin and Calcitonin Receptor Agonist Therapy.* Journal of Pharmacology and Experimental Therapeutics, 2020. **374**(1): p. 74-83.
707. Ravussin, É., et al., *Enhanced Weight Loss With Pramlintide/Metreleptin: An Integrated Neurohormonal Approach to Obesity Pharmacotherapy.* Obesity, 2009. **17**(9): p. 1736-1743.
708. Potes, C.S., et al., *Involvement of the Extracellular Signal-Regulated Kinase 1/2 Signaling Pathway in Amylin's Eating Inhibitory Effect.* Ajp Regulatory Integrative and Comparative Physiology, 2012. **302**(3): p. R340-R351.
709. Sanyal, A.J., et al., *Triple Hormone Receptor Agonist Retatrutide for Metabolic Dysfunction-Associated Steatotic Liver Disease: A Randomized Phase 2a Trial.* Nature Medicine, 2024. **30**(7): p. 2037-2048.
710. Kanu, C., et al., *Association Between Patient-reported Eating Behaviours and Weight Change: Secondary Analyses of a Randomized, Double-blind Trial Comparing Retatrutide and Placebo in People With Obesity or Overweight.* Diabetes Obesity and Metabolism, 2025. **27**(10): p. 6088-6091.
711. Bhattachar, S., et al., *Mazdutide Reduces Body Weight in Adults With Overweight or Obesity: A High-dose Phase 1 Trial.* Diabetes Obesity and Metabolism, 2025. **27**(11): p. 6460-6469.
712. Javor, E., D. Šarčević, and A. Rešić, *Metabolic Syndrome and Pharmacological Interventions in Clinical Development.* Diabetology, 2024. **5**(3): p. 300-320.
713. Psaltis, J.P., et al., *Incretin-based Therapies for the Management of Cardiometabolic Disease in the Clinic: Past, Present, and Future.* Medicinal Research Reviews, 2024. **45**(1): p. 29-65.

714. Tschöp, M.H., R. Nogueiras, and B. Åhrén, *Gut Hormone-Based Pharmacology: Novel Formulations and Future Possibilities for Metabolic Disease Therapy.* Diabetologia, 2023. **66**(10): p. 1796-1808.

715. Mathiesen, D.S., et al., *The Effects of Dual GLP-1/GIP Receptor Agonism on Glucagon Secretion—A Review.* International Journal of Molecular Sciences, 2019. **20**(17): p. 4092.

716. Wen, Y., et al., *Decreases in Circulating <scp>ANGPTL3</Scp> /8 Concentrations Following Retatrutide Treatment Parallel Reductions in Serum Lipids.* Diabetes Obesity and Metabolism, 2025. **27**(10): p. 5985-5995.

717. Först, T., et al., *Novel Pharmacotherapies for Weight Loss: Understanding the Role of Incretins to Enable Weight Loss and Improved Health Outcomes.* Diabetes Obesity and Metabolism, 2025. **27**(S2): p. 48-65.

718. Hong, S.h. and K.M. Choi, *Gut Hormones and Appetite Regulation.* Current Opinion in Endocrinology Diabetes and Obesity, 2024. **31**(3): p. 115-121.

719. Pratt, E., et al., *Orforglipron (<scp>LY3502970</Scp>), a Novel, Oral Non-peptide Glucagon-like Peptide-1 Receptor Agonist: A Phase 1a, Blinded, Placebo-controlled, Randomized, Single- and Multiple-ascending-dose Study in Healthy Participants.* Diabetes Obesity and Metabolism, 2023. **25**(9): p. 2634-2641.

720. Sloop, K.W., et al., *The Pharmacological Basis for Nonpeptide Agonism of the GLP-1 Receptor by Orforglipron.* Science Translational Medicine, 2024. **16**(778).

721. Sinha, B. and S. Ghosal, *Efficacy and Safety Of <scp>GLP</Scp> -1 Receptor Agonists, Dual Agonists, and Retatrutide for Weight Loss in Adults With Overweight or Obesity: A Bayesian <scp>NMA</Scp>*. Obesity, 2025. **33**(11): p. 2046-2054.

722. Alhomoud, I.S., et al., *Incretin Hormone Agonists: Current and Emerging Pharmacotherapy for Obesity Management.* Pharmacotherapy the Journal of Human Pharmacology and Drug Therapy, 2024. **44**(9): p. 738-752.

723. Jiang, Y., H. Zhu, and F. Gong, *Why Does <scp>GLP</Scp> -1 Agonist Combined With <scp>GIP</Scp> and/Or <scp>GCG</Scp> Agonist Have Greater Weight Loss Effect Than <scp>GLP</Scp> -1 Agonist Alone in Obese Adults Without Type 2 Diabetes?* Diabetes Obesity and Metabolism, 2024. **27**(3): p. 1079-1095.

724. Bhat, S., et al., *Efficacy and Safety of Incretin Co-Agonists: Transformative Advances in Cardiometabolic Healthcare.* World Journal of Cardiology, 2025. **17**(8).

725. Jiménez, B.R., et al., *Transforming body composition with semaglutide in adults with obesity and type 2 diabetes mellitus.* Frontiers in Endocrinology, 2024. **15**.

726. Kahn, S., et al., *Effect of Semaglutide on Regression and Progression of Glycemia in People With Overweight or Obesity but Without Diabetes in the SELECT Trial.* Diabetes Care, 2024. **47**: p. 1350-1359.

727. Rubino, D., et al., *Effect of Continued Weekly Subcutaneous Semaglutide vs Placebo on Weight Loss Maintenance in Adults With Overweight or Obesity: The STEP 4 Randomized Clinical Trial.* JAMA, 2021.

728. Bergmann, N., et al., *Semaglutide for the treatment of overweight and obesity: A review.* Diabetes, Obesity & Metabolism, 2022. **25**: p. 18-35.

729. Ryan, D., et al., *Long-term weight loss effects of semaglutide in obesity without diabetes in the SELECT trial.* Nature Medicine, 2024. **30**: p. 2049-2057.

730. Sokary, S. and H. Bawadi, *Exploring Beyond Numeric Weight Loss: The Metabolic Effects of Semaglutide.* Clinical nutrition ESPEN, 2025.

731. Xue, Q., et al., *2199-LB: Weight Loss Maintenance following Semaglutide Discontinuation—The Role of Concurrent Lifestyle Intervention.* Diabetes, 2025.
732. Yue, D., et al., *Development of a Risk Prediction Model for Gastrointestinal Adverse Events Associated With Semaglutide Administration in Patients With Type 2 Diabetes Mellitus.* Frontiers in Endocrinology, 2025. **16**.
733. Therapeutic Goods Administraltion, *Ozempic (semaglutide) supply information*. 2025, Commonwealth of Australia.
734. Medx, *What countries use Ozempic?: A Global Guide to Semaglutide Availability* 2025, Medx.
735. Sood, N. and R. Garg, *Global Rise of Compounded Weight-Loss Medicines: A Worrisome Trend.* Journal of the Endocrine Society, 2025. **9**(8): p. bvaf084.
736. Whitley, H., J. Trujillo, and J. Neumiller, *Special Report: Potential Strategies for Addressing GLP-1 and Dual GLP-1/GIP Receptor Agonist Shortages.* Clinical Diabetes : A Publication of the American Diabetes Association, 2023. **41**: p. 467-473.
737. Altabas, V., Z. Orlović, and M. Baretić, *Addressing the Shortage of GLP-1 RA and Dual GIP/GLP-1 RA-Based Therapies—A Systematic Review.* Diabetology, 2025.
738. Salvador, R., et al., *Semaglutide as a GLP-1 Agonist: A Breakthrough in Obesity Treatment.* Pharmaceuticals, 2025. **18**.
739. Bailey, C., P. Flatt, and J. Conlon, *An update on peptide-based therapies for type 2 diabetes and obesity.* Peptides, 2023. **161**.
740. Lu, J., G. Williams, and S. Fanning, *Reconsidering Semaglutide Use for Chronic Obesity in Patients of Asian Descent: A Critical Review.* Cureus, 2024. **16**.
741. Patoulias, D., et al., *Effect of semaglutide versus other glucagon-like peptide-1 receptor agonists on cardio-metabolic risk factors in patients with type 2 diabetes: A systematic review and meta-analysis of head-to-head, phase 3, randomized controlled trials.* Journal of diabetes and its complications, 2023. **37 8**: p. 108529.
742. Mahapatra, M., M. Karuppasamy, and B. Sahoo, *Therapeutic Potential of Semaglutide, a Newer GLP-1 Receptor Agonist, in Abating Obesity, Non-Alcoholic Steatohepatitis and Neurodegenerative diseases: A Narrative Review.* Pharmaceutical Research, 2022. **39**: p. 1233-1248.
743. Chiappini, S., et al., *PHARMACOVIGILANCE SIGNALS OF SEMAGLUTIDE AND OTHER GLP-1 RECEPTOR AGONISTS: AN ANALYSIS OF THE FOOD AND DRUG ADMINISTRATION (FDA) ADVERSE EVENTS REPORTING SYSTEM (FAERS) DATASET.* International Journal of Neuropsychopharmacology, 2025. **28**.
744. Du Soulier, N., et al., *Use and Potential Misuse of GLP-1 Receptor Agonists in France: a Nationwide Cohort Study.* Value in health : the journal of the International Society for Pharmacoeconomics and Outcomes Research, 2025.
745. Arillotta, D., et al., *GLP-1 Receptor Agonists and Related Mental Health Issues; Insights from a Range of Social Media Platforms Using a Mixed-Methods Approach.* Brain Sciences, 2023. **13**.
746. Drucker, D., *GLP-1-based therapies for diabetes, obesity and beyond.* Nature reviews. Drug discovery, 2025.
747. Alfadliah, R.S., S. Alasgah, and M. Kofi, *Semaglutide for Weight Loss in Diabetic and Non-Diabetic Patients: A Comprehensive Systematic Review of Efficacy and Safety.* Scientia. Technology, Science and Society, 2025.
748. Wilding, J., et al., *Once-Weekly Semaglutide in Adults with Overweight or Obesity.* The New England journal of medicine, 2021.

749. Gasoyan, H., et al., *Early-and <scp>later-stage</Scp> Persistence With <scp>antiobesity</Scp> Medications: A Retrospective Cohort Study.* Obesity, 2023. **32**(3): p. 486-493.
750. Barrett, T.S., et al., *Obesity Treatment With Bariatric Surgery vs GLP-1 Receptor Agonists.* Jama Surgery, 2025.
751. Semlitsch, T., et al., *Management of Overweight and Obesity in Primary Care—A Systematic Overview of International Evidence-based Guidelines.* Obesity Reviews, 2019. **20**(9): p. 1218-1230.
752. Rabbitt, L., et al., *Assessing the Financial Burden on Patients and Their Households Attending Hospital Clinics: A Pilot Cross-Sectional Study.* BMC Health Services Research, 2025. **25**(1).
753. Almohaileb, F.I., C.W.l. Roux, and M. Crotty, *Why Do Patients With Obesity Discontinue Glucagon-like Peptide 1 Analogues?* Diabetes Obesity and Metabolism, 2025. **27**(9): p. 5342-5345.
754. Gudzune, K.A. and R.F. Kushner, *Medications for Obesity.* Jama, 2024. **332**(7): p. 571.
755. Ullah, M.I. and S. Tamanna, *Obesity: Clinical Impact, Pathophysiology, Complications, and Modern Innovations in Therapeutic Strategies.* Medicines, 2025. **12**(3): p. 19.
756. Ngoc, D., et al., *GLP-1 Receptor Agonist Discontinuation Among Patients With Obesity and/or Type 2 Diabetes.* Jama Network Open, 2024. **7**(5): p. e2413172.
757. Gierlach, K., et al., *Critical Analysis of the Efficacy and Limitations of GLP-1 Pharmaceuticals in Obesity Management: A Comprehensive Literature Review.* Journal of Education Health and Sport, 2024. **55**: p. 87-103.
758. Goldkorn, M., B. Schwartz, and J. Monterosso, *Views Among the General Public on New Anti-Obesity Medications and on the Perception of Obesity as a Failure of Willpower.* Obesity Science & Practice, 2025. **11**(2).
759. Puhl, R.M. and S. Liu, *A National Survey of Public Views About the Classification of Obesity as a Disease.* Obesity, 2015. **23**(6): p. 1288-1295.
760. Puhl, R.M., M.S. Himmelstein, and R.L. Pearl, *Weight Stigma as a Psychosocial Contributor to Obesity.* American Psychologist, 2020. **75**(2): p. 274-289.
761. Robinson, K.M., et al., *Patient Perceptions of Weight Stigma Experiences in Healthcare: A Qualitative Analysis.* Health Expectations, 2024. **27**(5).
762. Puhl, R.M. and Y.J. Suh, *Health Consequences of Weight Stigma: Implications for Obesity Prevention and Treatment.* Current Obesity Reports, 2015. **4**(2): p. 182-190.
763. Kahan, S. and R.M. Puhl, *The Damaging Effects of Weight Bias Internalization.* Obesity, 2017. **25**(2): p. 280-281.
764. Ainz-Galende, A., M.J. Torres-Haro, and R.R. Puertas, *Binge Eating Disorder and Fatphobia: Social Stigma, Exclusion, and the Need for a New Perspective on Health.* Societies, 2025. **15**(5): p. 115.
765. Wang, Y., et al., *Systematic Literature Review on the Spread of Health-Related Misinformation on Social Media.* Social Science & Medicine, 2019. **240**: p. 112552.
766. Levi, J., et al., *Estimated Minimum Prices and Lowest Available National Prices for Antiobesity Medications: Improving Affordability and Access to Treatment.* Obesity, 2023. **31**(5): p. 1270-1279.
767. Quddos, F., et al., *Semaglutide and Tirzepatide Reduce Alcohol Consumption in Individuals With Obesity.* Scientific Reports, 2023. **13**(1).

768. Schoretsanitis, G., et al., *Disproportionality Analysis From World Health Organization Data on Semaglutide, Liraglutide, and Suicidality.* Jama Network Open, 2024. **7**(8): p. e2423385.
769. Aroda, V.R., et al., *PIONEER 1: Randomized Clinical Trial of the Efficacy and Safety of Oral Semaglutide Monotherapy in Comparison With Placebo in Patients With Type 2 Diabetes.* Diabetes Care, 2019. **42**(9): p. 1724-1732.
770. Hunt, B., et al., *Evaluation of the Cost Per Patient Achieving Treatment Targets With Oral Semaglutide: A Short-Term Cost-Effectiveness Analysis in the United States.* Advances in Therapy, 2019. **36**(12): p. 3483-3493.
771. Yamada, H., et al., *Retrospective Analysis of the Effectiveness of Oral Semaglutide in Type 2 Diabetes Mellitus and Its Effect on Cardiometabolic Parameters in Japanese Clinical Settings.* Journal of Cardiovascular Development and Disease, 2023. **10**(4): p. 176.
772. Bhatnagar, A., *Managing Blood Glucose With the Use of Oral Semaglutide and Life Style Modification Among Indian Patients.* Journal of Endocrinology and Metabolism Research, 2023.
773. Verma, S., et al., *Effects of Once-Weekly Semaglutide 2.4 mg on C-Reactive Protein in Adults With Overweight or Obesity (STEP 1, 2, and 3): Exploratory Analyses of Three Randomised, Double-Blind, Placebo-Controlled, Phase 3 Trials.* Eclinicalmedicine, 2023. **55**: p. 101737.
774. Williams, D.M., et al., *Real-World Clinical Experience of Oral Semaglutide in a Secondary Diabetes Clinic in the UK: A Retrospective Observational Study.* Diabetes Therapy, 2024. **15**(7): p. 1639-1646.
775. Smolderen, K.G., et al., *Lower Risk of Cardiovascular Events in Patients Initiated on Semaglutide 2.4 mg in the Real-world: Results From the <scp>SCORE</Scp> Study (Semaglutide Effects on Cardiovascular Outcomes in People With Overweight or Obesity in the Real World).* Diabetes Obesity and Metabolism, 2025. **27**(11): p. 6691-6704.
776. Janić, M., et al., *Efficacy, Safety, and Patient Satisfaction With Oral Semaglutide: First Single-Centre Clinical Experience.* Journal of International Medical Research, 2023. **51**(11).
777. Aroda, V.R., et al., *Efficacy and Safety of Oral Semaglutide by Subgroups of Patient Characteristics in The <scp>PIONEER</Scp> Phase 3 Programme.* Diabetes Obesity and Metabolism, 2022. **24**(7): p. 1338-1350.
778. Wing, R.R., et al., *Benefits of Modest Weight Loss in Improving Cardiovascular Risk Factors in Overweight and Obese Individuals With Type 2 Diabetes.* Diabetes Care, 2011. **34**(7): p. 1481-1486.
779. Lee, E.J. and T.N. Kim, *Pharmacological Management of Obesity in Patients With Type 2 Diabetes: An Update.* The Korean Journal of Obesity, 2016. **25**(3): p. 121-128.
780. Shin, Y.-l., et al., *Glucose Control in Korean Patients With Type 2 Diabetes Mellitus According to Body Mass Index.* Journal of Obesity & Metabolic Syndrome, 2023. **32**(1): p. 55-63.
781. Coleman, C.D., et al., *Comparative Effectiveness of a Portion-Controlled Meal Replacement Program for Weight Loss in Adults With and Without Diabetes/High Blood Sugar.* Nutrition and Diabetes, 2017. **7**(7): p. e284-e284.
782. Gregg, E.W., et al., *Association of the Magnitude of Weight Loss and Changes in Physical Fitness With Long-Term Cardiovascular Disease Outcomes in Overweight or Obese*

People With Type 2 Diabetes: A Post-Hoc Analysis of the Look AHEAD Randomised Clinical Trial. The Lancet Diabetes & Endocrinology, 2016. **4**(11): p. 913-921.

783. Sherr, J.L., et al., *Mitigating Meal-Related Glycemic Excursions in an Insulin-Sparing Manner During Closed-Loop Insulin Delivery: The Beneficial Effects of Adjunctive Pramlintide and Liraglutide.* Diabetes Care, 2016. **39**(7): p. 1127-1134.
784. Kaye, A.D., et al., *Glucagon-Like Peptide-1 Receptor Agonist Mediated Weight Loss and Diabetes Mellitus Benefits: A Narrative Review.* Cureus, 2024.
785. Dixon, J.B., *Obesity and Diabetes: The Impact of Bariatric Surgery on Type-2 Diabetes.* World Journal of Surgery, 2009. **33**(10).
786. Wing, R.R. and B. Marquez, *Behavioral Aspects of Weight Loss in Type 2 Diabetes.* Current Diabetes Reports, 2008. **8**(2): p. 126-131.
787. Wilding, J., *The Importance of Weight Management in Type 2 Diabetes Mellitus.* International Journal of Clinical Practice, 2014. **68**(6): p. 682-691.
788. Steffen, B.T., et al., *Cardiometabolic Health and Bariatric Surgery: A 25-Year Longitudinal Cohort Study in CARDIA Participants.* Annals of Surgery Open, 2025. **6**(3): p. e609.
789. Meyvis, K., C.D. Block, and L.F.V. Gaal, *Can Bariatric Surgery Be Considered Standard Therapy to Treat Type 2 Diabetes?* Us Endocrinology, 2013. **09**(02): p. 108.
790. Heerspink, H.J.L., et al., *Effects of Semaglutide on Albuminuria and Kidney Function in People With Overweight or Obesity With or Without Type 2 Diabetes: Exploratory Analysis From the STEP 1, 2, and 3 Trials.* 2023.
791. Bawazeer, N., et al., *Cost–Consequence Analysis of Semaglutide vs. Liraglutide for Managing Obese Prediabetic and Diabetic Patients in Saudi Arabia: A Single-Center Study.* Healthcare, 2025. **13**(14): p. 1755.
792. Karagiannis, T., et al., *Subcutaneously Administered Tirzepatide vs Semaglutide for Adults With Type 2 Diabetes: A Systematic Review and Network Meta-Analysis of Randomised Controlled Trials.* Diabetologia, 2024. **67**(7): p. 1206-1222.
793. Vosoughi, K., et al., *Association of Glucagon-Like Peptide 1 Analogs and Agonists Administered for Obesity With Weight Loss and Adverse Events: A Systematic Review and Network Meta-Analysis.* Eclinicalmedicine, 2021. **42**: p. 101213.
794. Wang, S., et al., *Glycemic Control, Weight Management, Cardiovascular Safety, and Cost-Effectiveness of Semaglutide for Patients With Type 2 Diabetes Mellitus: A Rapid Review and Meta-Analysis of Real-World Studies.* Diabetes Therapy, 2024. **15**(2): p. 497-519.
795. Τσάπας, A., et al., *Comparative Efficacy of Glucose-lowering Medications on Body Weight and Blood Pressure in Patients With Type 2 Diabetes: A Systematic Review and Network Meta-analysis.* Diabetes Obesity and Metabolism, 2021. **23**(9): p. 2116-2124.
796. Kieu, A., et al., *Benefits of the Addition of Continuous or Flash Glucose Monitoring Versus Standard Practice Using Self-Monitored Blood Glucose and Haemoglobin A1c in the Primary Care of Diabetes Mellitus: A Systematic Review Protocol.* BMJ Open, 2021. **11**(8): p. e050027.
797. Kassem, S., et al., *Efficacy, Adherence and Persistence of Various Glucagon-like Peptide-1 Agonists: Nationwide Real-life Data.* Diabetes Obesity and Metabolism, 2024. **26**(10): p. 4646-4652.
798. Stretton, B., et al., *Weight Loss With Subcutaneous Semaglutide Versus Other Glucagon-like Peptide 1 Receptor Agonists in Type 2 Diabetes: A Systematic Review.* Internal Medicine Journal, 2023. **53**(8): p. 1311-1320.

799. Rodriguez, P.J., et al., *Comparative Effectiveness of Semaglutide and Tirzepatide for Weight Loss in Adults With Overweight and Obesity in the US: A Real-World Evidence Study.* 2023.
800. Horii, T., et al., *Adherence and Treatment Discontinuation of Oral Semaglutide and Once-weekly Semaglutide Injection at 12 Month Follow-up: Japanese Real-world Data.* Journal of Diabetes Investigation, 2024. **15**(11): p. 1578-1584.
801. Talay, L., M. Vickers, and L. Ruíz-Cañas, *Effectiveness of an Email-Based, Semaglutide-Supported Weight-Loss Service for People With Overweight and Obesity in Germany: A Real-World Retrospective Cohort Analysis.* Obesities, 2024. **4**(3): p. 256-269.
802. McCrimmon, R.J., et al., *Effects of Once-Weekly Semaglutide vs Once-Daily Canagliflozin on Body Composition in Type 2 Diabetes: A Substudy of the SUSTAIN 8 Randomised Controlled Clinical Trial.* Diabetologia, 2020. **63**(3): p. 473-485.
803. Jastreboff, A.M., et al., *Tirzepatide Once Weekly for the Treatment of Obesity in People With Type 2 Diabetes (SURMOUNT-2): A Double-Blind, Randomised, Multicentre, Placebo-Controlled, Phase 3 Trial.* The Lancet, 2023. **402**(10402): p. 613-626.
804. Weiss, T., et al., *Real-World Weight Change, Adherence, and Discontinuation Among Patients With Type 2 Diabetes Initiating Glucagon-Like Peptide-1 Receptor Agonists in the UK.* BMJ Open Diabetes Research & Care, 2022. **10**(1): p. e002517.
805. Humphrey, C.D. and A. Lawrence, *Implications of Ozempic and Other GLP-1 Receptor Agonists for Facial Plastic Surgeons.* Facial Plastic Surgery, 2023. **39**(06): p. 719-721.
806. Sattar, N., et al., *Continued Treatment With Tirzepatide for Maintenance of Weight Reduction in Adults With Obesity.* Jama, 2024. **331**(1): p. 38.
807. Berg, S., et al., *Discontinuing Glucagon-like Peptide-1 Receptor Agonists and Body Habitus: A Systematic Review and Meta-analysis.* Obesity Reviews, 2025. **26**(8).
808. Jendle, J., et al., *Weight Loss With Liraglutide, a Once-daily Human Glucagon-like Peptide-1 Analogue for Type 2 Diabetes Treatment as Monotherapy or Added to Metformin, Is Primarily as a Result of a Reduction in Fat Tissue.* Diabetes Obesity and Metabolism, 2009. **11**(12): p. 1163-1172.
809. Cengiz, A., C.C. Wu, and S.D. Lawley, *Incretin Mimetics for Weight Loss Forgive Nonadherence.* 2025.
810. Shi, Q., et al., *Benefits and Harms of Drug Treatment for Type 2 Diabetes: Systematic Review and Network Meta-Analysis of Randomised Controlled Trials.* BMJ, 2023. **381**: p. e074068.
811. Tsukamoto, S., et al., *Effect of Tirzepatide on Glycaemic Control and Weight Loss Compared With Other Glucagon-like Peptide-1 Receptor Agonists in Japanese Patients With Type 2 Diabetes Mellitus.* Diabetes Obesity and Metabolism, 2023. **26**(1): p. 262-274.
812. Windram, M., et al., *Semaglutide, Tirzepatide, and Retatrutide Attenuate the Interoceptive Effects of Alcohol in Male and Female Rats.* 2025.
813. Huthmacher, J.A., J.J. Meier, and M.A. Nauck, *Efficacy and Safety of Short- And Long-Acting Glucagon-Like Peptide 1 Receptor Agonists on a Background of Basal Insulin in Type 2 Diabetes: A Meta-Analysis.* Diabetes Care, 2020. **43**(9): p. 2303-2312.
814. Pratt, E., et al., *Orforglipron (<scp>LY3502970</Scp>), a Novel, Oral Non-peptide Glucagon-like Peptide-1 Receptor Agonist: A Phase 1b, Multicentre, Blinded, Placebo-controlled, Randomized, Multiple-ascending-dose Study in People With Type 2 Diabetes.* Diabetes Obesity and Metabolism, 2023. **25**(9): p. 2642-2649.

815. Griffith, D.A., et al., *A Small-Molecule Oral Agonist of the Human Glucagon-Like Peptide-1 Receptor.* Journal of Medicinal Chemistry, 2022. **65**(12): p. 8208-8226.
816. Ono, R., et al., *A Phase 1 Study to Evaluate the Safety, Tolerability, Pharmacokinetics and Pharmacodynamics of Danuglipron (<scp>PF</Scp> -06882961), an Oral Small-molecule Glucagon-like Peptide-1 Receptor Agonist, in Japanese Adults With Type 2 Diabetes Mellitus.* Diabetes Obesity and Metabolism, 2022. **25**(3): p. 805-814.
817. Jastreboff, A.M. and R.F. Kushner, *New Frontiers in Obesity Treatment: GLP-1 and Nascent Nutrient-Stimulated Hormone-Based Therapeutics.* Annual Review of Medicine, 2023. **74**(1): p. 125-139.
818. Javeria, f., A. Kamal, and Z. Mohammadi, *Semaglutide: A Potential Treatment of Obesity in PCOD Patients.* 2023.
819. Wang, W., et al., *Associations of semaglutide with first-time diagnosis of Alzheimer's disease in patients with type 2 diabetes: target trial emulation using nationwide real-world data in the US.* Alzheimer's & Dementia, 2024. **20**(12): p. 8661-8672.
820. Frøssing, S., et al., *Effect of Liraglutide on Ectopic Fat in Polycystic Ovary Syndrome: <scp>A</Scp> Randomized Clinical Trial.* Diabetes Obesity and Metabolism, 2017. **20**(1): p. 215-218.
821. Aranäs, C., et al., *Semaglutide suppresses cocaine taking, seeking, and cocaine-evoked dopamine levels in the nucleus accumbens.* European Neuropsychopharmacology, 2025. **98**: p. 1-10.
822. Šalamun, V., et al., *Liraglutide Increases IVF Pregnancy Rates in Obese PCOS Women With Poor Response to First-Line Reproductive Treatments: A Pilot Randomized Study.* European Journal of Endocrinology, 2018. **179**(1): p. 1-11.
823. Abdalla, M., et al., *The Potential Role of Incretin-Based Therapies for Polycystic Ovary Syndrome: A Narrative Review of the Current Evidence.* Therapeutic Advances in Endocrinology and Metabolism, 2021. **12**.
824. Vergnaud, S., *Can You Get Pregnant While Taking Ozempic? How Weight-Loss Medications Affect Fertility*. 2024, GoodRx.
825. Ee, C. and C.T. Tay, *Pharmacological management of polycystic ovary syndrome.* Aust Prescr, 2024. **47**(4): p. 109-12.
826. Hendershot, C., *Human Laboratory Screening of Semaglutide for Alcohol Use Disorder*, A. National Institute on Alcohol and Alcoholism, Editors. 2022.
827. Sun, Z., et al., *GLP-1/GLP-1R Signaling Regulates Ovarian PCOS-Associated Granulosa Cells Proliferation and Antiapoptosis by Modification of Forkhead Box Protein O1 Phosphorylation Sites.* International Journal of Endocrinology, 2020. **2020**: p. 1-10.
828. Seino, Y., M. Fukushima, and D. Yabe, *GIP and GLP-1, the Two Incretin Hormones: Similarities and Differences.* Journal of Diabetes Investigation, 2010. **1**(1-2): p. 8-23.
829. Jall, S., et al., *Monomeric GLP-1/GIP/glucagon Triagonism Corrects Obesity, Hepatosteatosis, and Dyslipidemia in Female Mice.* Molecular Metabolism, 2017. **6**(5): p. 440-446.
830. Deacon, C.F., E. Mannucci, and B. Åhrén, *Glycaemic Efficacy of Glucagon-like Peptide-1 Receptor Agonists and Dipeptidyl Peptidase-4 Inhibitors as Add-on Therapy to Metformin in Subjects With Type 2 Diabetes—a Review and Meta Analysis.* Diabetes Obesity and Metabolism, 2012. **14**(8): p. 762-767.
831. Finan, B., et al., *Unimolecular Dual Incretins Maximize Metabolic Benefits in Rodents, Monkeys, and Humans.* Science Translational Medicine, 2013. **5**(209).

832. Pramanik, S. and S. Ray, *Next Step in Incretin-Based Therapy: From Single to Dual Agonism*. Emj Diabetes, 2022.
833. Véniant, M.M., et al., *A GIPR Antagonist Conjugated to GLP-1 Analogues Promotes Weight Loss With Improved Metabolic Parameters in Preclinical and Phase 1 Settings*. Nature Metabolism, 2024. **6**(2): p. 290-303.
834. Åhrén, B., Y. Yamada, and Y. Seino, *The Insulin Response to Oral Glucose in GIP and GLP-1 Receptor Knockout Mice: Review of the Literature and Stepwise Glucose Dose Response Studies in Female Mice*. Frontiers in Endocrinology, 2021. **12**.
835. Deacon, C.F. and B. Åhrén, *Physiology of Incretins in Health and Disease*. The Review of Diabetic Studies, 2011. **8**(3): p. 293-306.
836. Hansotia, T., et al., *Double Incretin Receptor Knockout (DIRKO) Mice Reveal an Essential Role for the Enteroinsular Axis in Transducing the Glucoregulatory Actions of DPP-IV Inhibitors*. Diabetes, 2004. **53**(5): p. 1326-1335.
837. Sztanek, F., et al., *New Developments in Pharmacological Treatment of Obesity and Type 2 Diabetes—Beyond and Within GLP-1 Receptor Agonists*. Biomedicines, 2024. **12**(6): p. 1320.
838. Gniuli, D., et al., *High-Fat Feeding Stimulates Endocrine, Glucose-Dependent Insulinotropic Polypeptide (GIP)-expressing Cell Hyperplasia in the Duodenum of Wistar Rats*. Diabetologia, 2010. **53**(10): p. 2233-2240.
839. Güemes, M., et al., *Enteroinsular Hormones in Two Siblings With Donohue Syndrome and Complete Leptin Deficiency*. Pediatric Diabetes, 2017. **19**(4): p. 675-679.
840. Hall, K.D. and S. Kahan, *Maintenance of Lost Weight and Long-Term Management of Obesity*. Medical Clinics of North America, 2018. **102**(1): p. 183-197.
841. Richards, R., et al., *Semaglutide and Tirzepatide in a Remote Weight Management Program: 12-Month Retrospective Observational Study*. Jmir Formative Research, 2025. **9**: p. e81912.
842. Budini, B., et al., *Trajectory of Weight Regain After Cessation of GLP-1 Receptor Agonists: A Systematic Review and Nonlinear Meta-Regression*. 2025.
843. Ross, K.M., *Mentor and Peer Support for Long-Term Weight Loss Maintenance*. Jama Internal Medicine, 2025. **185**(7): p. 776.
844. Dawwas, G.K., J.M. Samuels, and C. Stein, *Shifting Obesity Treatment Paradigms: Trends of Glucagon-like Peptide-1 Receptor Agonists and Bariatric Surgery in the United States*. Diabetes Obesity and Metabolism, 2025. **27**(10): p. 6023-6026.
845. Jensen, S.B.K., et al., *Protocol for a Randomised Controlled Trial of the Combined Effects of the GLP-1 Receptor Agonist Liraglutide and Exercise on Maintenance of Weight Loss and Health After a Very Low-Calorie Diet*. BMJ Open, 2019. **9**(11): p. e031431.
846. Ala, M. and S.P. Eftekhar, *Weight Loss Breaks the Bond Between Nonalcoholic Fatty Liver Disease and Cardiovascular Diseases: A Clinical and Epidemiological Perspective*. Obesity Reviews, 2023. **24**(6).
847. Brosnihan, P.J., et al., *Great Debates: Undergoing the Knife Versus Pill-Popping—The Comparative Efficacy and Cost-Effectiveness of Bariatric Surgery and GLP-1 Receptor Agonists in the Management of Obesity*. The American Surgeon, 2025. **91**(10): p. 1587-1593.
848. Heerspink, H.J.L., et al., *Effects of Tirzepatide Versus Insulin Glargine on Kidney Outcomes in Type 2 Diabetes in the SURPASS-4 Trial: Post-Hoc Analysis of an Open-*

Label, Randomised, Phase 3 Trial. The Lancet Diabetes & Endocrinology, 2022. **10**(11): p. 774-785.

849. Akwe, J., et al., *Medical vs. Surgical Obesity Management: A Narrative Review of Efficacy, Safety, and Long-Term Outcomes.* Cureus, 2025.
850. Georgiev, T. and P. Kabakchieva, *Weight Loss, but Not at Any Cost: Risks and Challenges in Patients With Osteoarthritis.* Mediterranean Journal of Rheumatology, 2025. **36**(1): p. 28.
851. Kim, D.D., J.H. Hwang, and A.M. Fendrick, *Balancing Innovation and Affordability in Anti-Obesity Medications: The Role of an Alternative Weight-Maintenance Program.* Health Affairs Scholar, 2024. **2**(6).
852. Alanazi, M., et al., *Effect of Semaglutide in Individuals With Obesity or Overweight Without Diabetes.* Cureus, 2024.
853. Quarenghi, M., et al., *Weight Regain After Liraglutide, Semaglutide or Tirzepatide Interruption: A Narrative Review of Randomized Studies.* Journal of Clinical Medicine, 2025. **14**(11): p. 3791.
854. Shannon, C.E., et al., *Precision Nutrition for Targeting Pathophysiology of Cardiometabolic Phenotypes.* Reviews in Endocrine and Metabolic Disorders, 2023. **24**(5): p. 921-936.
855. Berković, M.C., et al., *Saving Muscle While Losing Weight: A Vital Strategy for Sustainable Results While on Glucagon-Like Peptide-1 Related Drugs.* World Journal of Diabetes, 2025. **16**(9).
856. Cifuentes, L., et al., *Precision Medicine for Obesity.* Digestive Disease Interventions, 2021. **05**(03): p. 239-248.
857. Cirulli, E.T., et al., *Profound Perturbation of the Metabolome in Obesity Is Associated With Health Risk.* Cell Metabolism, 2019. **29**(2): p. 488-500.e2.
858. Rangel-Huerta, Ó.D., B. Pastor-Villaescusa, and Á. Gil, *Are We Close to Defining a Metabolomic Signature of Human Obesity? A Systematic Review of Metabolomics Studies.* Metabolomics, 2019. **15**(6).
859. Kelly, A.S., et al., *Working Toward Precision Medicine Approaches to Treat Severe Obesity in Adolescents: Report of an NIH Workshop.* International Journal of Obesity, 2018. **42**(11): p. 1834-1844.
860. Lee, S.H. and B.T. Kim, *Functional Approaches to Obesity Treatment Based on Phenotypes of Obesity.* Korean Institute for Functional Medicine, 2024. **7**(2): p. 46-52.
861. Napolsky, I.N. and P. Popova, *Personalized Nutrition for the Prevention and Treatment of Metabolic Diseases: Opportunities and Perspectives.* Russian Journal for Personalized Medicine, 2022. **2**(1): p. 15-34.
862. Pandey, A., et al., *Estimating the Lives That Could Be Saved by Expanded Access to Weight-Loss Drugs.* Proceedings of the National Academy of Sciences, 2024. **121**(43).
863. Woolf, E.K., et al., *Precision Prevention, Diagnostics, and Treatment of Obesity: Pipedream or Reality?* Obesity, 2025. **33**(11): p. 2029-2045.
864. O'Donovan, C.B., et al., *Can Metabotyping Help Deliver the Promise of Personalised Nutrition?* Proceedings of the Nutrition Society, 2015. **75**(1): p. 106-114.
865. Mayne, D. and R. McKenna, *Association Between Plausible Genetic Factors and Weight Loss From GLP-1 Receptor Agonists and Bariatric Surgery: A Review.* Dinkum Journal of Medical Innovations, 2025. **4**(7): p. 466.

866. Santos, R.L., et al., *Psychiatric Effects Associated With GLP-1 and Gip Agonists: A Review on Semaglutide and Tirzepatide*. Asclepius International Journal of Scientific Health Science, 2025. **4**(7): p. 509-518.
867. Garbuzova, E.V., et al., *Associations of Adipocytokines and Early Renal Dysfunction in Young People on the Background of Dyslipidemia*. Journal of Personalized Medicine, 2023. **13**(8): p. 1238.
868. Ramracheya, R., et al., *PYY-Dependent Restoration of Impaired Insulin and Glucagon Secretion in Type 2 Diabetes Following Roux-en-Y Gastric Bypass Surgery*. Cell Reports, 2016. **15**(5): p. 944-950.
869. Zhu, Y., et al., *Efficacy and Safety of GLP-1 Receptor Agonists in Patients With Type 2 Diabetes Mellitus and Non-Alcoholic Fatty Liver Disease: A Systematic Review and Meta-Analysis*. Frontiers in Endocrinology, 2021. **12**.
870. Nauck, M.A., et al., *Rapid Tachyphylaxis of the Glucagon-Like Peptide 1–Induced Deceleration of Gastric Emptying in Humans*. Diabetes, 2011. **60**(5): p. 1561-1565.

Index

A

B

C

D

E

F

G

H

I

K

L

M

N

O

P

R

S

T

V

W

Z

Made in United States
Cleveland, OH
06 November 2026

47787691R00211